Primary Care Urology

Guest Editors

KARL T. REW, MD
MASAHITO JIMBO, MD, PhD, MPH

PRIMARY CARE:
CLINICS IN OFFICE PRACTICE

www.primarycare.theclinics.com

Consulting Editor
JOEL J. HEIDELBAUGH, MD, FAAFP, FACG

September 2010 • Volume 37 • Number 3

SAUNDERS an imprint of ELSEVIER, Inc.

W.B. SAUNDERS COMPANY
A Division of Elsevier Inc.

1600 John F. Kennedy Boulevard, Suite 1800 ● Philadelphia, PA 19103-2899

http://www.theclinics.com

PRIMARY CARE: CLINICS IN OFFICE PRACTICE Volume 37, Number 3
September 2010 ISSN 0095-4543, ISBN-13: 978-1-4377-2489-9

Editor: Barbara Cohen-Kligerman
Developmental Editor: Donald Mumford

Primary Care: Clinics in Office Practice (ISSN: 0095–4543) is published quarterly by Elsevier Inc., 360 Park Avenue South, New York, NY 10010-1710. Months of issue are March, June, September, and December. Periodicals postage paid at New York, NY and additional mailing offices. Subscription prices are $190.00 per year (US individuals), $320.00 (US institutions), $96.00 (US students), $232.00 (Canadian individuals), $376.00 (Canadian institutions), $151.00 (Canadian students), $289.00 (international individuals), $376.00 (international institutions), and $151.00 (international students). Foreign air speed delivery is included in all *Clinics* subscription prices. All prices are subject to change without notice. POSTMASTER: Send address changes to *Primary Care: Clinics in Office Practice*, Elsevier Periodicals Customer Service, 11830 Westline Industrial Drive, St. Louis, MO 63146. Customer Service Health Sciences Division, Subscription Customer Service, 3251 Riverport Lane, Maryland Heights, MO 63043. **Customer Service: 1-800-654-2452 (U.S. and Canada); 314-447-8871 (outside U.S. and Canada). Fax: 314-447-8029. E-mail: journalscustomerservice-usa@elsevier.com (for print support); journalsonlinesupport-usa@elsevier.com (for online support).**

Reprints. For copies of 100 or more, of articles in this publication, please contact the Commercial Reprints Department, Elsevier Inc., 360 Park Avenue South, New York, NY 10010-1710. Tel. (212) 633-3812; Fax: (212) 482-1935; E-mail: reprints@elsevier.com.

Primary Care: Clinics in Office Practice is covered in *MEDLINE/PubMed (Index Medicus)* and *EMBASE/ Excerpta Medica, Current Contents/Clinical Medicine,* and *ISI/BIOMED.*

Printed and bound by CPI Group (UK) Ltd, Croydon, CR0 4YY

Transferred to Digital Print 2011

Contributors

CONSULTING EDITOR

JOEL J. HEIDELBAUGH, MD, FAAFP, FACG
Clinical Associate Professor, Departments of Family Medicine and Urology; Clerkship
Director, Department of Family Medicine, University of Michigan Medical School,
Ann Arbor, Michigan

GUEST EDITORS

KARL T. REW, MD
Clinical Instructor, Departments of Family Medicine and Urology, University of Michigan,
Ann Arbor, Michigan

MASAHITO JIMBO, MD, PhD, MPH
Associate Professor, Departments of Family Medicine and Urology, A. Alfred Taubman
Health Care Center, University of Michigan, Ann Arbor, Michigan

AUTHORS

ROLAND BRANDNER, MD
Department of Urology, New York University School of Medicine, New York
University Hospital, New York, New York

JOHN R. BRILL, MD, MPH
Associate Professor, Department of Family Medicine, University of Wisconsin School
of Medicine and Public Health, Milwaukee Academic Campus, Milwaukee, Wisconsin

JEREMY D. CLOSE, MD
Sports Medicine Fellow, Department of Family and Community Medicine, Jefferson
Medical College, Thomas Jefferson University, Philadelphia, Pennsylvania

VICTOR A. DIAZ Jr, MD
Assistant Professor, Department of Family and Community Medicine, Jefferson Medical
College, Thomas Jefferson University; Director of Quality Improvement, Jefferson
Family Medicine Associates, Philadelphia, Pennsylvania

BOB DJAVAN, MD, PhD
Professor and Director of the Department of Urology VA, New York University School
of Medicine, New York University Hospital, New York, New York

ELISABETH ECKERSBERGER, MPA
Urology Associates, Department of Urology, New York University School of Medicine,
New York University Hospital, New York, New York

GEOVANNI ESPINOSA, ND, LAc
Urology Associates, Department of Urology, New York University School of Medicine, New York University Hospital, New York, New York

GARY J. FAERBER, MD
Professor, Department of Urology, University of Michigan Medical School; Co-Director, Kidney Stone/Lithotriptor Program; Co-Director, Michigan Center for Minimally Invasive Urology, A. Alfred Taubman Health Care Center, Ann Arbor, Michigan

JULIA FINKELSTEIN, BSc
Urology Associates, Department of Urology, New York University School of Medicine, New York University Hospital, New York, New York

EVA FONG, MD
Department of Urology, NYU Langone Medical Center, New York, New York

KEITH A. FREY, MD, MBA
Professor, Department of Family Medicine, Mayo Clinic in Arizona, Scottsdale, Arizona

BRIAN H. HALSTATER, MD
Assistant Professor, Residency Program Director, Duke Family Medicine Residency Program, Division of Family Medicine, Department of Community and Family Medicine, Duke University, Duke University Medical Center, Durham, North Carolina

MASAHITO JIMBO, MD, PhD, MPH
Associate Professor, Departments of Family Medicine and Urology, A. Alfred Taubman Health Care Center, University of Michigan, Ann Arbor, Michigan

HERBERT LEPOR, MD
Professor and Martin Spatz Chairman, Urology Associates, Department of Urology, New York University School of Medicine, New York University Hospital, New York, New York

JANICE A. LITZA, MD
Assistant Professor, Department of Family Medicine, University of Wisconsin School of Medicine and Public Health, Milwaukee Academic Campus, Milwaukee, Wisconsin

MIKEL LLANES, MD
Resident Physician, Department of Family Medicine, University of Michigan, Ann Arbor, Michigan

VIVIANA MARTINEZ-BIANCHI, MD, FAAFP
Assistant Professor, Associate Residency Program Director, Duke Family Medicine Residency Program, Division of Family Medicine, Department of Community and Family Medicine, Duke University Medical Center, Duke University, Durham, North Carolina

VICTOR W. NITTI, MD
Professor of Urology; Director, Program in Voiding Dysfunction and Female Urology; Director, Fellowship in Female Pelvic Medicine and Reconstructive Surgery, Department of Urology, NYU Langone Medical Center, New York, New York

KALYANAKRISHNAN RAMAKRISHNAN, MD
Professor, Department of Family and Preventive Medicine, University of Oklahoma Health Sciences Center, Oklahoma City, Oklahoma

KARL T. REW, MD
Clinical Instructor, Departments of Family Medicine and Urology, University of Michigan,
Ann Arbor, Michigan

HELEN SADRI, MD
Urology Associates, Department of Urology, New York University School of Medicine,
New York University Hospital, New York, New York

ROBERT C. SALINAS, MD, CAQ
Geriatrics Medicine, Hospice and Palliative Medicine, Associate Professor,
Department of Family and Preventive Medicine, University of Oklahoma Health Sciences
Center, Oklahoma City, Oklahoma

GEORGE R. SCHADE, MD
Resident Surgeon, Department of Urology, University of Michigan Medical School,
A. Alfred Taubman Health Care Center, Ann Arbor, Michigan

OJAS SHAH, MD
Assistant Professor and Director of Endourology & Stone Disease; Urology Associates,
Department of Urology, New York University School of Medicine, New York University
Hospital, New York, New York

SAMIR S. TANEJA, MD
Department of Urology, New York University School of Medicine, New York
University Hospital, New York, New York

JULIAN WAN, MD
Associate Professor, Department of Urology, University of Michigan, Ann Arbor, Michigan

STEPHEN M. WAMPLER, MD
Associate Professor, Department of Family Medicine, University of Michigan, Ann Arbor,
Michigan

Contents

> Prostate specific antigen (PSA) screening is an integral part of current screening for prostate cancer. Together with digital rectal examinations, it is recommended annually by the American Cancer Society. PSA screening has resulted in a significant stage migration in the past decades. Different forms of PSA, including free PSA, volume adjusted, complexed, intact, or pro-PSA, are being used in the screening process. Other aspects of the screening process include age at diagnosis, survival, overdiagnosis, and overtreatment. Recent studies have cast doubt on whether PSA screening positively affects mortality and how the quality of life of patients may be affected by screening. Future considerations include the need for more longitudinal studies as well as further study of the PSA components that may become more relevant in the future.

> Causes of hematuria can range from benign conditions such as urinary tract infection to serious conditions such as bladder cancer. In evaluating a patient with hematuria, 3 questions must be answered by the primary care physician: (1) Is it really hematuria? (2) Should this patient with hematuria be worked up, and if so, how? (3) Should this patient with hematuria be referred, and if so, to which specialty? This article addresses these questions. Because uniformly high-quality studies are lacking, the recommendations included in this article are mostly based on expert consensus.

> Male sexual dysfunction is a common entity in primary care practice. The 3 most common types are erectile dysfunction, premature ejaculation, and decreased libido. Clinicians must be comfortable and skilled in taking a complete sexual, social, and medical history and performing a physical

examination in persons complaining of sexual dysfunction. Treatment of male sexual dysfunction may include medications and individual or couples psychotherapy. Treatment should be aimed at reducing emotional and physical morbidity in the patient and his partner.

Urinary tract infection (UTI) is the most common urologic disorder and one of the most common conditions for which physicians are consulted. Patients at increased risk for UTI include women; diabetics; the immuno-compromised; and those with anatomic abnormalities, impaired mobility, incontinence, advanced age, and instrumentation. Antibiotic therapy aims to relieve symptoms and prevent complications such as pyelonephritis and renal scarring. Distinguishing asymptomatic bacteriuria from a UTI can be difficult, especially in those with comorbidities. Most experts do not recommend screening for UTI, except in the first trimester of pregnancy.

Sexually transmitted infections (STIs) cause tremendous morbidity, great costs, and numerous avoidable deaths in the United States each year. STIs in men can present as discharge, ulcers, papules, infestations, or systemic disease, but most commonly STIs present without any symptoms. Molecular techniques, single-dose antibiotics and antivirals, and patient-administered therapies present opportunities for enhanced diagnosis and treatment. Screening for STIs should be part of all primary care practices, specifically targeting high-risk persons and those diagnosed with another STI.

Painful bladder syndrome or urologic chronic pelvic pain syndrome is a chronic condition that presents with lower urinary tract symptoms that include dysuria, urgency, frequent urination, and chronic pelvic pain. Diagnoses included in the painful bladder syndrome are interstitial cystitis and prostatodynia. The history, physical examination, and laboratory evaluation of patients with lower urinary tract symptoms are important in ruling out other diagnoses. Treatment options that are US Food and Drug Administration approved and evidence based are limited; however, many symptom-based treatment options can reduce symptoms and improve quality of life.

Prostatitis, one of the most common urological infections afflicting adult men, has recently been divided into 4 different categories based on the National Institutes of Health consensus classification: acute bacterial prostatitis, chronic bacterial prostatitis, chronic nonbacterial prostatitis and pelvic pain syndrome, and asymptomatic inflammatory prostatitis. Most patients with prostatitis are found to have either nonbacterial prostatitis or prostatodynia. Prostatitis poses an international health problem, with epidemiologic studies suggesting a worldwide prevalence of more than 10%. This article reviews current modes of diagnosis and therapy for acute and chronic prostatitis.

VISIT THE CLINICS ONLINE!

Access your subscription at:
www.theclinics.com

Foreword

A Primer for Primary Care Urology

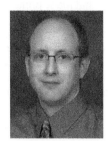

Joel J. Heidelbaugh, MD
Consulting Editor

The burden of urologic diseases is rapidly expanding in the United States with respect to physician office and hospital visits as well as to annual fiscal expenditures. Between 1994 and 2000, the number of outpatient visits with a complaint of lower urinary tract symptoms increased nearly 70%.[1] The cost of diagnosing and treating prostate cancer has more than doubled in the past decade.[1] Pharmacotherapy costs for erectile dysfunction in 2007 approached $1.5 billion.[2] As the US population ages, outpatient and hospital visits for seemingly benign urologic conditions will continue to escalate. With a paucity of time in medical student and primary care resident education dedicated to teaching the necessary skills to evaluate and treat common urologic conditions, will the next generation of physicians be equipped to treat and triage this burden?

This unique volume of reviews commences with perhaps the most controversial topic in primary care urology: prostate cancer screening. Dr Djavan and his colleagues have written an outstanding and timely review to aid readers through the challenges of choosing appropriate men to screen and to help understand the imperfections associated with the available tests for prostate cancer screening. Next, additional key urology topics in primary care are discussed, namely hematuria, erectile dysfunction, and urinary tract and sexually transmitted infections. These topics have significant importance given their high prevalence in primary care practices. Subsequent articles explore prostate issues, including benign prostatic hyperplasia and the ever-challenging acute versus chronic/infectious versus inflammatory prostatitis scenarios. As chronic prostatitis continues to perplex many clinicians, an excellent review by Drs Martinez-Bianchi and Halstater examines the challenges of treating chronic pelvic pain syndromes, an area that is poorly understood and often ignored in male patients.

Prim Care Clin Office Pract 37 (2010) xiii–xiv
doi:10.1016/j.pop.2010.05.005
0095-4543/10/$ – see front matter **primarycare.theclinics.com**

It has been suggested in many circles and across various cultures that men avoid going to a physician unless a urologic issue significantly worries them or their partner. Common testicular, scrotal, and penile issues are among the most anxiety-provoking issues that prompt men to see a physician and are presented in detailed reviews in this volume. Similarly, the topics of urinary tract stones and urinary incontinence are deftly presented in concise evidence-based reviews by experts in these areas. Lastly, male reproductive health and infertility are summarized, yet another topic that many primary care clinicians find challenging in daily practice.

I greatly commend my colleagues and friends, Drs Rew and Jimbo, on undertaking the arduous task of compiling this volume of evidence-based reviews on common urologic disorders in primary care. It is our collective hope that readers will greatly expand their knowledge base in urologic diseases and develop the skills to offer their patients more detailed initial work-ups and more appropriate specialist referrals with the goal of improving their quality of life.

Joel J. Heidelbaugh, MD
Departments of Family Medicine and Urology
University of Michigan Medical School
Ann Arbor, MI, and Ypsilanti Health Center
200 Arnet Suite 200, Ypsilanti, MI 48198, USA

E-mail address:
jheidel@umich.edu

REFERENCES

1. Litwin MS, Saigal CS, editors. Urologic diseases in America. Washington: US Department of Health and Human Services, Public Health Service, National Institutes of Health, National Institute of Diabetes and Digestive and Kidney Diseases, US Government Publishing Office; 2007. NIH Publication No. 07–5512.
2. Drug topics. Top 200 brand drugs by retail dollars in 2007. Available at: http://drug-topics.modernmedicine.com/drugtopics/data/articlestandard//drug-topics/102008/500221/article.pdf. Accessed May 10, 2010.

Preface

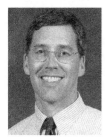 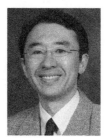

Karl T. Rew, MD   Masahito Jimbo, MD, PhD, MPH
Guest Editors

Primary care clinicians commonly encounter patients with urologic problems. Three challenging tasks they face are evaluating a urologic problem, treating it, and deciding whether or not and to whom to refer these patients.[1] Some lack of confidence in dealing with these challenges is not entirely surprising, because there is no minimum urology training time required in family medicine or internal medicine residency programs.[2,3]

The two of us and Consulting Editor Dr Joel J. Heidelbaugh all, family physicians, have been involved in a unique collaboration between the Department of Family Medicine and the Department of Urology at the University of Michigan. In this collaboration, we receive referrals from other physicians regarding evaluation and management of patients with commonly seen urologic problems that are treated, for the most part, nonsurgically. From this experience, we are convinced that many urologic problems can be competently managed by primary care clinicians.

The topics in this issue cover urologic problems commonly seen in a primary care office. Written by experts from primary care and urologic specialties, it is a practical guide that addresses the three key challenges noted in the first paragraph. We hope that readers find these reviews as useful in daily practice as we find them.

Prim Care Clin Office Pract 37 (2010) xv–xvi
doi:10.1016/j.pop.2010.05.004
0095-4543/10/$ – see front matter

Karl T. Rew, MD
Department of Family Medicine
University of Michigan Health System
24 Frank Lloyd Wright Drive
Lobby H, SPC 5795, Ann Arbor
MI 48106-5795, USA
Department of Urology
University of Michigan Health System
24 Frank Lloyd Wright Drive
Lobby H, SPC 5795
Ann Arbor, MI 48106-5795, USA

Masahito Jimbo, MD, PhD, MPH
Department of Family Medicine
University of Michigan
1018 Fuller Street
Ann Arbor, MI 48104-1213, USA
Department of Urology
University of Michigan
1018 Fuller Street, Ann Arbor
MI 48104-1213, USA

E-mail addresses:
karlr@med.umich.edu (K.T. Rew)
mjimbo@med.umich.edu (M. Jimbo)

REFERENCES

1. Resnick MI. Book review: urology for primary care physicians. N Engl J Med 1999; 341:2024–5.
2. ACGME program requirements for Graduate Medical Education in internal medicine. Available at: http://www.acgme.org/acWebsite/downloads/RRC_progReq/120pr07012007.pdf. Accessed March 23, 2010.
3. ACGME program requirements for Graduate Medical Education in internal medicine. Available at: http://www.acgme.org/acWebsite/downloads/RRC_progReq/140_internal_medicine_07012009.pdf. Accessed March 23, 2010.

Prostate-specific Antigen Testing and Prostate Cancer Screening

Bob Djavan, MD, PhD*, Elisabeth Eckersberger, MPA,
Julia Finkelstein, BSc, Helen Sadri, MD, Samir S. Taneja, MD,
Herbert Lepor, MD

KEYWORDS

• Prostate Cancer • PSA • Free PSA • Screening

Study	Level	Details
Catalona et al, 1993[30]	B	Nonrandomized, blinded
Bartsch et al, 2001[82]	B	RCT, blinded
PLCO, Andriole et al, 2009[84]	B	RCT, blinded
ERSPC, Schröeder et al, 2009[83]	B	RCT, blinded
McNaughton-Collins et al, 2008[87]	B	

Prostate cancer poses a significant problem for men's health, especially in Western societies. It has become the most common malignancy and the second most common cause of cancer death in American men. It is estimated that 1 in 6 men will be diagnosed with prostate cancer at some time in their lives; more than 30,000 men died of the disease in 2002.[1]

The advent of prostate-specific antigen (PSA) testing in the early 1980s revolutionized the diagnosis of prostate cancer, and the surge in the number of new prostate cancer cases identified by this tumor marker is unparalleled in oncological history. As is true for other common malignancies, such as breast and cervical cancer, the issue of population screening with PSA seems enticing. The American health care model provides us with some insight into this matter, with its advocated policy of screening since the early 1990s.

The current recommendation from the American Cancer Society is that PSA testing and digital rectal examination (DRE) should be offered annually to men more than

Conflict of interests: There is no conflict of interest for any of the authors, nor any funding source involved in the research mentioned.
Department of Urology, New York University School of Medicine (NYU), New York University Hospital, 150 East 32nd Street, New York, NY 10016, USA
* Corresponding author.
E-mail address: bdjavan@hotmail.com

50 years old who have a life expectancy of at least 10 years. Populations at higher risk, such as African American men or those who have a first-degree relative (father, brother, or son) with prostate cancer, should be offered testing beginning at 45 years of age.[2]

This review examines the international trends and patterns in the incidence of prostate cancer, with special attention on the United States and European populations, and discusses the widely debated issue of screening, including PSA testing and DRE. Three recent studies are discussed: the 2001 Tyrol Study, the European Randomized Study of Screening for Prostate Cancer (ERSPC) and the US-based Prostate, Lung, Colorectal, and Ovarian (PLCO) Cancer Screening Trial. Published in March 2009, the ERSPC and PLCO studies provide the most comprehensive and up-to-date information on prostate cancer screening available today. They have significantly contributed to our current knowledge and understanding of not only prostate cancer screening but also the difficulties and controversies associated with their ambiguous findings.

INCIDENCE OF PROSTATE CANCER

Prostate cancer is one of the few malignancies that display a wide geographic variation in incidences. Hsing and colleagues[3] classified 15 countries worldwide into high-risk (US, Canada, Sweden, Australia, and France), medium-risk (most other European countries), and low-risk (Asia) categories, and examined the trend in the incidences from 1973 to 1992. In the PSA era (1989–1992), the incidences in the high-risk countries ranged from 48.1 to 137 per 100,000 person years, whereas incidences in the low-risk countries were between 2.3 and 9.8 per 100,000 person years (**Table 1**). Generally, the incidences were increasing in all countries, and in the US they differed significantly between different populations (**Table 2**).

Statistics from the Surveillance, Epidemiology, and End Results Database

The most complete information available on prostate cancer epidemiology in the US is provided by the Surveillance, Epidemiology, and End Results (SEER) program of the National Cancer Institute.[4] The SEER incidence data for the years 1973 to 1999 can be divided into the pre-PSA and PSA eras, with the PSA era beginning in late 1980s. There was a gradual increase in prostate cancer incidence during the pre-PSA era that can be explained by an increase in transurethral resection of prostate, leading to a diagnosis of prostate cancer. As the PSA era began, an abrupt increase in prostate cancer incidence was observed, peaking in 1992 at 237 per 100,000 person years. A subsequent decline in the incidence followed until 1995, and was accounted for by the cull effect, whereby removal of detectable cases in prior years resulted in fewer available cases being found during repeated screening. A stable incidence was then observed between 1995 and 1999, but the rates were higher than they were before the PSA era. Rates have since fluctuated, falling to 169 per 100,000 in 1995, increasing again to 183.45 in 2001, and most recently falling again, showing rates of 152 and 163 per 100,000 for 2005 and 2006, respectively (**Fig. 1**).[5] Among the different ethnic groups in the US, African Americans have the highest prostate cancer incidences, followed by White Americans, Hispanic Americans, and Asian Americans.

Genetic and Environmental Factors

The worldwide and ethnic variations in prostate cancer incidence are caused by genetic and environmental factors. Genetic factors include variations in genetic

Table 1
Age-adjusted incidences (per 100,000 person years) of prostate cancer in 15 countries, 1973 to 1977, 1988 to 1992, and 2002

Countries	1973–1977[a]		1988–1992		% Change 1977–1992	2002[b]
	Total	Incidence	Total	Incidence		Incidence
High risk						
US total						124.8
US black	2664	79.9	7129	137.0	71.5	n/a
US white	24,192	47.9	66,227	100.8	110.4	n/a
Canada	3126	39.8	10,473	84.9	113.3	78.2
Sweden	16,556	44.4	25,253	55.3	24.5	90.9
Australia	3661	28.4	10,870	53.5	88.4	76.0
France	430	23.0	1502	48.1	109.1	59.3
Medium risk						
Denmark	3932	23.6	7392	31.0	31.4	39.9
England	5461	20.1	9529	29.3	45.8	52.2
Italy	219	22.8	884	28.2	23.7	56.3
Spain	291	17.6	641	27.2	54.5	35.9
Israel	1238	15.5	3147	23.9	54.2	46.8
Low risk						
Singapore	100	4.8	415	9.8	104.2	13.8
Japan	222	4.9	737	9.0	83.7	12.6
Hong Kong	268	5.1	1185	7.9	54.9	n/a
India	193	6.8	764	7.9	16.2	4.6
China	219	1.6	539	2.3	43.8	1.7

[a] Data from Hsing AW, Tsao L, Devesa SS. International trends and patterns of prostate cancer incidence and mortality. Int J Cancer 2000;85:61.
[b] Data from Ferlay J, Bray F, Pisani P, et al. GLOBOCAN 2002: Cancer incidence, mortality and prevalence worldwide; IARC CancerBase No. 5 version 2.0. Lyon (France): IARC Press; 2004. (Available at: http://www-dep.iarc.fr. Accessed April 29, 2010.)

Table 2
Incidence and mortality in the United States

Ethnicity	Incidence[a]	Mortality[a]
Total	159.3	25.6
White	153.0	23.6
Black	239.8	56.3
Asian/Pacific Islander	91.1	10.6
American Indian/Alaskan Native	76.1	20.0
Hispanic	133.4	19.6

[a] Per 100,000 men.

Data from Horner MJ, Ries LAG, Krapcho M, et al, editors. SEER Cancer Statistics Review, 1975–2006. National Cancer Institute. Bethesda (MD). Available at: http://seer.cancer.gov/csr/1975_2006/. Accessed June 10, 2010. Based on November 2008 SEER data submission, posted to the SEER Web site, 2009.

susceptibility or metabolism in high-risk and low-risk populations. It has been suggested that racial and ethnic variation in prostate cancer is partly caused by underlying differences in androgen secretions and metabolism. The activity of 5α reductase is crucial for converting testosterone to dihydrotestosterone, the principal nuclear androgen in the prostate. Ross and colleagues[6] suggested a difference in the activity of this enzyme between Western and Asian men.[7] Polymorphism of the SRD5A2 gene, which codes for 5α reductase, may account for these differences. Makridakis and colleagues[8] reported an association of missense substitution in the gene (alanine residue at codon 49 replaced with threonine) with the risk of developing prostate cancer in African American and Hispanic American men. The variant allele conferred greater risks of developing localized and advanced prostate cancer, especially in African Americans. A shorter androgen receptor cystosine adenine guanine CAG repeat length has also been reported to be more prevalent in African American men than in European American men, accounting for the increased risk for development of prostate cancer.[9,10] Recently, a variant CYP3A4 gene (coding for an enzyme involved in the oxidation of testosterone) was found to be associated with adverse clinical parameters of prostate cancer such as Gleason score, stage, and PSA.[11] More importantly, the allele frequency of the variant, G, is differentially distributed

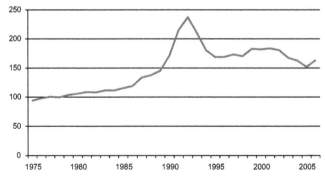

Fig. 1. Prostate cancer incidence, 1975 to 2006 (per 100,000). (*Data from* Horner MJ, Ries LAG, Krapcho M, et al. SEER Cancer Statistics Review, 1975–2006, National Cancer Institute. Bethesda (MD). Available at: http://seer.cancer.gov/csr/1975_2006/. Accessed June 10, 2010. Based on November 2008 SEER data submission, posted to the SEER Web site, 2009.)

across racial and ethnic groups, with the highest frequency found in African American men.

Environment plays an important role in prostate cancer risk. Higher animal fat intake in Western society has been reported as a risk factor.[12] In contrast, the Asian dietary intake of soy, seaweed, rice, shiitake mushrooms, fish, and greens may exert some protective effects against prostate cancer.[13] The observation that Chinese Americans and Japanese Americans have higher incidences than their counterparts in China and Japan further supports the role of environmental factors in prostate cancer development. In low-risk countries where PSA screening was not prevalent, prostate cancer incidence is also increasing.[3] In these populations, an increasing prevalence of Westernization accompanied by potential risk factors such as dietary fat, obesity, and low physical activity have been postulated to be among the causes for the increasing incidence of prostate cancer.[14,15]

Immunology and Inflammatory Responses

The immunology and inflammatory responses of the prostate are correlated with carcinogenesis. Inflammation of the prostate is closely linked to the development of prostate cancer, and most resected prostate cancer tissues show signs of an inflammatory reaction. Several types of inflammation exist, and must be distinguished as to the distribution and location of leukocytes and the histology of the prostate tissue. A relationship between T cell infiltration and stromal proliferation has been shown, and there is evidence that estrogen plays an additional role.[16]

PROSTATE CANCER SCREENING AND EARLY DETECTION WITH PSA

The ideal screening test is minimally invasive, easily available and performed, acceptable to the general population, has a low rate of false-negative results, and can significantly affect the outcome of the disease, such as mortality. During the past 15 years, PSA has become an indispensable marker for diagnosis and follow-up of prostate cancer patients.[17] PSA remains the most clinically relevant tumor marker in human oncology. PSA, which is encoded by an androgen-responsive gene located on chromosome 19q13.3 to 13.4,[18] is secreted from prostate epithelial cells. PSA screening has been advocated in the US since the early 1990s, and many studies have evaluated PSA as a screening test. Because recent studies have found that prostate cancer screening may not reduce mortality (see the ERSPC and PLCO trials), using PSA for early detection may be an additional option, which is defined as looking for cancer in a preselected population, as opposed to screening a whole population.

The measurement of serum prostate-specific antigen (tPSA) and DRE are standard procedures in clinical practice when screening for prostate cancer. If suspect results are found, they are followed by an aggressive biopsy policy.[19] PSA is a valuable tool for cancer detection using age-related cutoff reference serum levels. However, the specificity of this serum marker is limited, and patients must be aware of pros as well as cons (**Table 3**).[20] A summary of PSA testing, as well as different methods of measurement, is given in **Table 4**.

PSA at Diagnosis

The level of PSA at diagnosis is a general surrogate of tumor volume or cancer burden. Studies have shown a decrease in PSA levels at diagnosis over time.[17,21] The median PSA at the time of diagnosis decreased from 11.8 ng/dL in 1990 to 6.3 ng/dL in 1998.[17] Currently the upper limit of normal PSA is between 3 and 4 ng/dL[22,23]; if it is more than this, further testing is needed. Normal values for PSA include anything less than these

Table 3
Pros and cons of PSA screening

Pros	Cons
Stage migration: more localized disease, and less advanced/metastatic disease	Incidence of indolent tumors
Earlier age at diagnosis	Problems associated with overdiagnosis and overtreatment
Lower PSA at diagnosis	Lead-time and length-time biases in survival rates in PSA era
Improved survival in the PSA era	Ideal PSA cutoff for screening unknown

cutoffs, and change in the PSA value over time is often a better disease indicator than 1 static measurement. Uniformity in this cutoff has not yet been established, but because pretreatment PSA is an important predictor of the final pathologic stage[24] and disease recurrence after radical prostatectomy,[25] conformal radiotherapy,[26] and brachytherapy (BT),[27] it is important to direct further studies in this direction. Generally, a lower PSA at diagnosis is associated with better pathologic outcomes and longer disease-free survival.

Among patients in a PSA range between 4.0 and 10 ng/mL (the diagnostic gray zone), the positive predictive value is only 18% to 25% (mean 21%).[28–30] Thus, the ability of PSA to distinguish prostate cancer from benign conditions such as benign prostatic hyperplasia and prostatitis is not convincing. This may cause unnecessary anxiety and morbidity of patients undergoing prostate biopsies. Another emerging issue is the increasing incidence of clinically relevant prostate cancers in patients with low PSA serum levels (<4.0 ng/mL). An incidence of prostate cancer from 24% to 26.3% (mean 20.5%) was found when serum PSA levels were between 2.5 and 4.0 ng/mL.[31–34] Catalona and colleagues[32] found that 19% of detected prostate cancers with low PSA were not organ confined. Among 42 specimens from patients who had radical prostatectomy after a serum PSA of 2.6 to 4.0 ng/mL, only 17% were clinically insignificant.[26] We conclude that most cancers in men with PSA levels less than 4.0 ng/mL can be considered clinically significant.

These findings suggest that there is a need for new tools to improve the specificity of PSA determination in the diagnostic gray zone and the detection of cancer in men with low PSA levels. Currently it is not possible to use PSA to differentiate between clinically significant and insignificant prostate cancer. For better follow-up, to reduce unnecessary biopsies, and to select patients suitable for appropriate therapy, new molecular markers are urgently required. Novel urinary diagnostic tests are potentially interesting screening tools for this disease. For example, uPM3 is a recently developed urine-based test for detecting prostate cancer. It is a specific biomarker that is effective for diagnosing cancers of all stages.[35]

Stage Migration

One of the most significant changes in the PSA era has been stage migration, the downward shift in the stage at which prostate cancer is discovered and treated, as a result of earlier detection through the use of PSA. Catalona and colleagues[30] first reported a decrease in advanced prostate cancer in the screened population in 1993. They found that 70% of the prostate cancers they detected with PSA screening were pathologically organ confined, in contrast to 51% in the referred population from the same institution. According to the Center for Prostate Disease Research (CPDR)

Table 4
Summary of PSA measurements

	Benefits	Disadvantages
PSA at diagnosis and stage migration	Important indicator, lower cutoffs show cancer at earlier stages than before[17,21,30]	Diagnostic gray zone between 4 and 10 ng/mL only has a predictive value of 21%[28–30] PSA cannot differentiate between clinically significant and insignificant tumors[26]
Percentage free/total PSA (%fPSA)	Ratio of free/total PSA has been shown to be lower in men with prostate cancer[23]	Optimal threshold has yet to be determined; instability currently hampers practical use[32]
Volume adjusted (PSA, PSA density [PSAD] and PSA density of transitional zone)	PSAD is involved in the enlargement of the transitional zone and can help to avoid negative biopsies in other areas[39–41]	Limited use in prostates of 30 cm^3 and less and the effect of interexaminer differences in ultrasound measurement[37,45]
PSA velocity (PSAV)	Annual increase of PSAV has been reported to identify men who have increased risk of, or already have, prostate cancer[46,47]	Individual biologic variability and interassay variability can hamper usefulness[48,49]
Complexed PSA (cPSA)	Can be superior to tPSA in men with more than 4 ng/mL[56]	Results similar to f/t PSA ratio, and superior results not always found in repeat studies[57,58]
Intact PSA (iPSA) and nicked PSA (nPSA)	Higher ration of i/fPSA found in some prostate cancer patients, and higher n/tPSA ratio in men without prostate cancer[61,63]	Low specificity of the test, and hampered by the test's occasional inability to distinguish benign lesions[64]
Benign PSA (bPSA)	Median values of b/tPSA were higher in those patients with benign prostatic hypertrophy (BPH)[66]	BPH can coexist in men with prostate cancer, rendering bPSA an inexact measure[65]
Pro-PSA (pPSA)	Shown to have higher cancer specificity of pPSA in ratio with fPSA[72]	Highly specific immunoassays necessary, and more studies needed[70,71]

database, the percentage of patients presenting with metastatic disease decreased from 19.8% in 1989 to 3.3% in 1998.[36] Data from other American registries also documented age-adjusted incidences of distant metastasis being reduced by approximately 50%.[37] It is believed that a decrease in the rate of distant metastasis will precede a decrease in mortality, as there is no cure for metastatic disease. Roehl and colleagues[23] showed that more than 60% of the prostate cancers in the PSA era were clinical T1c tumors, compared with more than 70% clinical T2 tumors in the pre-PSA era.[23] The overall temporal trend in stage at diagnosis has moved toward earlier-stage disease.

Free PSA, Percentage Free/Total PSA

Studies have shown that the ratio of free PSA/total PSA (f/tPSA) was lower in men with prostate cancer. In 1998, the role of percentage free/total PSA (%fPSA) as a screening tool was reported by Catalona and colleagues.[22] This multicenter study evaluated men with benign prostate hypertrophy and total PSA (tPSA) serum levels between 4 and 10 ng/mL. A %fPSA of less than 25% showed a sensitivity of 95% at a specificity improvement of 20% compared with tPSA. %fPSA was found to be the most important predictor of prostate cancer in first and repeat biopsies if the volume of the entire prostate gland was less than 30 cm^3.[38,39] These findings are of growing importance, because an increasing number of younger patients with smaller glands are investigated in clinical practice. It was also found that an f/tPSA ratio cutoff of 0.1 to 0.2 detected 33% to 56% of prostate cancers among men with a PSA of 2.5 to 4.0 ng/mL.[33] In an identical group of men with tPSA of 2.1 to 4.0 ng/mL, Catalona and colleagues[32] found that all advanced, non–organ-confined, large-volume tumors were identified, and 80% of tumors deemed insignificant with the use of f/tPSA of 0.1 to 0.15. However, the use of f/tPSA could be limited by the stability of fPSA. The optimal threshold for %fPSA remains to be determined, and its inherent instability will hamper its practical use.

Volume-adjusted PSA: PSA Density and PSA Density of Transitional Zone

PSA density (PSAD) is the serum PSA level divided by the prostate volume. PSAD and PSA density of transitional zone (PSAD-TZ) have been reported to offer significant enhancement in cancer detection since 1992. Most of the prostate volume in benign prostatic hypertrophy (BPH) is involved in the enlargement of the transitional zone.[40–42] The specificity of PSAD was reported to be 20% to 37% at sensitivity rates greater than 90% using a cutoff of 0.10 ng/mL/cm^3. Evaluating the PSAD avoided 20% to 37% of negative biopsies with a maximum undetected cancer rate of 10%.[43–45] Djavan and colleagues[38] found improvement in the effectiveness of PSAD-TZ compared with PSAD in men with tPSA between 4.0 and 10.0 ng/mL. The use of a PSAD-TZ cutoff of 0.25 resulted in a specificity of 47% with a sensitivity of 95%. Multivariate analysis showed that PSAD-TZ and %fPSA were the most powerful and highly significant predictors of prostate cancer. However, the main problem of this measurement is related to the effect of interexaminer differences in ultrasound measurement, and it is of limited usefulness in men with prostate volumes of less than 30 cm^3.[37,46] Therefore, PSAD-TZ has been recommended for use in prostate cancer screening in men with low PSA and prostate volumes greater than 30 cm^3. Djavan and colleagues[38] found that PSAD-TZ was an important predictor on repeat biopsy in a prospective study of 1051 cases. Repeat biopsies are recommended in men with PSA levels between 4.0 and 10.0 ng/mL if the PSAD-TZ is more than 0.26 ng/mL/cm^3 or fPSA less than 30%. PSAD-TZ also proved to be useful in the PSA range between 2.5 and 4.0 ng/mL.

PSA Velocity

Data on the value of PSA velocity (PSAV) have so far been controversial. It has been reported that an annual increase of 0.75 ng/mL/y in serum PSA can identify men who have increased risk of, or already have, prostate carcinoma.[47,48] Other studies debate the usefulness of PSAV, because there can be significant individual (biologic) variability and interassay (analytical) variability between PSA tests and low-end PSA values, particularly with shorter intervals between tests.[49,50] Furthermore, the accurate measurement of PSAV requires longitudinal checking over many years.

Complexed PSA

Most PSA in men with prostate cancer is complexed to protease inhibitors, including α_1-antichymotrypsin (ACT) and α_2-macroglobulin,[51] the measurement of which has been hampered by the nonspecific binding of complexed PSA (cPSA).[51,52] An immunoassay using a monoclonal antibody was recently developed (Immuno 1 system, Bayer Diagnostics, New York) to detect all complexed forms except PSA complexed to α_1-macroglobulin. Studies have shown the superiority of cPSA compared with tPSA in men with tPSA more than 4 ng/mL, but results were similar compared with f/tPSA ratio.[20,53–57] Djavan and colleagues[57] found that cPSA cutoff values of 3.06 ng/mL and 2.52 ng/mL resulted in 90% and 95% sensitivity for detecting prostate cancer, and helped avoid unnecessary biopsies in 20.3% and 9.1% of cases, respectively. In contrast, Okihara and colleagues[58] and Stamey and Yemoto[59] were not able to show significant improvement in the specificity for cPSA relative to tPSA. A recent prospective study of 831 patients by Partin and colleagues[60] revealed a significant enhancement in specificity of cPSA compared with tPSA of 6.2% to 7.9% within the tPSA range from 2.0 ng/mL to 10 ng/mL. With a cPSA cutoff value of 2.1 ng/mL, Horninger and colleagues[61] achieved a sensitivity and specificity of 86% and 34.2% respectively for cancer detection in men with tPSA of 2.0 to 4.0 ng/mL. The cPSA immunoassay seems to be a useful tool in the early detection of prostate cancer because of its marked improvement of specificity in patients with low tPSA levels in the range from 2 ng/mL to 4.0 ng/mL. It is a potential new marker for prostate cancer detection and screening.

Intact PSA and Nicked PSA

Intact PSA (iPSA) has been introduced as a molecular subfraction of fPSA that is not internally cleaved. Nurmikko and colleagues[62] developed a novel fPSA antibody, which failed to recognize fPSA that was internally cleaved at Lys145-Lys146. This antibody only measured intact single-chain forms of fPSA (iPSA), such as mature inactive PSA and pro-PSA (pPSA).[63] This trial showed a significantly higher ratio of iPSA/fPSA in prostate cancer patients, compared with patients with benign prostatic disease. Conversely, a higher nicked PSA (nPSA)/tPSA ratio in men without prostate cancer was seen.[64] The investigators suggested using a combination of iPSA, fPSA, and tPSA to more accurately detect prostate cancer. This test is hampered by its low specificity, and the measurements are biased to some extent, because uncleaved PSA (at the position Lys145-Lys146) produced by benign lesions, is also included in the calculation.[65]

Benign PSA

Benign PSA (bPSA) is a fraction of inactive fPSA with a characteristic clip at Lys182. Mikolajczyk and colleagues[66] first found an increased tissue level of bPSA within the transitional zone and in the seminal plasma of patients with nodular BPH. A study by Linton and colleagues[66] showed that bPSA represents a significant percentage of about 50% of fPSA in BPH serum but not in control serum. bPSA was low or undetectable in the control group, consisting of urologic patients not suspected to have BPH or prostate cancers, young and healthy men and women, and patients after radical prostatectomy. The median bPSA/tPSA values were significantly higher in the BPH group, compared with the cancer group. However, BPH may coexist in men with prostate cancer, and this may explain why serum bPSA was not significantly lower in the prostate cancer group in this study.

pPSA

pPSA is a precursor form of PSA enriched in tumors compared with benign prostate tissues.[67–70] It comprises native pPSA ([−7] pPSA) as well as truncated proleader peptides containing 2 or 4 amino acids, [−2] pPSA and [−4] pPSA respectively. With the development of highly specific research immunoassays for pPSA, multiple recent studies have been conducted to establish the clinical usefulness of pPSA in cancer detection compared with the currently used PSA assays.[71,72] Catalona and colleagues[73] established the higher cancer specificity of pPSA in a ratio with fPSA (%pPSA) compared with fPSA and cPSA in PSA ranges 2 to 4 ng/mL and 4 to 10 ng/mL. Immunoassays for all 3 types of pPSA were used and the [−2] pPSA assay outperformed the other 2 assays in cancer detection.

ASPECTS OF SCREENING
Age of Diagnosis

The mean and median ages of men at diagnosis have decreased significantly in the PSA era.[38] The SEER database documented a decline in age at diagnosis from 72 to 69.4 years from 1990 to 1994 (**Table 5**).[18] Theoretically, the younger patients are at the time of diagnosis, the earlier they are in the course of their disease. Carter and colleagues[74] investigated the influence of age on the chance of curable prostate cancer among men with nonpalpable disease. Younger age was found to be associated with greater probability of curable cancer, and was more likely to lead to a decrease in prostate cancer mortality. Similarly, Smith and colleagues[75] showed that younger age at diagnosis is an independent predictor of better prognosis. The earlier age at diagnosis and stage migration with the advent of PSA screening have introduced a lead time of at least 3 to 5 years. This lead-time bias is an important consideration in studies that show improved survival in the PSA era.

Indolent Tumors

Earlier detection of prostate cancer introduces the problem of detection and treatment of indolent tumors. Indolent tumors are generally defined as small tumors (<0.5 cm^3), that are well differentiated (Gleason grade 1 or 2) or noninvasive, and lack the propensity to penetrate beyond the prostatic capsule. In a prospective study by Humphrey and colleagues,[76] 68% of prostate cancers detected by PSA screening were larger

Table 5
Age of diagnosis in the United States, 2002 to 2006

Age at Diagnosis (y)	Total Incidence (%)
<20	0.0
20–34	0.0
35–44	0.6
45–54	8.7
55–64	29.0
65–74	35.6
74–84	21.4
85+	4.7

Data from Horner MJ, Ries LAG, Krapcho M, et al, editors. SEER Cancer Statistics Review, 1975–2006, National Cancer Institute. Bethesda (MD). Available at: http://seer.cancer.gov/csr/1975_2006/, based on November 2008 SEER data submission, posted to the SEER Web site, 2009. Accessed July 2009.

than 0.5 cm^3, and 94% of them had a Gleason score more than 4. The investigators concluded that most prostatic carcinomas detected via PSA screening did not resemble those of autopsy cancers, and that most prostatic cancers detected in the screening programs were likely to be clinically important. Several epidemiologic studies have also shown that moderately differentiated (Gleason score 5–7) tumors predominate in the PSA era.[15,18,24] Although the definitions of indolent tumors differed between studies, it is estimated that up to 30% of all cases of PSA-detected (stage T1c) prostate cancer were indolent tumors.[77]

Prostate Cancer Survival

Survival is an important end point in prostate cancer, and several studies in the PSA era have shown improved survival after the advent of PSA. Gilliland and colleagues[78] found that the 5-year survival rate for prostate cancers diagnosed from 1989 to 1995 was significantly better (92%) than the survival rates from 1974 to 1977 (67%) and 1980 to 1982 (73%). Similar findings were reported by CPDR.[79] In a multivariate analysis by Roehl and colleagues,[23] the era of treatment (1983–1991 vs 1992–2003) was independently associated with biochemical progression-free survival. However, given the prolonged natural history of prostate cancer and the inherent delay in measurement of treatment effects on mortality, it is unlikely that the influence of earlier treatment on the mortality of PSA-detected cancers has yet been fully realized. The favorable era effects seen in these studies are probably caused by a combination of earlier detection (especially detection of advanced disease followed by immediate administration of hormonal therapy), more effective treatment, lead-time and possibly length-time bias, and shorter follow-up during the PSA screening era.

Overdiagnosis and Overtreatment

There are issues of overdiagnosis and overtreatment with PSA screening. Increases in overdiagnosis and overtreatment are related to several factors: (1) the prolonged natural history of prostate cancer, with death of the host from prostate cancer possibly occurring decades from the time of diagnosis, whether or not treatment is undertaken; (2) the generally older age of men when diagnosed with prostate cancer, with the effect of competing causes of death from other comorbidities; (3) the detection of indolent tumors in the general population. Albertson and colleagues[80] showed that many pre–PSA era patients, when followed without treatment, were destined to die of non–prostate cancer causes. Reviewing the SEER data, the increasing gap between the incidence and mortalities in the PSA era indicates increasing rates of overdiagnosis. The declines in mortality are small compared with the large number of men diagnosed with and treated for prostate cancer. This implies that, even if prostate cancer mortality could be eradicated, it would be accomplished at the expense of substantial overtreatment. Recent studies have shown an additional worrying side effect of overdiagnosis of prostate cancer; the effects of this diagnosis on the patients' quality of life (QOL). Even patients with clearly indolent cancers suffer greatly from the diagnosis, and their most important reason for seeking and undergoing active treatment is anxiety, not disease progression.[81]

RECENT FINDINGS ON SCREENING AND PSA
Mortalities in the Tyrol Study

Bartsch and colleagues[82] conducted a study in the federal state of Tyrol, Austria, where PSA testing has been freely available since 1993. When more than two-thirds of the suitable men in Tyrol had been tested at least once, the reduction in mortality (42%) in Tyrol was significantly greater than in the rest of Austria. The investigators noted that most of the decline was likely caused by aggressive down-staging and successful treatment, and they stressed that any contribution from detecting early cancers by PSA testing would only become apparent in the years to come.

Mortalities in the ERSPC Study

The European Randomized Screening for Prostate Cancer (ERSPC) study[83] used data from 7 centers in different countries, with a total of 167,387 men undergoing random-ization. Of these, 72,952 underwent screening, and 89,245 were assigned to the control group. With average and median follow-up times of 8.8 and 9.0 years respec-tively, there were 214 prostate cancer deaths in the screening group and 326 in the control group. This finding results in an unadjusted rate ratio for death in the screening group of 0.80 (95% confidence interval [CI], 0.67–0.95; $P = .01$), and after adjusting of 0.80 (95% CI, 0.65–0.98; $P = .04$). This result means that, to prevent 1 prostate cancer–related death, 1410 (95% CI, 1132–1721) people would need to be screened, and 48 treated (**Table 6**). After adjusting for noncompliance, 1068 would need to be treated; the rate ratio after 9 years was 0.73 (95% CI, 0.56–0.90). The investigators concluded that the population that did benefit from screening was restricted to men between the ages of 55 and 69 years at the start of the trial, and that other age groups did not show any reduction in mortality through screening.

Mortalities in the PLCO Trial

The American PLCO[84] Cancer Screening Trial used the end point of mortality. 76,639 men at 10 study centers in the United States were included; the screening group consisted of 38,343 men, with a control group of 38,350. The incidence of death per 10,000 person years was 2.0 (50 deaths) in the screening group and 1.7 (44 deaths) in the control group (rate ratio, 1.13; 95% CI, 0.75–1.70) (**Table 7**). Most cancers found were diagnosed at stage II, nearly all were adenocarcinomas, and more than 50% had a Gleason score of 5 to 6. These findings did not differ between the screening and control groups. More advanced stage cancers (stage III or IV) were also similar between the 2 groups, although cancers with Gleason scores of 8 to 10 were higher in the control group (341) than in the screening group (289). These results show that, after an average of 7 years of follow-up, the mortality did not significantly differ between the 2 groups. So far in this study, screening is not associated with mortality (rate ratio, 1.13); however, the CIs are wide. It is additionally believed that the effects of any screening of the control group performed outside the study may have obscured the effects of the annual tests within the screening group.

Table 6 Results of ERSPC study	
Rate/ratio for death (95% CI, 0.65–0.98)	0.80
Absolute risk/1000	0.71
Men screened to prevent 1 death	1410
Men screened to prevent 1 death, adjusted	1068
Men treated to prevent 1 death	48

Data from Schroeder FH, Hugosson J, Roobol MJ, et al, for the ERSPC Investigators. Screening and Prostate-Cancer Mortality in a Randomized European Study. N Engl J Med 2009;360:1320–8.

Table 7	
Results of PLCO study (death rates from prostate cancer per 10,000 person years at 10 years)	
Rate/ratio for death (95% CI, 0.83–1.50)	1.11
Number of deaths in screening group	92
Number of deaths in control group	82

Data from Andriole GL, Crawford ED, Grubb RL 3rd, et al; PLCO Project Team. Mortality results from a randomized prostate-cancer screening trial. N Engl J Med 2009 Mar 26;360(13):1316.

False-positive Results

The problem of false positives was also examined with the data from the PLCO trial. Increased prostate screening causes a high rate of false positives; 15.0% of DRE and 10.4% of PSA tests had false-positive results.[85] Rates of overdiagnosis in the PLCO trial were shown to be as high as 50%, whereby men would not show clinical symptoms during their lifetimes.[86] False-positive results have a clear psychological cost and can have a serious effect on patient health. McNaughton-Collins and colleagues[87] showed that 49% of men who initially received a false positive, but later received a confirmed normal result, thought about prostate cancer a lot or some of the time, compared with only 18% of those with a normal PSA (P<.001). This finding raises several questions regarding treatment options, effects on the patients' overall health and well-being, and the costs of screening and treatment caused by overdiagnosis.

QOL Studies

The ERSPC and PLCO reports mention the need for further studies regarding the relationship between prostate cancer screening, treatment, and QOL. If results continue to show that screening has little effect on mortality, the effect on other areas of patients' lives will become more important. For example, a study comparing radical retropubic prostatectomy (RRP) with permanent BT for prostate cancer showed that the choice of method can affect patient QOL. Kobuke and colleagues[88] found that RRP patients scored better in overall QOL, except for 1 month after surgery. Studies like this could be used as a starting point for monitoring patients' QOL throughout screening, diagnosis, and treatment, as well as after treatment.

Future Developments

Although the longitudinal ERSPC and PLCO trials are a start, they need to be examined further. Because of the difficulties associated with using mortality as an end point in prostate cancer, the studies need to be extended and the patients' follow-up times increased. The ERSPC trial[83] noted that the rates of death from prostate cancer between the screening and control groups only began to diverge after 7 to 8 years, and that this diversion continued to grow with time, showing a clear need for longer follow-up times. The ERSPC trial additionally noted that the benefit from screening was present only in the 55- to 69-year-old age group. However, it did not evaluate between centers and between age subgroups, which may be an important next step for evaluating screening methods. Additional studies of options other than screening for those less than 55 and more than 69 years old are also needed, to look for ways to improve their mortalities. As the 2 latest trials show, there is also a need for more uniformity within and between studies.

Risk categories can be predicted using a tool (PROSTATE Px+, Aureon Laboratories, USA) that combines histologic, molecular, and clinical parameters. Histologically, it quantitatively captures and analyzes cellular features. Multiple molecular layers are assessed for comprehensive protein analysis. This information is then combined with clinical and biochemical parameters (PSA, Gleason score) to improve the prediction of cancer outcomes. Cordon-Cardo and colleagues[89] reported improved prediction of prostate cancer recurrence using this tool. The model predicted recurrence with high accuracy, as indicated by a concordance index in the validation set of 0.82, sensitivity of 96%, and specificity of 72%. They then extended this approach, using quantitative multiplex immunofluorescence on an expanded cohort, with sensitivity of 77% and specificity of 72%.

SUMMARY

Prostate cancer is the most common malignancy in men in Western societies, and the incidence of prostate cancer is rapidly increasing in other lower-risk countries. The question of using PSA as a screening tool for prostate cancer detection is often debated, but PSA remains the gold standard in prostate cancer screening. However, improving the specificity and sensitivity of this screening method is imperative. Novel markers for prostate cancer detection, staging, and monitoring are required. The new molecular forms of pPSA are exciting, but further studies are required to validate its clinical application. Initial results show that uPM3 may be an effective noninvasive tool for prostate cancer detection. Currently, the most promising new marker is cPSA. Measurement of cPSA seems to be more stable than fPSA. Therefore, it could improve early diagnosis of prostate cancer, especially in patients with low serum PSA levels. The question of prostate cancer mortality reduction will be addressed in the 2 ongoing trials: ERSPC and PLCO. Based on evidence from studies in the PSA era, PSA testing can be recommended to the patient, but the pros and the cons must be mentioned in the discussion. In the latest recommendation by the American Cancer Society, PSA testing is called for when the patient is undecided.[90]

REFERENCES

1. Greenlee RT, Hill-Harmon MB, Murray T, et al. Cancer statistics 2001. CA Cancer J Clin 2001;51:15–37.
2. Eyre H, Kahn R, Robertson RM, et al. Preventing cancer, cardiovascular disease, and diabetes. A common agenda for the American Cancer Society, the American Diabetes Association, and the American Heart Association. Circulation 2004;109: 3244–55.
3. Hsing AW, Tsao L, Devesa SS. International trends and patterns of prostate cancer incidence and mortality. Int J Cancer 2000;85:60–7.
4. Stephenson RA. Prostate cancer trends in the era of prostate specific antigen: an update of incidence, mortality, and clinical factors from the SEER database. Urol Clin North Am 2002;29:173–8.
5. Horner MJ, Ries LAG, Krapcho M, et al. SEER Cancer Statistics Review, 1975–2006. National Cancer Institute. Bethesda (MD). Available at: http://seer.cancer.gov/csr/1975_2006/. Accessed June 10, 2010. Based on November 2008 SEER data submission, posted to the SEER Web site, 2009.
6. Ross RK, Bernstein L, Lobo RA, et al. 5-Alpha-reductase activity and risk of prostate cancer among Japanese and US white and black males. Lancet 1992;339: 887–9.
7. Ross RK, Coetzee GA, Reichardt J, et al. Does the racial-ethnic variation in prostate cancer risk have a hormonal basis? Cancer 1995;75:1778–92.

8. Makridakis NM, Ross RK, Pike MC, et al. Association of mis-sense substitution in SRD5A2 gene with prostate cancer in African American and Hispanic men in Los Angeles. Lancet 1999;354:975–8.

9. Hardy DO, Scher HI, Bogenreider T, et al. Androgen receptor CAG repeat lengths in prostate cancer: correlation with age of onset. J Clin Endocrinol Metab 1996; 81:4400–5.

10. Ross RK, Henderson BE. Do diet and androgen alter prostate cancer risk via a common etiologic pathway? J Natl Cancer Inst 1994;86:252–4.

11. Paris PL, Kupelian PA, Hall JM, et al. Association between CYP3A4 genetic variant and clinical presentation in African American prostate cancer patients. Cancer Epidemiol Biomarkers Prev 1998;8:901–5.

12. Kolonel LN, Nomura AM, Cooney RV. Dietary fat and prostate cancer: current status. J Natl Cancer Inst 1999;91:414–28.

13. Denis L, Morton MS, Griffiths K. Diet and its preventive role in prostatic disease. Eur Urol 1999;35:377–87.

14. Hsing AW, Devesa SS, Jin F, et al. Rising incidence of prostate cancer in Shanghai. Cancer Epidemiol Biomarkers Prev 1998;7:83–4.

15. Paeratakul S, Popkin BM, Keyou G, et al. Changes in diet and physical activity affect the body mass index of Chinese adults. Int J Obes Relat Metab Disord 1998;22:424–31.

16. Djavan B, Eckersberger E, Espinosa G, et al. Complex mechanisms in prostatic inflammatory response. Eur Urol 2009;8(13):872–8.

17. Margreiter M, Stangelberger A, Valimberti E, et al. Biomarkers for early prostate cancer detection. Minerva Urol Nefrol 2008;60:51–60.

18. Riegman PH, Vlietstra RJ, Klaassen P, et al. The prostate-specific antigen gene and the human glandular kallikrein-1 gene are tandemly located on chromosome 19. FEBS Lett 1989;247(1):123–6.

19. Boccon-Gibod L. Rising PSA with negative biopsy. Eur Urol 2001;40(Suppl 2):3–8.

20. Brawer MK, Cheli CD, Neaman IE, et al. Complexed prostate specific antigen provides significant enhancement of specificity compared with total prostate specific antigen for detecting prostate cancer. J Urol 2000;163:1476–80.

21. Schwartz KL, Grignon DJ, Sakr WA, et al. Prostate cancer histologic trends in the Metropolitan Detroit area, 1982 to 1996. Urology 1999;53:769–74.

22. Catalona WJ, Partin AW, Slawin KM, et al. Use of percentage of free prostate specific antigen to enhance differentiation of prostate cancer from benign prostatic disease: a prospective multicenter clinical trial. JAMA 1998;279:1542–7.

23. Roehl KA, Han M, Ramos CG, et al. Cancer progression and survival rates following anatomical radical retropubic prostatectomy in 3,478 consecutive patients: long-term results. J Urol 2004;172:910–4.

24. Partin AW, Mangold LA, Lamm DM, et al. Contemporary update of prostate cancer staging nomograms (Partin tables) for the new millennium. Urology 2001;58:843–8.

25. Kattan MW, Eastham JA, Stapleton AM, et al. A preoperative nomogram for disease recurrence after radical prostatectomy for prostate cancer. J Natl Cancer Inst 1998;90:766–71.

26. Kattan MW, Zelefsky MJ, Kupelian PA, et al. Pretreatment nomogram for predicting the outcome of three-dimensional conformal radiotherapy in prostate cancer. J Clin Oncol 2000;18:3352–9.

27. Kattan MW, Potters L, Blasko JC, et al. Pretreatment nomogram for predicting freedom from recurrence after permanent prostate brachytherapy in prostate cancer. Urology 2001;58:393–9.

28. Catalona WJ, Smith DS, Ratliff TL, et al. Measurement of prostate specific antigen in serum as a screening test for prostate cancer. N Engl J Med 1991;324: 1156–61.
29. Bretton PR. Prostate specific antigen and digital rectal examination in screening for prostate cancer: a community based study. South Med J 1994;87:720–3.
30. Catalona WJ, Smith DS, Ratliff TL, et al. Detection of organ confined prostate cancer is increased through prostate specific antigen based screening. JAMA 1993;270:948–54.
31. Catalona WJ, Smith DS, Ornstein DK. Prostate cancer detection in men with serum PSA concentrations of 2.6 to 4.0 ng/ml and benign prostate examination. Enhancement of specificity with free PSA measurements. JAMA 1997;277:1452–5.
32. Catalona WJ, Partin AW, Finlay JA, et al. Use of percentage of free prostate specific antigen to identify men at high risk of prostate cancer when PSA levels are 2.51 to 4 ng/ml and digital rectal examination is not suspicious for prostate cancer: an alternative model. Urology 1999;54:220–4.
33. Djavan B, Zlotta A, Kratzik C, et al. PSA, PSA density, PSA density of transitional zone, free/total PSA ratio, and PSA velocity for early detection of prostate cancer in men with serum PSA 2.5 to 4.0 ng/ml. Urology 1999;54:517–22.
34. Babaian RJ, Fritsche H, Ayala A, et al. Performance of a neural network in detecting prostate cancer in the prostate-specific antigen reflex range of 2.5 to 4.0 ng/ml. Urology 2000;56:1000–6.
35. Bostwick DG, Gould VE, Qian J, et al. Prostate cancer detected by uPM3: radical prostatectomy findings. Mod Pathol 2006;19(5):630–3.
36. Sun L, Gancarczyk K, Paquette EL, et al. Introduction to the Department of Defense Center for Prostate Disease Research Multicenter National Prostate Cancer Database and analysis in the PSA era. Urol Oncol 2001;203–9.
37. Stephenson RA, Stanford JL. Population-based prostate cancer trends in the United States: patterns of change in the era of prostate specific antigen. World J Urol 1997;15:331–5.
38. Djavan B, Zlotta AR, Byttebier G, et al. Prostate specific antigen density of the transitional zone for early detection of prostate cancer. J Urol 1998;160:411–9.
39. Djavan B, Zlotta A, Remzi M, et al. Optimal predictors of prostate cancer on repeat prostate biopsy: a prospective study of 1051 patients. J Urol 2000;163: 1144–9.
40. Stamey TA, Yang N, Hay AR, et al. Prostate specific antigen as a serum marker for adenocarcinoma of the prostate. N Engl J Med 1987;317:909–16.
41. Babaian RJ, Fritsche HA, Evans RB. Prostate specific antigen and prostate gland volume: correlation and clinical application. J Clin Lab Anal 1990;4:135–7.
42. Benson MC, Whang IS, Olsson CA, et al. The use of prostate specific antigen density to enhance the predictive value of intermediate levels of serum prostate specific antigen. J Urol 1992;147:817–21.
43. Morote J, Raventos CX, Lorente JA, et al. Comparison of percent free prostate specific antigen and prostate specific antigen density as methods to enhance prostate specific antigen specificity in early prostate cancer detection in men with normal rectal examination and prostate specific antigen between 4.1 and 10 ng/ml. J Urol 1997;158:502–4.
44. Kuriyama M, Uno H, Watanabe H, et al. Determination of reference values for total PSA, F/T and PSAD according to prostatic volume in Japanese prostate cancer patients with slightly elevated serum PSA levels. Jpn J Clin Oncol 1999;29:617–22.
45. Reissigl A, Horninger W, Fink K, et al. Prostate cancer screening in the county of Tyrol, Austria: experience and results. Cancer 1997;80:1818–29.

46. Borer JG, Sherman J, Solomon MC, et al. Age specific prostate specific antigen reference ranges: population specific. J Urol 1998;159:444–8.

47. Schmid HP, McNeal JE, Stamey TA. Observations on the doubling time of prostate cancer. The use of serial prostate-specific antigen in patients with untreated disease as a measure of increasing cancer volume. Cancer 1993;71(6):2031–40.

48. Carter HB, Morrell CH, Pearson JD, et al. Estimation of prostatic growth using serial prostate-specific antigen measurements in men with and without prostate disease. Cancer Res 1992;52(12):3323–8.

49. Ornstein DK, Smith DS, Rao GS, et al. Biological variation of total, free and percent free serum prostate specific antigen levels in screening volunteers. J Urol 1997;157(6):2179–82.

50. Nixon RG, Wener MH, Smith KM, et al. Day to day changes in free and total PSA: significance of biological variation. Prostate Cancer Prostatic Dis 1997;1(2):90–6.

51. Porter JR, Hayward R, Brawer MK. The significance of short term PSA change in men undergoing ultrasound guided prostate biopsy. J Urol 1994;264(Suppl): 239A.

52. Nixon RG, Meyer GE, Blase AB, et al. Comparison of three investigational assays for the free form of prostate specific antigen. J Urol 1998;160:420–5.

53. Brawer MK, Meyer GE, Letran JL, et al. Measurement of complexed PSA improves the specificity for early detection of prostate cancer. Urology 1998; 52:372–8.

54. Okegawa T, Noda H, Nutahara K, et al. Comparison of two investigational assays for the complexed prostate specific antigen in total prostate specific antigen between 4.0 and 10.0 ng/ml. Urology 2000;55:700–4.

55. Mitchell ID, Croal BL, Dickie A, et al. A prospective study to evaluate the role of complexed prostate specific antigen and free/total prostate specific antigen ratio for the diagnosis of prostate cancer. J Urol 2001;165:49–53.

56. Miller MC, O'Dowd GJ, Partin AW, et al. Contemporary use of complexed PSA and calculated per cent free PSA for early detection of prostate cancer: impact of changing demographics. Urology 2001;57:1105–11.

57. Djavan B, Remzi M, Zlotta AR, et al. Complexed prostate specific antigen, complexed prostate specific antigen density of total and transitional zone, complexed/total prostate specific antigen ratio, free-to-total prostate specific antigen ratio, density of total and transition zone prostate specific antigen: results of the prospective multicenter European trial. Urology 2002;60:4–9.

58. Okihara K, Cheli CD, Partin AW, et al. Comparative analysis of complexed prostate specific antigen, free prostate specific antigen, and their ratio in detecting prostate cancer. J Urol 2002;167:2017–23.

59. Stamey TA, Yemoto CE. Examination of the 3 molecular forms of serum prostate specific antigen for distinguishing negative from positive biopsy: relationship to transitional zone volume. J Urol 2000;163:119–24.

60. Partin AW, Brawer MK, Bartsch G, et al. Complexed prostate specific antigen improves the specificity for prostate cancer detection: results of a prospective multicenter clinical trial. J Urol 2003;170:1787–91.

61. Horninger W, Cheli CD, Babaian RJ, et al. Complexed prostate-specific antigen for early detection of prostate cancer in men with serum prostate-specific antigen levels of 2 to 4 nanograms per milliliter. Urology 2002;60(4 Suppl 1):31–5.

62. Nurmikko P, Vaisanen V, Piironen T, et al. Production and characterization of novel anti-prostate specific antigen (PSA) monoclonal antibodies that do not detect the internally cleaved Lys145-Lys146 inactive PSA. Clin Chem 2000; 46:1610–8.

63. Nurmikko P, Pettersson K, Piironen T, et al. Discrimination of prostate cancer from benign disease by plasma measurement of intact, free prostate specific antigen lacking an internal cleavage site at Lys145-Lys146. Clin Chem 2001; 47:1415–23.
64. Steuber T, Nurmikko P, Haese A, et al. Discrimination of benign from malignant prostatic disease by selective measurements of single chain, intact free prostate specific antigen. J Urol 2002;168:1917–22.
65. Linton HJ, Marks LS, Millar LS, et al. Benign prostate specific antigen (BPSA) in serum is increased in benign prostate disease. Clin Chem 2003;49:253–9.
66. Mikolajczyk SD, Millar LS, Marker KM, et al. Seminal plasma contains "BPSA", a molecular form of prostate specific antigen that is associated with benign prostatic hyperplasia. Prostate 2000;45:271–6.
67. Mikolajczyk SD, Millar LS, Wang TJ, et al. A precursor form of prostate specific antigen is highly elevated in prostate cancer compared with benign transitional zone prostate tissue. Cancer Res 2000;60:756–9.
68. Mikolajczyk SD, Grauer LS, Millar LS, et al. A precursor form of PSA (pPSA) is a component of the free PSA in prostate cancer serum. Urology 1997;50:710–4.
69. Mikolajczyk SD, Marker KM, Millar LS, et al. A truncated precursor form of prostate specific antigen is a more specific serum marker of prostate cancer. Cancer Res 2001;61:6958–63.
70. Peter J, Unverzagt C, Krogh TN, et al. Identification of precursor forms of free prostate specific antigen in serum of prostate cancer patients by immunosorption and spectrometry. Cancer Res 2001;61:957–62.
71. Mikolaiczyk SD, Rittenhouse HG. Pro PSA: a more cancer specific form of prostate specific antigen for the early detection of prostate cancer. Keio J Med 2003; 52:86–9.
72. Sokoll LJ, Chan DW, Mikolajczyk SD. Proenzyme PSA for the early detection of prostate cancer in the 2.5–4.0 ng/ml total PSA range: preliminary analysis. Urology 2002;59:261–5.
73. Catalona WJ, Bartsch G, Rittenhouse HG, et al. Serum pro prostate specific antigen improves cancer detection compared to free and complexed prostate specific antigen in men with prostate specific antigen 2.4–4 ng/ml. J Urol 2003; 170:2181–5.
74. Carter HB, Epstein JI, Partin AW. Influence of age and prostate specific antigen on the chance of curable prostate cancer among men with nonpalpable disease. Urology 1999;53:126–30.
75. Smith CV, Bauer JJ, Connelly RR, et al. Prostate cancer in men age 50 years or younger: a review of the Department of Defense Center for Prostate Disease Research multicenter prostate cancer database. J Urol 2000;164:1964–7.
76. Humphrey PA, Keetch DW, Smith DS, et al. Prospective characterization of pathological features of prostatic carcinomas detected via serum prostate specific antigen based screening. J Urol 1996;155:816–20.
77. Anast JW, Andriole GL, Bismar TA, et al. Relating biopsy and clinical variables to radical prostatectomy findings: can insignificant and advanced prostate cancer be predicted in a screened population? Urology 2004;64:544–50.
78. Gilliland FD, Hunt WC, Key CR. Improving survival for patients with prostate cancer diagnosed in the prostate specific antigen era. Urology 1996;48:67–71.
79. Paquette EL, Connelly RR, Sesterhenn IA, et al. Improvements in pathologic staging for African American men undergoing radical retropubic prostatectomy during the prostate specific antigen era: implications for screening a high-risk group for prostate carcinoma. Cancer 2001;92:2673–9.

80. Albertson PC, Fryback DG, Storer BE, et al. Long term survival among men with conservatively treated localized prostate cancer. JAMA 1995;274:626–31.
81. Canfield S. Commentary; annual screening for prostate cancer did not reduce mortality from prostate cancer. Evidence Based Med 2009;150:4–5.
82. Bartsch G, Horninger W, Klocker H, et al. Prostate cancer mortality after introduction of prostate specific antigen mass screening in the federal state of Tyrol, Austria. Urology 2001;58:417–24.
83. Schröder FH, Hugosson J, Roobol MJ, et al. Screening and prostate-cancer mortality in a randomized European study. N Engl J Med 2009;360:1320–8.
84. Andriole GL, Crawford ED, Grubb RL 3rd, et al. Mortality results from a randomized prostate-cancer screening trial. N Engl J Med 2009;360:1310–9.
85. Croswell JM, Kramer BS, Kreimer AR, et al. Cumulative incidence of false-positive results in repeated, multimodal cancer screening. Ann Fam Med 2009;7:212–22.
86. Draisma G, Boer R, Otto SJ, et al. Lead times and overdetection due to prostate-specific antigen screening: estimates from the European Randomized Study of Screening for Prostate Cancer. J Natl Cancer Inst 2003;95:868–78.
87. McNaughton-Collins M, Fowler FJ, Caubet JF, et al. Psychological effects of a suspicious prostate cancer screening test followed by a benign biopsy result. Am J Med 2004;117:719–25.
88. Kobuke M, Saika T, Nakanishi Y. Prospective longitudinal comparative study of health-related quality of life in patients with radical prostatectomy or permanent brachytherapy for prostate cancer. Acta Med Okayama 2009;63:129–35.
89. Cordon-Cardo C, Kotsianti A, Verbel DA, et al. Improved prediction of prostate cancer recurrence through systems pathology. J Clin Invest 2007;117:1876–83.
90. Smith RA, Von Eschenbach AC, Wender R, et al. American cancer society guidelines for early detection of cancer: Update of early detection guidelines for prostate, colorectal and endometrial cancers. CA Cancer J Clin 2001;51:38–75.

Evaluation and Management of Hematuria

Masahito Jimbo, MD, PhD, MPH[a,b,*]

KEYWORDS

- Hematuria • Microscopic hematuria • Gross hematuria
- Urinalysis • Management

DEFINITION OF HEMATURIA

Hematuria is defined as the presence of an abnormal quantity of red blood cells (RBCs) in the urine. Clinically, it can be classified as either gross or microscopic hematuria.

Gross Hematuria

Gross hematuria is defined as urine that is visibly discolored by blood. It may occur with as little as 1 mL of blood in 1 L of urine. Because the patients can recognize the abnormal color of the urine, they typically present to their physician soon after the episode. Gross hematuria must be differentiated from other causes of discolored urine.[1] The causes of abnormal urine color are shown in **Table 1**.

Microscopic Hematuria

Definitions of microscopic hematuria vary, ranging from 1 to more than 10 RBCs per high-power field (400× magnification). Therefore, making a clear-cut recommendation for the evaluation of microscopic hematuria based on past studies is difficult.[2] In this article, the American Urological Association's definition is used: the presence of 3 or more RBCs per high-powered field, in 2 of 3 properly collected urine samples.[3] Microscopic hematuria is typically differentiated into glomerular (hematuria from the glomeruli, suggesting a nephrological disease) and nonglomerular (hematuria from

This work was supported by the Family Medicine Educational Scholars Program of the University of Michigan, Department of Family Medicine.

[a] Department of Family Medicine, University of Michigan, 1018 Fuller Street, Ann Arbor, MI 48104, USA

[b] Department of Urology, 1500 East Medical Center Drive, A. Alfred Taubman Health Care Center, Room 3875, University of Michigan, Ann Arbor, MI 48109-0330, USA

* Department of Family Medicine, University of Michigan, 1018 Fuller Street, Ann Arbor, MI 48104.

E-mail address: mjimbo@med.umich.edu

Prim Care Clin Office Pract 37 (2010) 461–472

doi:10.1016/j.pop.2010.04.006

Table 1
Causes of abnormal urine color

Color	Foods	Drugs	Others

Red/Brown	Beets
	Blackberries
	Rhubarb
	Fava beans
	Aloe
		Laxatives (eg, Ex-Lax,
		    phenolphthalein)
		Tranquilizers (eg,
		    chlorpromazine,
		    thioridazine, propofol)
			Porphyrin (eg, lead,
			    mercury poisoning)
			Globins (eg, hemoglobin,
			    myoglobin)

Orange	Carotene-
	    containing foods
	    (eg, carrots,
	    winter squash)
		Beta-carotene
		    supplements
		Vitamin B supplements
		Warfarin
		Rifampin
		Pyridium
			Urochrome (eg,
			    dehydration)

Green/Blue	Asparagus	Amitriptyline Indomethacin Cimetidine Promethazine	
Black		Methyldopa	

Data from Sokolosky MC. Hematuria. Emerg Med Clin North Am 2001;19:621–32.

nonglomerular sites, such as renal pelvis, ureter, and bladder, suggesting a urological disease).

EPIDEMIOLOGY OF HEMATURIA
Prevalence of Hematuria

The prevalence of microscopic hematuria in the general population ranges from 0.19% to 16.1%, with 2 out of 6 studies showing a lower prevalence among men.[2–4] The variation in prevalence is because of the heterogeneity of the populations studied. When the population studied more closely resembles the adult primary care population, the prevalence is less variable, ranging from 2.5% to 4.3%.[5–7] Transient microscopic hematuria may occur in 6% to 39% of the population studied, but persistent microscopic hematuria in 3 or more consecutive urinalyses occurs less often, and is seen in 0.5% to 2% of the population under study.[8,9] Causes of transient hematuria may include vigorous exercise, sexual intercourse, mild trauma, and menstrual contamination. In the prevalence of underlying urinary tract disease, there is no clear difference between patients with transient microscopic hematuria and those with persistent microscopic hematuria.[2]

Screening for Hematuria

At present, routine screening for microscopic hematuria is not advocated by any professional organization, including the American Urological Association.[10] The United States Preventive Services Task Force recommends against routine screening for bladder cancer, including urinalysis to check for microscopic hematuria, as do the Canadian Task Force on Preventive Health Care and the American Academy of Family Physicians.[11] The American Cancer Society notes that certain high-risk people, such as those with a previous diagnosis of bladder cancer, certain birth defects of the bladder, or a history of work-related exposure (particularly in the dye or rubber industries) may be screened.[12] However, in reality patients often get screened for hematuria through urinalysis during a routine checkup, as part of hospital admission laboratory set, and as part of the school or work screening done in some countries such as Japan. Thus, it is not unusual for a patient to present to the physician's office with an abnormal urinalysis result, including a positive dipstick and positive microscopic examination for hematuria.

Causes of Hematuria

Sixteen studies looked at the causes of asymptomatic hematuria.[5,7,13–26] Underlying causes were found in 32% to 100% of the population studied. Moderately significant disease (stones, inflammation, and anatomic abnormalities) was noted in 3.4% to 27%, and highly significant disease (malignancy) was noted in 0% to 26% of the population studied. These studies were heterogeneous in patient age and gender, and whether the patient groups were referral- or population-based. In the 6 studies that were population-based, the prevalence of moderately or highly significant disease was lower, at 0.6% to 16.1%.

An extrarenal site is responsible for more than 60% of cases of hematuria.[27] Of these, the most important underlying disease is malignancy. In the primary care population, about 5% of patients with microscopic hematuria will have a urinary tract malignancy, mainly of the bladder or prostate.[2] Urinary tract malignancies are more common in men, with an incidence twice that of women,[28] even if one excludes prostate cancer. In particular, gross hematuria is associated with a urinary tract malignancy in up to 22% of the cases, so a full urological workup with cystoscopy and upper urinary tract imaging is needed in these patients.[29,30] The most common nonmalignant causes of extrarenal hematuria are infections, such as cystitis, prostatitis, and urethritis.[2]

Regarding renal causes of microscopic hematuria, the most common cause of isolated glomerular hematuria (without significant proteinuria) is IgA nephropathy, followed by thin basement membrane disease, hereditary nephritis (Alport syndrome), and mild focal glomerulonephritis of other causes. Other common renal causes of nonglomerular hematuria include renal stones, pyelonephritis, polycystic kidney disease, and renal cell carcinoma.[2] Hematuria is a less reliable indicator of renal disease than proteinuria, and hematuria does not correlate with the degree or progression of the renal disease. The common causes of hematuria, classified by location and mechanism, are shown in **Table 2**.

CLINICAL EVALUATION
History

Because microscopic hematuria has a benign cause in many patients, particularly in younger women, careful history-taking is essential. Particular attention should be paid to any history that suggests a benign cause, such as menstruation, recent exercise, sexual activity, viral infection, or trauma. If any of these conditions are found and the patient has no other risk factors, urinalysis may be repeated 48 hours after stopping these activities, and further workup can be stopped if the result is negative.[30]

Certain factors raise the risk of significant disease as the cause of microscopic hematuria. Factors include age greater than 40 years; tobacco use; occupational exposure to chemicals or dyes (benzenes or aromatic amines); history of gross hematuria, urologic disorder or disease, irritative voiding symptoms, urinary tract infection, or pelvic irradiation; and analgesic abuse.[30] In such situations, the presence of microscopic hematuria in just one properly obtained urine sample may be a valid trigger for further workup. The exception may be a young woman with symptoms and urinary findings suggestive of urinary tract infection. In this case, if urine culture is positive,

Table 2
More common causes of microscopic hematuria

Site	Malignancy	Inflammation	Stones	Anatomic Abnormality	Other
Kidney	Renal cell carcinoma Renal transitional cell carcinoma Renal lymphoma	IgA nephropathy[a] Hereditary nephritis[a] Other glomerulopathies[a] Pyelonephritis Renal tuberculosis	Renal stones	Thin basement membrane disease[a] Polycystic kidney disease Medullary sponge kidney Hydronephrosis	Hypercalciuria Hyperuricosuria Renal trauma Papillary necrosis Sickle cell disease/trait Renal infarction
Ureter	Ureteral transitional cell carcinoma		Ureteral stones	Ureteral stricture	
Bladder	Bladder cancer	Bacterial cystitis Tuberculous cystitis Radiation cystitis *Schistosoma haematobium*	Bladder stones	Vesicoureteral reflux Cystocele Bladder papilloma Trabeculated bladder	
Prostate	Prostate cancer	Prostatitis	Prostate stones	Benign prostate hypertrophy	
Other	Urethral cancer Penile cancer Metastatic cancer	Urethritis		Urethral stricture	Abdominal aortic aneurysm Over-anticoagulation

[a] Denotes glomerular disease.
Data from Cohen RA, Brown RS. Microscopic hematuria. N Engl J Med 2003;348:2330–8; and Grossfeld GD, Litwin MS, Wolf JS, et al. Evaluation of asymptomatic microscopic hematuria in adults: the American Urological Association best practice policy—part I: definition, detection, prevalence, and etiology. Urology 2001;57:599–603.

she may be treated with an appropriate antibiotic, and repeat urinalysis is performed 6 weeks after the treatment. If the subsequent result is negative, no further workup is necessary.[30] Therefore, eliciting the presence of these risk factors would be paramount when taking history from patients with documented hematuria.

Certain tools aid in obtaining an appropriate history, particularly regarding irritative voiding symptoms. The American Urology Association Symptom Index, which assesses the severity of irritative and obstructive voiding symptoms, is a validated questionnaire that can be completed by the patient.[31] This index grades the severity of the following 7 symptoms from 0 to 5: incomplete emptying, frequency, intermittency, urgency, weak stream, straining, and nocturia. The total maximum score possible is 35, and the severity is classified as mild (0–7), moderate (8–19), or severe (20–35). The actual template is presented by Djavan and colleagues elsewhere in this issue for further exploration of this topic, and is readily available online.

Because a glomerular cause may be a possibility, premature focus on the genitourinary system may cause diagnostic errors. Attention to medical history, medication use, family history, and a review of the systems can help in finding the potential underlying disease that may cause secondary glomerulopathy. The patient should also be asked about any symptoms of chronic kidney disease, such as edema and other signs of volume overload.

Physical Examination

When a urological condition is suspected, a detailed genitourinary examination is essential, which is discussed by Martinez-Bianchi and Halstater elsewhere in this issue for further exploration of this topic. When a nephrological condition (such as glomerular hematuria) is suspected, checking the blood pressure and performing a detailed cardiovascular examination are important.[27]

LABORATORY EVALUATION
Urinalysis

Urinalysis is a simple and efficient tool to diagnose renal and urological diseases. Typically, the urine dipstick test for blood initially identifies patients with microscopic hematuria. The sensitivity of a urine dipstick test for blood varies from 91% to 100%, and the specificity varies from 65% to 99%.[29] The test detects the peroxidase activity of RBCs, so hemoglobin and myoglobin can cause a false-positive result. Other causes of false-positive results include dehydration, exercise, povidone-iodine, and oxidizing agents.[27] Causes of false-negative results include vitamin C (a reducing agent) and air exposure.[27]

The urine dipstick is sensitive enough to detect 1 to 2 RBCs per high-power field. Because of its high sensitivity, a urine dipstick test is generally sufficient to rule out hematuria. However, because of its variable specificity, a positive dipstick test should be verified with urine microscopy. A midstream clean-catch technique usually provides uncontaminated urine from men and women; cleansing of the external genitalia has no proven benefit.[29,32] When performing urine microscopy, proper care should be taken in preparing the sample. A fresh sample of 10 to 15 mL of urine should be centrifuged at 1500 to 3000 rpm for 5 minutes. The supernatant is then decanted and the sediment is agitated in the remaining supernatant. A single drop is applied to a clean glass slide, and a coverslip is applied.[33]

The urine microscopic evaluation not only confirms hematuria but also helps differentiate glomerular from nonglomerular sources of bleeding. In glomerular hematuria, the RBCs are exposed to large changes in pH and osmotic pressure as they go through the renal tubules, making them dysmorphic.[34] In nonglomerular hematuria, the RBCs tend to be homogeneous and normal in shape. The presence of proteinuria of 2+ or greater by dipstick also suggests glomerular hematuria, because hematuria alone does not result in such a large protein excretion.[29] Blood clots do not occur in glomerular hematuria, because of the presence of urokinase and tissue-type plasminogen activators in the glomerular filtrate.[27] RBC casts are virtually pathognomonic for glomerular hematuria, because the matrix of the cast is Tamms-Horsfall protein, which is secreted by the distal tubule.

One situation for which urine dipstick is more accurate than urine microscopy is when the urine is very dilute, with specific gravity of less than 1.007. In this urine environment, RBCs may lyse and not be visible, causing the urine microscopic examination to be falsely negative for hematuria.[35]

Urine Cytology

Checking voided urine for abnormal cells is not very sensitive (66%–79%), but is highly specific (95%–100%) for bladder cancer.[2,30,36] Obtaining 3 consecutive first-morning-voided urine samples for cytologic analysis increases sensitivity.[37] Its sensitivity is higher for high-grade bladder tumors and lower for low-grade tumors; only 15% of patients with "atypical and/or suspicious" cytologic findings may have underlying urinary tract malignancy.[38]

Urine Tumor Markers

Urine tumor marker tests detect antigens and other substances unique to cancer cells, mostly of the bladder, including the bladder tumor antigen (BTA) test, nuclear matrix protein 22 (NMP22), carcinoembryonic antigen (CEA), cytokeratin tissue polypeptide-specific antigen (TPS), fluorescence in situ hybridization (FISH) assay, Lewis X antigen, telomerase activity, and urinary bladder cancer tumor marker (UBCTM) tests.[36,39] Although these tests potentially hold promise in complementing or supplanting urine cytology, none is widely used at present.[36,39]

Urine Culture

It is prudent to obtain a urine culture in patients with hematuria, particularly from those with irritative voiding symptoms or a history of urinary tract infection.

Serum Creatinine and Calculation of Glomerular Filtration Rate

If the clinical evaluation and urinalysis suggest a glomerular (nephrological) cause of hematuria, then renal function should be measured. Glomerular filtration rate (GFR) is the most reliable estimate of the renal function, and is the foundation of the chronic kidney disease staging system used by the National Kidney Foundation Kidney Disease Outcomes Quality Initiative (NKF-KDOQUI).[40] GFR cannot be measured directly, so it is estimated using the urinary clearance of a filtration marker. Clearance is the rate at which a substance is cleared from the plasma by excretion in the urine.

Serum creatinine is the most commonly used endogenous filtration marker. Creatinine is an amino acid derivative that is freely filtered by the glomerulus. Creatinine has all the characteristics of an ideal filtrate, except that it is actively secreted in the renal tubule, and active secretion proportionately increases as renal function declines.[40] Thus, creatinine clearance overestimates GFR, particularly as the renal dysfunction progresses. Also, serum creatinine is affected by factors such as age, sex, and lean body mass, with higher creatinine levels seen in those who are younger, male, and more muscular. Equations that estimate GFR from serum creatinine at least partially overcome the inaccuracy of creatinine clearance and the inconvenience of collecting urine over 24 hours. The 2 widely used equations are the Cockcroft-Gault equation and the MDRD (Modification of Diet in Renal Disease) equation **(Box 1)**.[41,42] The National Kidney Foundation has a link in their Web site where the GFR can be quickly calculated using either equation: http://www.kidney.org/professionals/kdoqi/gfr_calculator.cfm.

NKF-K/DOQUI has developed a staging scheme in which chronic kidney disease is classified into 5 stages based on GFR (Stage 1: GFR ≥90; Stage 2: GFR 60–89; Stage 3: GFR 30–59; Stage 4: GFR 15–29; Stage 5: GFR <15 mL/min per body surface area [BSA] 1.73 m^2 or dialysis). Treatment recommendations are then tailored based on the stage.[43]

Other Blood Tests

When suspecting a nephrological disease, other tests to consider would include complete blood count, blood urea nitrogen, coagulation studies, and serologic studies such as complement levels, antinuclear antibody (ANA), hepatitis B and C titers, antiglomerular basement membrane antibody, antineutrophilic cytoplasmic antibody (ANCA), antistreptolysin O titer (ASO), and cryoglobulin assay.[27]

IMAGING STUDIES

Numerous radiographic methods are available for anatomic and functional assessment of the kidneys and urinary tract.[44] Deciding on which modality to use initially depends on whether a urological or a nephrological cause for the hematuria is suspected. At present, the 3 imaging modalities used are ultrasonography (US), intravenous urography (IVU), and computed tomography (CT).

Ultrasonography

For evaluation of renal disease, US offers an accurate, noninvasive approach to rule out obstructive uropathy, determine renal size and cortical thickness, and look for masses or cysts. The availability of color duplex to assess renal vascular flow and resistance provides additional information regarding renal parenchyma. US is the first choice among the imaging studies to evaluate a patient with deterioration in renal function, because it does not involve the usage of nephrotoxic contrast media. US is the imaging test to consider in patients with suspected glomerular hematuria, as manifested by dysmorphic RBCs, proteinuria of at least 2+, and RBC casts.[45,46] Because radiation is not involved, US is safe in pregnant patients as well. It is less accurate in detecting ureteral lesions such as nonobstructing stones (sensitivity 19%), and thus may not be the first choice for evaluating a suspected urological cause

---

Box 1
Formulas for calculating GFR from creatinine

Cockcroft-Gault equation

$$GFR\ (mL/min) = \frac{[140 - Age\ (years)] \times Weight\ (kg) \times 0.85\ (if\ female)}{72 \times Serum\ Creatinine\ (mg/dL)}$$

MDRD study equation

$$GFR\ (mL/min/1.73m^2) = 186 \times Serum\ Creatinine^{-1.154}\ (mg/dL)$$
$$\times Age^{-0.203}\ (years) \times 0.742\ (if\ female)$$
$$\times 1.212\ (if\ African\ American)$$

of hematuria.[47] For the radiologic evaluation of hematuria, the American College of Radiology (ACR) gives US an appropriateness rating of 6, with 8 being the highest and 2 being the lowest.[46]

Intravenous Urography

IVU (also known as intravenous pyelography, or IVP) has been the traditional imaging modality of choice for evaluating hematuria. IVU is widely available and most cost-efficient in most centers.[30] Indeed, it scores the highest ACR appropriateness rating of 8.[46] However, IVU may miss smaller renal masses, with sensitivity of 21%, 52%, and 85% for masses less than 2 cm, 2 cm to 3 cm, and greater than 3 cm, respectively, when compared with contrast-enhanced CT.[48] IVU also cannot distinguish between solid from cystic masses, requiring another imaging modality such as US or CT for further lesion characterization.[30] Finally, IVU has relatively low sensitivity of 52% to 59% for detecting urinary tract stones.[47]

Computed Tomography

CT of the kidneys and urinary tract is better than US in detecting stones in patients with hematuria,[2] and it has the highest sensitivity, at 94% to 98%.[47] Noncontrast helical CT is excellent for detection of urinary stones. CT urography has been increasingly supplanting IVU when a urological cause for hematuria is suspected, as a result of its higher accuracy in detecting lesions in the renal parenchyma and the rest of the urinary tract.[46] CT urography involves the injection of iodinated contrast media, with subsequent high-resolution nephrogenic phase and delayed phase imaging to evaluate the renal pelvis, ureter, and bladder. CT urography also scores 8 in the ACR appropriateness rating.

TIMING OF REFERRAL

The evaluation methods for hematuria discussed earlier are well within the scope of practice for primary care physicians. However, certain patients will require a referral to a urologist or a nephrologist for further evaluation.

When to Refer to a Urologist

Urological referral for hematuria is indicated when the workup has identified a urological disease, or when the risk profile of the patient with a negative workup is such that cystoscopy should be considered.

Except for low-risk patients with benign causes of transient hematuria or uncomplicated urinary tract infection, patients with microscopic hematuria should first have upper tract imaging and cytology. Imaging should be with CT urography in most patients, renal US for those suspected of glomerular hematuria or who are pregnant, and noncontrast CT if a urinary tract stone is strongly suspected. Cytology should be performed on 3 consecutive first-morning samples of voided urine.[2,30] If an abnormality is noted, with the possible exception of urinary tract stones of 4 mm or less, for which spontaneous passage can be expected with medical management, the patient should see a urologist.

When this workup is negative, urological referral is indicated for patients with high-risk factors (eg, age >40 years, tobacco use) mentioned earlier in this article in the History section. Also, patients who have experienced gross hematuria should be referred to a urologist, unless the discoloration of urine was definitely caused by a drug, food, or other causes (see **Table 1**).

Cystoscopy

Cystoscopy is the best way to evaluate the lower urinary tract, including the bladder, urethra, and urethral orifice. Initial diagnostic cystoscopy can be performed in the urologist's office using a flexible cystoscope under local anesthesia; this is a quick procedure that does not require sedation. Flexible cystoscopy has diagnostic accuracy equal or superior to rigid cystoscopy.[30] Flexible cytoscopy is superior to rigid cytoscopy in the evaluation of the anterior bladder neck.[49,50] However, if a lesion is detected that requires a biopsy, a rigid cystoscopy will be needed.

When to Refer to a Nephrologist

If the urinalysis is strongly suggestive of glomerular hematuria (with dysmorphic RBCs, proteinuria 2+ or greater, or RBC casts), the patient needs further workup for nephrological causes. In the absence of significant proteinuria and RBC casts, recognizing glomerular hematuria based solely on RBC dysmorphism may be difficult. The percentage of dysmorphic RBCs required to classify the hematuria as glomerular has not been adequately defined. A urinalysis with presence of dysmorphic RBCs of at least 80% suggests glomerular hematuria, and one with normal RBCs of at least 80% suggests nonglomerular hematuria. However, there can be an overlap, and accurate assessment of RBC dysmorphism through careful urine microscopic examination may be beyond the scope of a busy primary care physician.[30] Therefore, the patients may undergo urological workup with urinary tract imaging and urine cytology, and may also have cystoscopy if indicated. However, the presence of elevated blood pressure and decreased GFR increases the suspicion that the patient may have a nephrological cause of hematuria.[43]

Nephrological referral should be strongly considered in the following situations:

1. Acute renal failure, defined as an increase in the serum creatinine level of 0.5 mg per dL, a 50% increase in the serum creatinine level above baseline, a 50% decrease in the baseline calculated GFR, or the need for acute dialysis.[51]
2. Significantly diminished renal function (GFR <60 mL/min per BSA 1.73 m^2) of chronic or unknown duration.
3. Possible indication for renal biopsy, including persistent proteinuria of 2+ or greater by urine dipstick, hematuria with persistent proteinuria, or persistent isolated glomerular hematuria for more than 1 year with negative urological workup.
4. Underlying cause of hematuria unclear.
5. For management of a nephrological cause (such as primary glomerulopathy).[52]

FOLLOW-UP OF PATIENTS WITH A NEGATIVE WORKUP

Initial workup may fail to reveal the underlying cause of hematuria in at least 8% to 10% of cases.[53] Because urologic malignancy is subsequently found in 1% to 3% of those with asymptomatic microscopic hematuria and most lesions are discovered within 3 years of the initially negative findings, a case can be made to follow these patients for 3 years. However, there is no strong evidence that a particular interval or test modality is superior to another. The following monitoring plan is based on expert consensus: urinalysis, voided urine cytology, and blood pressure determination at 6, 12, 24, and 36 months.[30] The urinalysis is to detect for hematuria and possible new onset of proteinuria. The cytology (a single voided urine sample, not 3) is to check for high-grade tumors and carcinoma, whereby the test has its greatest utility. The blood pressure measurement is to detect elevation early that might suggest a nephrological cause.

If abnormal cytology is found, or if gross hematuria or irritative voiding symptoms without urinary tract infection occurs, the patient should be referred back to urology. If none of these occur within 3 years, further monitoring may be stopped.[30] Patients with persist hematuria, development of proteinuria, evidence of glomerular hematuria, new onset of hypertension, or decreased GFR all warrant a referral to a nephrologist.

SUMMARY

Hematuria is a common complaint in the primary care patient population. Hematuria is generally benign in younger patients with no risk factors, particularly women. However, older individuals, particularly men, should be evaluated for potentially serious urologic conditions such as malignancy. Whereas most patients with hematuria will undergo urological workup to some degree, it is important to efficiently recognize those at minimal risk of serious underlying urologic condition for whom detailed workup is not necessary; those at high risk for whom a complete workup with cystoscopy is warranted; and those with likely nephrological causes for whom a nephrological referral is prudent.

REFERENCES

1. Sokolosky MC. Hematuria. Emerg Med Clin North Am 2001;19:621–32.
2. Cohen RA, Brown RS. Microscopic hematuria. N Engl J Med 2003;348:2330–8.
3. Grossfeld GD, Litwin MS, Wolf JS, et al. Evaluation of asymptomatic microscopic hematuria in adults: the American Urological Association best practice policy—part I: definition, detection, prevalence, and etiology. Urology 2001;57:599–603.
4. Woolhandler S, Pels RJ, Bor DH, et al. Dipstick urinalysis screening of asymptomatic adults for urinary tract disorders. JAMA 1989;262:1214–9.
5. Ritchie CD, Bevan EA, Collier SJ. Importance of occult haematuria found at screening. Br Med J 1986;292:681–3.
6. Hiatt RA, Ordenez JD. Dipstick urinalysis screening, asymptomatic microhematuria, and subsequent urological cancers in a population-based sample. Cancer Epidemiol Biomarkers Prev 1994;3:439–43.
7. Thompson IM. The evaluation of microscopic hematuria: a population-based study. J Urol 1987;138:1189–90.
8. Fromm P, Ribak J, Benbassat J. Significance of microhaematuria in young adults. Br Med J 1984;288:20–2.
9. Mohr DN, Offord KP, Owen RA, et al. Asymptomatic microhematuria and urologic disease: a population-based study. JAMA 1986;256:224–9.
10. Kryszczuk K, Kelsberg G, Rich J. Should we screen adults for asymptomatic microhematuria? J Fam Pract 2004;53:150–3.
11. United States Preventive Services Task Force. Screening for bladder cancer in adults. Available at: http://www.ahrq.gov/clinic/3rduspstf/bladder/blacanrs.htm. Accessed March 1, 2010.
12. American Cancer Society. Bladder cancer screening. Available at: http://www.cancer.org/docroot/CRI/content/CRI_2_4_3X_Can_bladder_cancer_be_found_early_44.asp?sitearea=. Accessed March 1, 2010.
13. Bard RH. The significance of asymptomatic microhematuria in women and its economic implications: a ten-year study. Arch Intern Med 1988;148:2629–32.
14. Britton JP, Dowell AC, Whelan P. Dipstick hematuria and bladder cancer in men over 60: results of a community study. Br Med J 1989;299:1010–2.
15. Britton JP, Dowell AC, Whelan P, et al. A community study of bladder cancer screening by the detection of occult urinary bleeding. J Urol 1992;148:788–90.

16. Carson CC, Segura JW, Greene LF. Clinical importance of microhematuria. JAMA 1979;241:149–50.
17. Davides KC, King LM, Jacobs D. Management of microscopic hematuria: twenty-year experience with 150 cases in a community hospital. Urology 1986;28:453–5.
18. Fracchia JA, Motta J, Miller LS, et al. Evaluation of asymptomatic microhematuria. Urology 1995;46:484–9.
19. Greene LF, O'Shaughnessy EJ, Hendricks ED. Study of five hundred patients with asymptomatic microhematuria. JAMA 1956;161:610–2.
20. Golin AL, Howard RS. Asymptomatic microscopic hematuria. J Urol 1980;124: 389–91.
21. Jones DJ, Langstaff RJ, Holt SD, et al. The value of cystourethroscopy in the investigation of microscopic haematuria in adult males under 40 years: a prospective study of 100 patients. Br J Urol 1988;62:541–5.
22. Mariani AJ, Mariani MC, Macchioni C, et al. The significance of adult hematuria: 1,000 hematuria evaluations including a risk-benefit and cost-effectiveness analysis. J Urol 1989;141:350–5.
23. Messing EM, Young TB, Hunt VB, et al. The significance of asymptomatic microhematuria in men 50 or more years old: findings of a home screening study using urinary dipsticks. J Urol 1987;137:919–22.
24. Messing EM, Young TB, Hunt VB, et al. Urinary tract cancers found by homescreening with hematuria dipsticks in healthy men over 50 years of age. Cancer 1989; 164:2361–7.
25. Messing EM, Young TB, Hunt VB, et al. Home screening for hematuria: results of a multiclinic study. J Urol 1992;148:289–92.
26. Murakami S, Igarashi T, Hara S, et al. Strategies for asymptomatic microscopic hematuria: a prospective study of 1,034 patients. J Urol 1990;144:99–101.
27. Ahmed Z, Lee J. Asymptomatic urinary abnormalities. Med Clin North Am 1997; 81:641–52.
28. Jemal A, Siegel R, Ward E, et al. Cancer statistics, 2006. CA Cancer J Clin 2006; 56:106–30.
29. Simerville JA, Phira JJ. Urinalysis: a comprehensive review. Am Fam Physician 2005;71:1153–62.
30. Grossfeld GD, Litwin MS, Wolf JS, et al. Evaluation of asymptomatic microscopic hematuria in adults: the American Urological Association best practice policy—part II: patient evaluation, cytology, voided markers, imaging, cystoscopy, nephrology evaluation, and follow-up. Urology 2001;57:604–10.
31. American Urological Association. Guideline on the management of benign prostatic hyperplasia 2003. Available at: http://www.auanet.org/content/guidelines-and-quality-care/clinical-guidelines/main-reports/bph-management/preface_toc. pdf. Accessed March 1, 2010.
32. Lifshitz E, Kramer L. Outpatient urine culture: does collection technique matter? Arch Intern Med 2000;160:2537–40.
33. Fogazzi GB, Garigali G. The clinical art and science of urine microscopy. Curr Opin Nephrol Hypertens 2003;12:625–32.
34. Silkensen JR, Kasiske BL. Laboratory assessment of kidney disease: clearance, urinalysis, and kidney biopsy. In: Brenner BM, editor. Brenner and Rector's the kidney. 7th edition. Philadelphia: Saunders; 2004. p. 1107–50.
35. Vaughan ED Jr, Wyker AW Jr. Effect of osmolality on the evaluation of microscopic hematuria. J Urol 1971;105:709–11.
36. Rodgers MA, Hempel S, Aho T, et al. Diagnostic tests used in the investigation of adult haematuria: a systematic review. BJU Int 2006;98:1154–60.

37. Badalament RA, Hermansen DK, Kimmel M, et al. The sensitivity of bladder wash flow cytometry, bladder wash cytology, and voided cytology in the detection of bladder carcinoma. Cancer 1987;60:1423–7.
38. Novicki DE, Stern JA, Nemec R, et al. Cost-effective evaluation of indeterminate urinary cytology. J Urol 1998;160:734–6.
39. Grossfeld G, Carroll P. Evaluation of asymptomatic microscopic hematuria. Urol Clin North Am 1998;25:661–76.
40. Stevens LA, Levey AS. Measurement of kidney function. Med Clin North Am 2005; 89:457–73.
41. Cockcroft D, Gault M. Prediction of creatinine clearance from serum creatinine. Nephron 1976;16:31–41.
42. Levey A, Bosch J, Lewis J, et al. A more accurate method to estimate glomerular filtration rate from serum creatinine: a new prediction equation. Ann Intern Med 1999;130:461–70.
43. Levey AS, Coresh J, Balk E, et al. National Kidney Foundation practice guidelines for chronic kidney disease: evaluation, classification, and stratification. Ann Intern Med 2003;139:137–47.
44. Kellert MJ. The genitourinary tract: methods of investigation. In: Grainger RG, Allison DJ, Adam A, et al, editors. Grainger & Allison's diagnostic radiology: a textbook of medical imaging. 4th edition. New York: Churchill Livingstone; 2001. p. 1489–97.
45. Webb JAW, Maisey MN, Reidy JF. Renal failure and transplantation. In: Grainger RG, Allison DJ, Adam A, et al, editors. Grainger & Allison's diagnostic radiology: a textbook of medical imaging. 4th edition. New York: Churchill Livingstone; 2001. p. 1671–92.
46. Choyke PL. Radiologic evaluation of hematuria: guidelines from the American College of Radiology's appropriateness criteria. Am Fam Physician 2008;78: 347–52.
47. Fielding JR, Silverman SG, Samuel S, et al. Unenhanced helical CT of ureteral stones: a replacement for excretory urography in planning treatment. Am J Roentgenol 1998;171:1051–3.
48. Warshauer DM, McCarthy SM, Street L, et al. Detection of renal masses: sensitivities and specificities of excretory urography/linear tomography, US, and CT. Radiology 1988;169:363–5.
49. Clayman RV, Reddy P, Lange PH. Flexible fiberoptic and rigid-rod lens endoscopy of the lower urinary tract: a prospective controlled comparison. J Urol 1984;131:715–6.
50. Pavone-Macaluso M, Lamartina M, Pavone C, et al. The flexible cystoscope. Int Urol Nephrol 1992;24:239–42.
51. Needham E. Management of acute renal failure. Am Fam Physician 2005;72: 1739–46.
52. Snyder S, Pendergraph B. Detection and evaluation of chronic kidney disease. Am Fam Physician 2005;72:1723–32.
53. Sutton JM. Evaluation of hematuria in adults. JAMA 1990;263:2475–80.

Male Sexual Dysfunction

Victor A. Diaz Jr, MD[a,b,*], Jeremy D. Close, MD[a]

KEYWORDS

- Male sexual dysfunction • Premature ejaculation
- Decreased libido • Hypoactive sexual desire disorder
- Erectile dysfunction • Sexual history • Partner
- Psychotherapy

PREMATURE EJACULATION

Premature ejaculation (PE) is the most common type of male sexual dysfunction. Most clinicians use the broad definition of PE as ejaculation occurring sooner than desired (before or shortly after penetration), causing distress to one or both partners. No strict time parameters have been defined, but an intravaginal ejaculatory latency time (IELT; ie, penetration to ejaculation) of less than 2 minutes is generally accepted as defining PE.[1] Use of this broad definition has contributed to the large range in prevalence, from 5% to 30%.[2] New definitions for PE are being considered for the Diagnostic and Statistical Manual, Fifth Edition (DSM-V) and International Classification of Diseases (ICD)-11. PE can be divided into primary PE, which begins when the patient becomes sexually active, and secondary PE, which is acquired later in life.[3] Additional subclasses include global and situational PE. Global PE is present in all circumstances, whereas situational PE occurs only with certain partners and situations.[4]

Physiology and Pathophysiology of Ejaculation

There are 3 distinct components to antegrade, or normal, ejaculation: emission, ejaculation, and orgasm. Emission is the contraction of seminal vesicles and the prostate with expulsion of sperm and seminal fluid into the posterior urethra. The ejaculation phase involves relaxation of the external urinary sphincter and pulsatile contractions of the bulbocavernosus and pelvic floor muscles. Ejaculatory inevitability, or the point at which ejaculation cannot be stopped, occurs in response to distention of the

[a] Department of Family and Community Medicine, Jefferson Medical College, Thomas Jefferson University, 401 Curtis Building, 1015 Walnut Street, Philadelphia, PA 19107, USA
[b] Jefferson Family Medicine Associates, 833 Chestnut Street East, Suite 301, Philadelphia, PA 19107, USA
* Corresponding author. Department of Family and Community Medicine, Jefferson Medical College, Thomas Jefferson University, 401 Curtis Building, 1015 Walnut Street, Philadelphia, PA 19107.
E-mail address: victor.diaz@jefferson.edu

Prim Care Clin Office Pract 37 (2010) 473–489
doi:10.1016/j.pop.2010.04.002   **primarycare.theclinics.com**

posterior urethra. The ejaculatory phase may or may not be followed by orgasm, defined as the centrally experienced conclusion of sexual excitation.[4] The intricacies of these biologic sequences have made it difficult to understand the pathophysiology of PE.

Historically, PE has been attributed to psychological causes such as early sexual experience, sexual conditioning, sexual technique, frequency of sex, and anxiety. Newer research is focused on neurobiological explanations, such as hyposensitivity of 5-hydroxytryptamine 2C (5-HT$_{2c}$) receptors or hypersensitivity of 5-HT$_{1a}$ receptors. Men with low 5-HT levels reach the ejaculatory threshold earlier, resulting in more rapid ejaculation, whereas men with high 5-HT levels may have delayed or absent ejaculation. This idea is supported by the successful use of selective serotonin reuptake inhibitor (SSRIs), which increase 5-HT levels, in patients with PE. It has also been suggested that men with PE have a hyperexcitable ejaculatory reflex that prevents them from controlling ejaculation.[4]

Diagnosis

PE often goes undiagnosed because many men are reluctant to discuss sexual issues, and clinicians generally do not initiate these conversations. Time constraints and provider uneasiness with the topic compound the problem.[5] The importance of dialog cannot be overemphasized, given that the diagnosis of PE is mostly based on sexual history. Many men do not realize that loss of erection after ejaculation is normal. Some men confuse PE with erectile dysfunction (ED). However, a skilled interviewer can help the patient clearly describe his true concerns. Including the partner in the discussion is often helpful, but this should be the patient's choice.

PE is difficult to diagnosis because there is no universally accepted definition. The American Urological Association (AUA) recommends that PE be diagnosed wholly on sexual history. Four key factors need to be considered when making the diagnosis. The first factor is decreased IELT. IELT refers to the time between vaginal insertion of the penis and the start of intravaginal ejaculation. IELT has been assessed by patient and partner recall, and by stopwatch evaluation. Men with PE have a shortened or nonexistent IELT, tending to ejaculate in a few seconds to minutes. Normal IELT values have been somewhat difficult to define, as there is substantial variation in patient and partner recall, leading to self-reported IELTs that are inaccurately longer than actual stopwatch times.[6] One multinational study of men without PE revealed self-reported times ranging from nearly 7 minutes in Germany to more than 13 minutes in the United States.[7] There appears to be considerable overlap in times between PE and non-PE groups, suggesting that, until better normative values are available, the diagnosis cannot be made on an individual's IELT alone.

Three additional self-reported factors that may be present include poor control over ejaculation, dissatisfaction with intercourse by the patient or partner, and perceived distress about the condition by the patient or partner. Not all of these factors need to be present to identify PE. A focused sexual history will help elicit many of these complaints to establish a diagnosis.[8]

Sexual history should include questions regarding frequency and duration of PE (primary vs acquired) and relationship to specific partners (global vs situational). It should be determined whether PE occurs with all or some sexual attempts, and what degree of stimulus results in PE. Inquiries about the type and frequency of current and past sexual activity (eg, foreplay, masturbation, intercourse, use of visual clues) should include feelings toward these behaviors, to help elucidate any underlying guilt or poor sexual education that may be playing a role. It is also important to explore the effect of PE on current and past sexual activity, types and quality of personal relationships, and general quality of life, as well as aggravating or alleviating factors and any relationship to drug use or abuse. Awareness of the issues surrounding PE may affect treatment considerations and, ultimately, treatment success.

Physical examination should include a complete general examination and a genital examination. The provider should always be reassuring when normal findings are present. The examiner should look for signs of underlying chronic disease or endocrine dysfunction (eg, gynecomastia, muscle wasting). Laboratory evaluation is rarely necessary in men with lifelong PE, unless there are complicating factors or concerning physical examination findings.[9] Secondary PE may need additional laboratory work, specifically focused on risk factors such as vascular disease, obesity, diabetes, and depression.

Specific attention should be given to the possibility of underlying ED. Recent data show that almost half of men with PE also have ED.[10] Men with ED may hurry their sexual experience to prevent loss of erection, leading to rapid ejaculation. This behavior may inappropriately lead to the diagnosis of PE, when ED may be the true diagnosis.

Treatment

Options for treatment of PE include pharmacologic, psychological, and behavioral therapies. The primary goal should be patient and partner satisfaction and should not focus on the IELT. Options should be discussed with the patient (and partner) to best fit their desired outcome, and should include discussion of how common and treatable PE is, to help normalize this problem. Each treatment modality can be used individually or in combination with others.

Oral agents

Antidepressant medications have been the most studied, because their well-known side effects, including anorgasmia and delayed ejaculation, make them ideal for treating PE. The most commonly used agents are the SSRIs. Tricyclic antidepressants (TCAs), such as clomipramine, have also been used, but TCAs have fallen out of favor because of safety concerns, especially in the elderly. Options include once-daily dosing or situational dosing regimens. Daily dosing increases IELT more than situational dosing. Dosing routines should be selected on a case-by-case basis after discussion of risks and benefits with the patient and his partner.

The most common SSRIs used for PE are fluoxetine, paroxetine, sertraline, fluvoxamine, and citalopram. Fluoxetine doses range from 5 to 20 mg/d and can be increased slowly to reach the desired response. Sertraline can be given in daily doses of 25, 50, 100, or 200 mg, or as a situational dose of 50 mg daily. Paroxetine dosing can be 10, 20, or 40 mg/d, increasing to the desired effect, or as a situational dose of 20 mg, 3 to 4 hours before sexual activity.[1,11,12] Most evidence for paroxetine treatment suggests that a dosing regimen of 20 mg/d is the most effective.[9] Paroxetine seems to exert the strongest ejaculatory delay, increasing IELT approximately 8.8-fold compared with the baseline in one study.[13] The effects of SSRI medications, measured by ejaculatory delay, tend to occur 5 to 10 days after initiation, but may occur earlier.[14]

Ejaculoselective serotonin transport inhibitors (ESSTIs), which are not yet approved in the United States, are currently being tested for on-demand use in PE treatment. Dapoxetine is structurally similar to fluoxetine but, because of its pharmacokinetics, it is more successful in situational dosing. It has shown improvement in IELT and is well tolerated by men from the Asia-Pacific area.[15] A dose of 60 mg of dapoxetine can increase IELT by 50% compared with placebo, when taken on demand.[16]

Topical agents

Topical agents are intended to decrease penile sensation and prolong IELT. These agents are usually applied 10 to 30 minutes before sexual activity. The most common such agent is a mixture of lidocaine and prilocaine, available in cream and aerosol. Both formulations have been shown to improve IELT compared with baseline.[17,18] There are numerous other non–FDA-approved topical treatments that contain a variety of ingredients. These should not be recommended to patients, because their safety profiles have not yet been fully established.

The most common side effect of topical medications is penile numbness, which can result in loss of erection. Like all topical medications, there is always a risk of local burning, irritation, or allergic reaction. An additional concern is partner numbness, which can reduce partner sexual satisfaction. Condoms have also been used to reduce penile sensation, with and without the use of additional topical agents.[19]

Psychological treatment

Counseling alone is rarely successful in treating lifelong PE. Therapy is more likely to be successful in patients with acquired PE, especially those with situational PE. Psychosexual therapy is best used to help the patient cope with the stress and relationship problems that develop secondary to sexual dysfunction.[19] Psychosexual therapies use behavioral interventions to educate the patient on how to control or delay his ejaculation, and assist him in reestablishing confidence and lessening performance anxiety. Psychosexual therapy has the best success when combined with pharmacologic therapies.[20]

PE causes significant stress on relationships, and therapy should involve the patient and his partner. Frequently, neither partner is comfortable discussing sexual dysfunction, likely because of poor communication skills, frustration, and embarrassment. Psychotherapy promotes open discussion between sexual partners, education about the condition, and expression of physical and emotional concerns.[20]

Behavioral techniques

Behavioral techniques were once the mainstay of treatment of PE. The 2 most commonly used techniques involve penile manipulation; squeezing the glans when ejaculation is imminent (the squeeze technique) or attempting a program of intermittent cessation of penile thrusting during intercourse (the stop/start technique).[21] The popularity of these practices has declined because of their lack of reproducible success and their intrusiveness in normal sexual activity.

Treatment considerations

Most patients will have tried a variety of behavioral and over-the-counter treatments before meeting with their clinician. In addition, some men masturbate before sexual intercourse to desensitize the penis and delay subsequent ejaculations. This technique may have benefit for younger men, but can be detrimental to older patients secondary to prolonged refractory periods. In general, self-help techniques may have temporary benefit, but usually provide no long-term benefit and may complicate the problem in the long-term.[7] Asking about previously tried self-help techniques may help in guiding future treatment. Care providers should be aware of the abundance of misinformation on the Internet. Providing evidence-based education to the patient and his partner can help prevent them from engaging in detrimental actions and behaviors that can cause setbacks in treatment and their relationship.

Summary

PE is a common, but complex, disease process that needs to be better defined to facilitate research and treatment. Proper focus and comfort with taking sexual history, and an understanding of current and future treatments will lead to success in treatment of PE.

DECREASED LIBIDO

Decreased libido, also known as hypoactive sexual desire disorder (HSDD), is an area lacking substantial research, particularly in men. It is more common in women, and most research is in female subjects. However, decreased libido is still encountered to a certain degree in the male population. The Diagnostic and Statistical Manual, Fourth Edition, Text Revision (DSM-IV-TR) lists 3 diagnostic components for HSDD:

1. Persistently or recurrently deficient (or absent) sexual fantasies and desire for sexual activity. The judgment of deficiency or absence is made by the clinician, taking into account factors that affect sexual functioning, such as age and the context of the person's life.
2. The disturbance causes marked distress or interpersonal difficulty.
3. The sexual dysfunction is not better accounted for by another Axis I disorder (except another sexual dysfunction) and is not caused exclusively by the direct physiologic effects of a substance (eg, a drug of abuse, a medication) or a general medical condition.[22]

There are several subtypes of decreased libido. Lifelong decreased libido is usually present at the start of puberty, and it is uncommon. More frequently, the disorder develops in adulthood, after a period of adequate sexual interest. The loss of sexual desire may be generalized or situational, depending on psychosocial or relationship factors. A situational pattern of loss of sexual desire occurs in some individuals in relation to problems with intimacy and commitment. The course can be consistent or periodic, and can recur after periods of normal sexual desire. Recurrence is usually secondary to the return of life or relationship stressors.[23]

The lack of research on decreased libido in men has made the determination of prevalence difficult. This is compounded by societal and cultural pressures that make men unlikely to complain of decreased libido. One study found a prevalence of decreased libido ranging from 13% to 17% among men aged 18 to 59 years and showed that it became more common with increasing age.[24]

Diagnosis

Decreased libido can have multiple causes, and the key to making the diagnosis is taking a thorough history. Specific attention should be paid to sexual, psychosocial, and medical history.[5] To facilitate disclosure, the interviewer should be aware of personal, social, and cultural sensitivities.[25]

Men with lifelong decreased libido should be questioned on sexual experiences before sexual maturity. Some individuals may have experienced sexual trauma (eg, rape, incest) or physical discomfort with initial sexual experiences that may have precluded them from developing a normal libido.

The psychosocial history should focus on possible underlying depression, which is closely correlated with decreased libido.[26] Numerous causes of depression, including work, family, and relationship stressors, need to be explored as possible causes of decreased libido. Loss of sexual desire may also worsen an underlying depression. Other considerations include socioeconomic status (poor men have a higher prevalence), marital status (single men have more problems with decreased desire than married men), and education level attained (those with less education have a higher prevalence).[24]

Clinicians should take into account both partners' willingness for sexual activity as they age. Men and women experience a decline in sexual desire as they age, but the effect tends to be larger in women.[27] Exploring sexual interest and discussing the normal aging process with the couple may help guide treatment decisions. Decreased libido may only be affecting 1 partner and may not be of concern to the other.

Medication history is important in the diagnosis of decreased libido. Antidepressants are well known to affect libido, especially SSRIs, which are the most widely prescribed antidepressants and have significant effects on arousal and orgasm.[28] Antihypertensive medications such as centrally acting antihypertensive agents (methyldopa, clonidine), nonselective β-adrenergic blockers (propranolol), and potassium-sparing diuretics (spironolactone) can decrease libido.[29,30] Opioid medications can decrease libido, especially with prolonged use.[31] Use of recreational drugs (including anabolic steroids) and alcohol should also be assessed as potential causes of decreased libido.[32] New attention has been given to occupational exposures and the risk of developing sexual dysfunction. Bisphenol-A (BPA), a chemical used in some plastics, has been linked to an increase in self-reported decreased libido.[33]

Underlying medical conditions can decrease libido as a result of the medications used to treat the disease, symptoms related to the ailment, psychological stressors of illness, and general concerns regarding health and safety with sexual activity. Symptoms of hypogonadism may include lack of male hair growth, gynecomastia, anosmia (Kallmann syndrome), headaches, or vision changes (pituitary tumors). A history of orchitis (such as from mumps) can cause testicular atrophy.

The physical examination should include an assessment of body habitus and secondary sexual characteristics (such as for Klinefelter syndrome), and assessment of the cardiovascular, neurologic, and genitourinary systems, including penile, testicular, and rectal examinations. Blood pressure and heart rate should be measured. The patient should be examined for signs of hypogonadism. Laboratory work should be focused on concerns of any underlying disease process.[32] Laboratory examination should include evaluation for underlying disease and age-appropriate screening tests based on the medical history and physical examination findings. A morning blood draw may help avoid the daily cycle in hormonal levels. Tests may include fasting glucose, lipids, testosterone and free testosterone, luteinizing hormone, and estradiol (in obese patients).[25]

Treatment

Because of the many causes of decreased libido, diagnosis can be imprecise, and initial treatment may not be successful. Medical, social, and psychological treatment options should be presented and initiated on the preference of the patient and partner. Any underlying medical problems, (eg, hypertension, diabetes) should be treated.[34] Specific attention should be paid to the treatment of depression. Therapy should be initiated to see whether libido improves, with the understanding that many antidepressant medications can decrease libido.[28]

Despite lack of evidence, many clinicians recommend individual or couples' psychotherapy as a treatment option for decreased libido. Therapy may be able to reveal the stressors and concerns contributing to the problem. Decreased libido can be the result of, or the cause of, significant stress. Exploring fears, concerns, and misconceptions of sexual function with the couple may aid in treatment.

There is a paucity of medication trials related to male decreased libido, and there are no FDA-approved medications for decreased libido in men or women. Medication treatment should initially be directed toward underlying medical conditions (eg, diabetes, hypothyroidism, hypertension) to determine whether adequate treatment improves sexual desire.

Testosterone levels decrease as men age, and some older men exhibit serum total testosterone levels that are less than the normal range for younger men.[35] Testosterone therapy has been used off-label for years in women with decreased libido, especially in postmenopausal women.[36–38] Men with decreased libido and low testosterone levels tend to improve with testosterone supplementation.[39] However, there are no good studies of supplementation in men with normal testosterone levels. Testosterone supplementation should be used with caution, because long-term effects have not been well studied. Initiation of treatment should include a thorough discussion of risks and benefits.

Summary

Decreased libido is not yet well understood or researched in men. Underlying medical conditions and medications should be reviewed to assess their contribution to loss of libido. Depression should always be considered in the evaluation. Psychotherapy may be helpful. No FDA-approved medications exist for decreased libido. Further research is needed to see whether testosterone supplementation can benefit men with normal testosterone levels but decreased libido.

ED
Definition

ED is the persistent inability to attain or maintain a penile erection sufficient for satisfactory sexual performance.[40] The term ED is preferable to impotence because the latter has pejorative implications. ED also describes the problem more accurately, because it is possible to maintain sexual libido, reach orgasm, and ejaculate, despite the inability to achieve or maintain an erection.[41] There is no consensus on how often, or for what length of time, the problem has to occur to meet this definition. A duration of greater than 3 months has been suggested as a reasonable clinical guideline.[42]

The DSM-IV-TR suggests the following diagnostic criteria for male erectile disorder:

1. There is a persistent or recurrent inability to attain, or to maintain until completion of the sexual activity, an adequate erection.
2. The disturbance causes marked distress or interpersonal difficulty.
3. The ED is not otherwise accounted for by another Axis I disorder (other than a sexual dysfunction) and is not caused exclusively by the direct physiologic effects of a substance (eg, a drug of abuse, a medication) or a general medical condition.[22]

Anatomy and Physiology of Erection

The male sexual cycle can be considered to have 4 phases: sexual desire (libido), arousal (erection), ejaculation (orgasm), and detumescence (penile flaccidity).[43] Erections usually begin with sexual stimulation and subside with ejaculation or after stimulation ends. The subsequent flaccid state remains until the next sexual stimulation or nocturnal erection occurs.

Psychogenic and reflexogenic mechanisms play a role in this chain of events. Psychogenic erections are triggered centrally in response to visual, auditory, olfactory, or imaginary stimuli. Reflexogenic erections are brought on peripherally by stimulation of sensory receptors on the penis, involving somatic and parasympathetic efferent actions via spinal pathways.[44] On a biochemical level, the parasympathetic activity sets off the release of nitric oxide (NO), eventually resulting in increased levels of the intracellular mediator cyclic guanosine monophosphate (cGMP), which in turn causes penile vascular and trabecular smooth muscle relaxation.[44]

In the flaccid state, the penis maintains a balance between the blood flowing into the corpora cavernosa and the corpus spongiosum and the blood flowing out via postcavernous venules that eventually drain into the deep dorsal vein. During an erection, the blood flowing into the erectile tissue increases considerably, compressing the venules and restricting venous outflow, and eventually resulting in full penile rigidity.[44] The mechanisms responsible for penile flaccidity are as important as those that promote erections, and both play critical roles in ED.[45]

Classification

ED may be classified as organic or psychogenic in nature. According to the 1992 National Institutes of Health (NIH) Consensus Conference on Impotence, up to 80% of ED cases may have an organic cause that can be further categorized into vascular, neurogenic, anatomic, and hormonal subtypes. ED has also been categorized as mild, moderate, or complete, but these terms have yet to be clearly defined.[44] The DSM-IV-TR suggests 3 additional distinctions: lifelong versus acquired, generalized versus situational, and resulting from psychological factors versus combined factors.[22]

Epidemiology

In 1995, studies suggested that more than 152 million men experienced ED worldwide. That number may reach 322 million by 2025, because life expectancy and the prevalence of chronic illnesses are expected to increase.[45] In the United States, 10 to 20 million men have ED. In 1994, The Massachusetts Male Aging Study determined that 52% of men between the ages of 40 and 70 years reported some ED. This landmark study also established that ED is an age-dependent disorder. By the age of 70 years, only 32% of men described themselves as having no ED.[46] Another similar survey of approximately 1400 men aged 18 to 59 years showed a 31% prevalence of male sexual dysfunction.[46] Other studies reported a prevalence of ED ranging from 15% in Brazil to 74% in Finland.[47]

Despite these accounts, the true prevalence of ED may be much higher. Factors such as low health literacy, social stigma, cultural taboos, and ethnic differences often lead to under-reporting.[47] Men with ED may wait for years before consulting a health professional. Despite growing public awareness and media attention, fewer than half of affected men seek medical treatment.[48]

Pathology and Associated Conditions

Any condition that interferes with the blood flow or the neural pathways of penile erectile tissue can cause ED. Vascular disease is, by far, the leading organic cause of ED, with arterial or inflow disorders being much more common than venous or outflow problems. Vascular causes include hypertension, cerebrovascular disease, coronary artery disease, and congestive heart failure. Common neurogenic causes include spinal cord injury, herniated disc disease, Parkinson disease, and multiple sclerosis. Anatomic abnormalities associated with ED include Peyronie disease. Typical hormonal causes include hypogonadism, hyperprolactinemia, adrenal disease, and thyroid abnormalities.[44,45] ED is also a common complaint in men with diabetes because of the adverse effects on vascular and autonomic function.[44]

Other conditions associated with ED include benign prostatic hyperplasia (BPH), prostate cancer, dyslipidemias, liver disease, renal failure, chronic alcohol abuse, cigarette smoking, obesity, sedentary lifestyle, pelvic radiation, pelvic trauma, and postoperative complications of pelvic surgery.[41,44,46]

Some investigators have suggested bicycling as another risk factor for ED. One study reported that nocturnal erections decreased with increased perineal pressure from the bicycle's saddle.[49] Some bicyclists have numbness of the perineum after riding, suggesting perineal nerve compression or vascular ischemia, but this link is controversial and more research is needed.[50]

Psychogenic Causes

Many studies have documented an association between clinical depression and ED. Men with high scores on depression inventories are more likely to experience ED than those with lower scores. Some suggest that a depressed mood has a negative effect on arousal, thus affecting erectile function. The same has been proposed for anxiety disorder and certain social stressors.[51]

Two models have been proposed to explain how depression promotes the development of ED. According to the behavior-based model, men with depression engage in behaviors or thoughts that negatively affect arousal, thus decreasing libido and sexual pleasure. Eventually this leads to less sexual activity, less stimulation, and, eventually, ED. According to the biologic model, the stress of depression adversely affects the hypothalamic-pituitary-adrenocortical axis, leading to excess catecholamine production, cardiovascular disease, and consequently poor cavernosal muscle relaxation and ED.[51]

Similarly, ED and sleep disorders have psychogenic and vascular factors in common. A proposed mechanism links the nocturnal hypoxia and raised acetylcholine of sleep apnea with the peripheral nerve dysfunction, decreased NO production, and vasoconstriction that lead to ED.[52]

Medications and ED

Primary care clinicians are likely to encounter male patients who complain of ED or decreased libido in association with certain medications, especially those that interfere with the mechanisms involved in penile smooth muscle control. Common among these are antihypertensives (diuretics, α-blockers, β-blockers, central agents) and antidepressants (tricyclics, monoamine oxidase [MAO] inhibitors, SSRIs).[28,44] One report cites as many as 25% of cases of ED being related to medication side effects. Other potential agents include benzodiazepines, antipsychotics, antiandrogens, digoxin, H2-receptor blockers, excessive amounts of alcohol, hypoglycemics, phenytoin, phenobarbital, ketoconazole, and niacin.[44,47,48]

Diagnosis

The office evaluation of ED starts with a comprehensive history. Clinicians and patients may be reluctant to bring up sexual issues, for various reasons. However, most patients acknowledge that it is appropriate for their clinician to raise the topic, and they are often relieved when these issues are brought to light.[44] Because these men are often embarrassed and in need of reassurance, questions should be asked in a respectful and culturally sensitive manner, using appropriate layman's terminology while avoiding gestures or body language that might be misinterpreted.[46]

Many clinicians prefer to use patient questionnaires such as the International Index of Erectile Function (IIEF), which is used not only in diagnosing ED but in determining the effectiveness of treatment.[53] The IIEF contains 15 items divided into 5 domains: Erectile Function, Intercourse Satisfaction, Orgasmic Function, Sexual Desire, and Overall Satisfaction, as shown in **Table 1**. Patients are asked to respond to each item based on their sexual experiences during the past 4 weeks. The lower the total score, the more severe the ED.[53] This questionnaire has been successfully validated in 32 languages and is considered culturally appropriate. Limitations include that it takes 10 to 15 minutes to administer, it only assesses a patient's sexual experience during the

Table 1
IIEF questionnaire

Precede all questions with the phrase, "Over the past 4 weeks, . . ." Use the scale to the right of each question in determining response.

Questions	Response Options	Questions	Response Options
Q1. How often were you able to get an erection during sexual activity?	0 = No sexual activity 1 = Almost never/never 2 = A few times (much < half the time) 3 = Sometimes (about half the time) 4 = Most times (much more than half the time) 5 = Almost always/always	**Q8.** How much have you enjoyed sexual intercourse?	0 = No intercourse 1 = No enjoyment 2 = Not very enjoyable 3 = Fairly enjoyable 4 = Highly enjoyable 5 = Very highly enjoyable
Q2. When you had erections with sexual stimulation, how often were your erections hard enough for penetration?		**Q9.** When you had sexual stimulation or intercourse, how often did you ejaculate?	0 = No sexual stimulation/intercourse 1 = Almost never/never 2 = A few times (< half the time) 3 = Sometimes (about half the time) 4 = Most times (more than half the time) 5 = Almost always/always
Q3. When you attempted sexual intercourse, how often were you able to penetrate (enter) your partner?	0 = Did not attempt intercourse 1 = Almost never/never 2 = A few times (much < half the time) 3 = Sometimes (about half the time) 4 = Most times (much more than half the time) 5 = Almost always/always	**Q10.** When you had sexual stimulation or intercourse, how often did you have the feeling of orgasm or climax?	
Q4. During sexual intercourse, how often were you able to maintain your erection after you had penetrated (entered) your partner?		**Q11.** How often have you felt sexual desire?	1 = Almost never 2 = A few times (< half the time) 3 = Sometimes (about half the time) 4 = Most times (more than half the time) 5 = Almost always/always
Q5. During sexual intercourse, how difficult was it to maintain your erection	0 = Did not attempt intercourse 1 = Extremely	**Q12.** How would you rate your level of sexual desire?	1 = Very low/none at all 2 = Low 3 = Moderate 4 = High 5 = Very high

Table 1
(continued)

to completion of intercourse?	difficult 2 = Very difficult 3 = Difficult 4 = Slightly difficult 5 = Not difficult	**Q13.** How satisfied have you been with your overall sex life?	1 = Very dissatisfied 2 = Moderately dissatisfied 3 = About equally satisfied and dissatisfied 4 = Moderately satisfied 5 = Very satisfied
Q6. How many times have you attempted sexual intercourse?	0 = No attempts 1 = 1–2 attempts 2 = 3–4 attempts 3 = 5–6 attempts 4 = 7–10 attempts 5 = More than 11 attempts	**Q14.** How satisfied have you been with your sexual relationship with your partner?	
Q7. When you attempted sexual intercourse, how often was it satisfactory to you?	0 = Did not attempt intercourse 1 = Almost never/never 2 = A few times (< half the time) 3 = Sometimes (about half the time) 4 = Most times (more than half the time) 5 = Almost always/always	**Q15.** How do you rate your confidence that you could get and keep an erection?	1 = Very low 2 = Low 3 = Moderate 4 = High 5 = Very high

Scoring

Domain:	Erectile Function	Intercourse Satisfaction	Orgasmic Function	Sexual Desire	Overall Satisfaction
Questions:	1._____ 2._____ 3._____ 4._____ 5._____ 15._____	6._____ 7._____ 8._____	9._____ 10._____	11._____ 12._____	13._____ 14._____
Total score	_____ (1-30)	_____ (0-15)	_____ (0-10)	_____ (2-10)	_____ (2-10)

Reprinted from Rosen RC, Riley A, Wagner G, et al. The International Index of Erectile Function (IIEF): a multidimensional scale for assessment of erectile dysfunction. Urology 1997;49:829–30; with permission.

past 4 weeks, and it is not meant to replace the level of information that can only be obtained by performing a thorough sexual, psychosocial, and medical history.[54]

A modified version of the IIEF, known as the Sexual Health Inventory for Men (SHIM), is used by many clinicians to assess ED. The SHIM is a 5-item questionnaire that asks about erectile function during the previous 6 months. The SHIM consists of questions 2, 4, 5, 7, and 15 from the IIEF, along with their respective Likert scale responses, to yield the following possible results:

Score of 22 to 25: no ED
Score of 17 to 21: mild ED
Score of 12 to 16: mild to moderate ED
Score of 8 to 11: moderate ED
Score of 0 to 7: severe ED.[54]

In many cases, the SHIM has replaced the need for vascular testing; however, it is not to be used as a predictor of outcomes.[46] Neither the IIEF nor the SHIM was designed to assess for sexual dysfunctions other than ED, but their scores can be influenced by factors other than erectile function. For example, low scores may reflect a lack of sexual opportunities, decreased libido, or the partner's sexual dysfunctions, so clinicians will need to rule out these possibilities.[54] These instruments can also help uncover potentially serious coexisting medical conditions that might otherwise be missed.[46]

Because ED is an early marker for cardiovascular disease, the social history should explore for the possibilities of smoking, physical inactivity, and alcohol abuse. Further workup should include documentation of the body mass index and vital signs, along with a focused physical examination of the thyroid, lymph glands, breasts, abdomen, penis, testicles, secondary sexual characteristics, and lower-extremity pulses. A digital rectal examination of the prostate may be useful, especially when considering testosterone therapy in the management of ED.[41] Recommended laboratory testing begins with a fasting morning blood draw of total and free testosterone, prolactin, luteinizing hormone, glucose, and lipids. Additional testing may include urinalysis, blood count, thyroid stimulating hormone, serum creatinine, and prostate-specific antigen (PSA).[45,46] Other helpful diagnostic techniques may include duplex ultrasonography, penile tumescence studies, RigiScan (a device for recording nocturnal erections), test injections of intracavernous alprostadil, audio-visual stimulation, and penile brachial blood pressure index measurements.[45]

Treatment

Therapy for ED includes risk factor modification, followed by counseling and, when necessary, medication. Lifestyle interventions such as healthy eating, weight loss, smoking cessation, moderation of alcohol intake, and increased physical activity have been shown to benefit men with ED by reducing the markers of inflammation and improving endothelial function.[55]

Regardless of the primary cause of ED, there is often a coexisting psychological element. Education, support, and reassurance may be all that is needed to restore sexual function. However, for some depressed men with ED, referral to a mental health professional may be warranted.[41] When using antidepressant medications, clinicians must balance effectiveness of treatment with the potential sexual side effects of the medication. SSRIs are more likely to cause ED, whereas dopamine and norepinephrine enhancers (eg, bupropion) are less likely to do so. Among SSRIs, paroxetine is most likely to cause ED, followed by sertraline, fluvoxamine, and fluoxetine. Citalopram has the most favorable profile. Strategies for minimizing ED among patients who take SSRIs include reducing the dose, switching to another SSRI, or switching to another class of antidepressant. Use of phosphodiesterase type 5 inhibitors remains the most common tactic for dealing with these side effects.[51]

Oral medications

Phosphodiesterase type 5 (PDE5) inhibitors (sildenafil, tadalafil, and vardenafil) are currently preferred by most clinicians and patients as the first line of pharmacotherapy for ED. The advent of PDE5 inhibitors has revolutionized the management of ED, allowing for accessible treatment in the primary care setting.[45] They work by preventing the breakdown of cGMP and enhancing vasodilation of the penile erectile tissue. Their overall efficacy rate is about 60% to 70%, although efficacy rates are lower in patients with more severe neurologic or vascular disease. Contraindications include concomitant nitrate use, concomitant α-blocker therapy, a history of retinitis pigmentosa, and conditions that can predispose to priapism, such as leukemia or multiple myeloma.[56] Patients with cardiovascular disease who engage in sexual activity have a slightly increased risk for myocardial infarction, regardless of ED treatment.[46]

Trazodone hydrochloride, an antidepressant with anxiolytic and sedative effects that can cause priapism as one of its adverse reactions, is not recommended for use in ED. Neither is yohimbine, a drug similar to reserpine, which was used frequently for ED before the arrival of PDE5 inhibitors. Yohimbine can cause unsafe increases of blood pressure and heart rate, and can increase irritability. Similarly, testosterone is not recommended in men with ED who have normal testosterone levels, but may be considered in men who have been diagnosed with hypogonadism.[41,46]

Herbal remedies and alternative medicine

Although many herbal therapies are used for ED, their efficacy and safety have yet to be properly validated, and they are not clinically approved in the United States. Some studies have suggested that Korean red ginseng is a promising herbal therapy for ED.[41,57] Other studies have conferred similar properties to mountain (Panax) ginseng,[58] Crocus sativus (saffron),[59] Lepidium meyenii (Maca) extract,[60] fermented Rubus coreanus (Korean black raspberry),[61] and xanthones from Securidaca longipedunculata,[62] but until the clinical efficacy of these products are authenticated by larger trials, the AUA recommends against herbal remedies for ED.[41]

A recent South Korean study systematically reviewed the feasibility of acupuncture as an alternative treatment of ED, but found insufficient evidence to suggest it as an effective intervention and recommended further research on its potential benefits.[63]

Local therapies

Intracavernous and intraurethral pharmacotherapy with alprostadil can be tried in men who do not respond to oral agents. Alprostadil is generally used as monotherapy; there is an increased risk of priapism if used in combination with other treatments, such as PDE5 inhibitors. Local pain is the most common side effect. Priapism and fibrosis are rare complications. In contrast to men taking PDE5 inhibitors, patients using alprostadil do not need sexual stimulation to achieve an erection.[56]

Mechanical devices

Vacuum constriction devices, also known as vacuum erection devices, provide an affordable and noninvasive alternative to pharmacotherapy, although they can be used in combination with PDE5 inhibitors. The tube-shaped device is placed over the penis and uses subatmospheric pressure to draw blood flow into the cavernosal structures until achieving the desired effect. A constricting band is then placed on the base of the penis to keep the blood in place. The penis will seem cooler than usual.

The major disadvantage is that these devices can be cumbersome to use. To prevent injury, only devices that use a vacuum limiter should be used.[48] Various devices are available with or without a prescription.

Surgery

Surgical placement of penile prostheses or implants is an option when other treatments have failed. These appliances can be semirigid, malleable (containing a system of stacked discs), or inflatable. A 3-piece inflatable device typically includes a pump in the scrotum, a reservoir in the pelvis, and 2 cylinders that replace the corpora cavernosa. Inflatable devices provide flaccidity and rigidity, and have high rates of patient and partner satisfaction. Disadvantages include the need for surgery, mechanical failure, tissue breakdown, infection, and local pain.[48]

Vascular surgery remains controversial and is rarely carried out. Penile arterial reconstructive surgery should only be performed on men with acutely acquired ED caused by a focal arterial occlusion without evidence of generalized vascular disease. Penile venous reconstructive surgery is not recommended by the AUA.[41]

Other treatments

Clinicians should consider the possibility of a coexisting sleep disorder when evaluating patients with ED, especially in those who are refractory to routine therapy. A sleep study can easily detect for the presence of sleep apnea. Indeed, studies have shown that men with ED who are successfully treated for sleep apnea may also see improvements in erectile function.[52]

Several other new agents are in development, including selective dopamine, glutamate, serotonin, and melanocortin receptor agonists; guanylate cyclase activators; rho-kinase inhibitors; and hexarelin analogs. Gene therapy trials and tissue engineering for reconstruction of corporal tissue are in their preliminary phases.[56]

Summary

ED is common throughout the world and increases in prevalence with aging. Clinicians are encouraged to inquire about patients' sexual health during routine history taking. Patients with undiagnosed cardiovascular disease often present initially with symptoms of ED. The clinician needs to bear this strong association in mind and order the appropriate tests when evaluating these patients. In most cases, an underlying organic cause can be identified, but there is usually a coexisting psychological component that should be addressed. The importance of lifestyle modification in the treatment of ED cannot be overemphasized. Many therapies are available for the management of ED, but patients should be aware that no ideal treatment exists. However, there is evidence that the most successful outcomes occur when the partner is included in the evaluation and treatment process.

REFERENCES

1. Waldinger MD, Berendsen HH, Blok BF, et al. Premature ejaculation and serotonergic antidepressants-induced delayed ejaculation: the involvement of the serotonergic system. Behav Brain Res 1998;92(2):111–8.
2. Waldinger MD. Premature ejaculation: state of the art. Urol Clin North Am 2007; 34(4):591–9, vii–viii.
3. Godpodinoff ML. Premature ejaculation: clinical subgroups and etiology. J Sex Marital Ther 1989;15(2):130–4.
4. Donatucci CF. Etiology of ejaculation and pathophysiology of premature ejaculation. J Sex Med 2006;3(Suppl 4):303–8.

5. Nusbaum MR, Hamilton CD. The proactive sexual health history. Am Fam Physician 2002;66(9):1705–12.
6. Waldinger MD, Zwinderman AH, Olivier B, et al. Proposal for a definition of lifelong premature ejaculation based on epidemiological stopwatch data. J Sex Med 2005;2(4):498–507.
7. Sotomayor M. The burden of premature ejaculation: the patient's perspective. J Sex Med 2005;2(Suppl 2):110–4.
8. Shabsigh R. Diagnosing premature ejaculation: a review. J Sex Med 2006; 3(Suppl 4):318–23.
9. Montague DK, Jarow J, Broderick GA, et al. AUA guideline on the pharmacologic management of premature ejaculation. J Urol 2004;172(1):290–4.
10. Laumann EO, Nicolosi A, Glasser DB, et al. Sexual problems among women and men aged 40–80 y: prevalence and correlates identified in the global study of sexual attitudes and behaviors. Int J Impot Res 2005;17(1):39–57.
11. Waldinger MD, Hengeveld MW, Zwinderman AH. Paroxetine treatment of premature ejaculation: a double-blind, randomized, placebo-controlled study. Am J Psychiatry 1994;151(9):1377–9.
12. Waldinger MD, Hengeveld MW, Zwinderman AH. Ejaculation-retarding properties of paroxetine in patients with primary premature ejaculation: a double-blind, randomized, dose-response study. Br J Urol 1997;79(4):592–5.
13. Waldinger MD. Towards evidence-based drug treatment research on premature ejaculation: a critical evaluation of methodology. Int J Impot Res 2003;15(5): 309–13.
14. McMahon CG. Treatment of premature ejaculation with sertraline hydrochloride: a single-blind placebo controlled crossover study. J Urol 1998;159(6): 1935–8.
15. McMahon C, Kim SW, Park NC, et al. Treatment of premature ejaculation in the Asia-Pacific region: results from a phase III double-blind, parallel-group study of dapoxetine. J Sex Med 2010;7(1 Pt 1):256–68.
16. Pryor JL, Althof SE, Steidle C, et al. Efficacy and tolerability of dapoxetine in treatment of premature ejaculation: an integrated analysis of two double-blind, randomised controlled trials. Lancet 2006;368(9539):929–37.
17. Busato W, Galindo CC. Topical anaesthetic use for treating premature ejaculation: a double-blind, randomized, placebo-controlled study. BJU Int 2004;93(7): 1018–21.
18. Dinsmore WW, Hackett G, Goldmeier D, et al. Topical eutectic mixture for premature ejaculation (TEMPE): a novel aerosol-delivery form of lidocaine-prilocaine for treating premature ejaculation. BJU Int 2007;99(2):369–75.
19. Palmer NR, Stuckey BG. Premature ejaculation: a clinical update. Med J Aust 2008;188(11):662–6.
20. Althof S. The psychology of premature ejaculation: therapies and consequences. J Sex Med 2006;3(Suppl 4):324–31.
21. Shindel A, Nelson C, Brandes S. Urologist practice patterns in the management of premature ejaculation: a nationwide survey. J Sex Med 2008;5(1):199–205.
22. American Psychiatric Association. Diagnostic and statistical manual of mental disorders. Text Revision DSM-IV-TR. 4th edition. Washington, DC: American Psychiatric Association; 2000.
23. Hatzimouratidis K, Hatzichristou D. Sexual dysfunctions: classifications and definitions. J Sex Med 2007;4(1):241–50.
24. Laumann EO, Paik A, Rosen RC. Sexual dysfunction in the United States: prevalence and predictors. JAMA 1999;281(6):537–44.

25. Hatzichristou D, Rosen RC, Broderick G, et al. Clinical evaluation and management strategy for sexual dysfunction in men and women. J Sex Med 2004;1(1):49–57.
26. Bonierbale M, Lancon C, Tignol J. The ELIXIR study: evaluation of sexual dysfunction in 4557 depressed patients in France. Curr Med Res Opin 2003;19(2):114–24.
27. Beutel ME, Stobel-Richter Y, Brahler E. Sexual desire and sexual activity of men and women across their lifespans: results from a representative German community survey. BJU Int 2008;101(1):76–82.
28. Kennedy SH, Rizvi S. Sexual dysfunction, depression, and the impact of antidepressants. J Clin Psychopharmacol 2009;29(2):157–64.
29. Weiss RJ. Effects of antihypertensive agents on sexual function. Am Fam Physician 1991;44(6):2075–82.
30. Fogari R, Zoppi A, Corradi L, et al. Sexual function in hypertensive males treated with lisinopril or atenolol: a cross-over study. Am J Hypertens 1998;11(10):1244–7.
31. Katz N, Mazer NA. The impact of opioids on the endocrine system. Clin J Pain 2009;25(2):170–5.
32. Lue TF, Giuliano F, Montorsi F, et al. Summary of the recommendations on sexual dysfunctions in men. J Sex Med 2004;1(1):6–23.
33. Li D, Zhou Z, Qing D, et al. Occupational exposure to bisphenol-A (BPA) and the risk of self-reported male sexual dysfunction. Hum Reprod 2010;25(2):519–27.
34. Basson R, Schultz WW. Sexual sequelae of general medical disorders. Lancet 2007;369(9559):409–24.
35. Harman SM, Metter EJ, Tobin JD, et al. Longitudinal effects of aging on serum total and free testosterone levels in healthy men. Baltimore longitudinal study of aging. J Clin Endocrinol Metab 2001;86(2):724–31.
36. Davis SR. Should women receive androgen replacement therapy, and if so, how? Clin Endocrinol (Oxf) 2010;72(2):149–54.
37. Krapf JM, Simon JA. The role of testosterone in the management of hypoactive sexual desire disorder in postmenopausal women. Maturitas 2009;63(3):213–9.
38. Snabes MC, Simes SM. Approved hormonal treatments for HSDD: an unmet medical need. J Sex Med 2009;6(7):1846–9.
39. Gruenewald DA, Matsumoto AM. Testosterone supplementation therapy for older men: potential benefits and risks. J Am Geriatr Soc 2003;51(1):101–15 [discussion: 115].
40. Anonymous. NIH Consensus Conference. Impotence. NIH Consensus Development Panel on Impotence. JAMA 1993;270(1):83–90.
41. Montague DK, Jarow J, Broderick GA, et al. AUA guideline on the management of erectile dysfunction: diagnosis and treatment recommendations. American Urological Association Education and Research, Inc. New York (NY): Elsevier; 2005.
42. Feldman HA, Goldstein I, Hatzichristou DG, et al. Impotence and its medical and psychosocial correlates: results of the Massachusetts Male Aging Study. J Urol 1994;151(1):54–61.
43. Bella A, Lue T. Male sexual dysfunction. In: Tanagho E, editor. Smith's general urology. 17th edition. New York: Lange/McGraw-Hill; 2008. p. 589–610.
44. Miller TA. Diagnostic evaluation of erectile dysfunction. Am Fam Physician 2000;61:95–104 109–10.
45. Tsertsvadze A, Yazdi F, Fink HA, et al. Diagnosis and treatment of erectile dysfunction. Evidence report/technology assessment no.171 (prepared by the

University of Ottawa Evidence-based Practice Centre (UO-EPC) under contract no. 290-02-0021). AHRQ publication no. 08(09)-E016. Rockville (MD): Agency for Healthcare Research and Quality; 2009.

46. Seftel AD, Miner MM, Kloner RA, et al. Office evaluation of male sexual dysfunction. Urol Clin North Am 2007;34:463–82.

47. Manolis A, Doumas M. Sexual dysfunction: the 'prima ballerina' of hypertension-related quality-of-life complications. J Hypertens 2008;26:2074–84.

48. Steggall MJ. Erectile dysfunction: physiology, causes and patient management. Nurs Stand 2007;21(43):49–56.

49. Goldstein I, Lurie AL, Lubisich JP. Bicycle riding, perineal trauma, and erectile dysfunction: data and solutions. Curr Urol Rep 2007;8:491–7.

50. Asplund C, Barkdull T, Weiss BD. Genitourinary problems in bicyclists. Curr Sports Med Rep 2007;6:333–9.

51. Makhlouf A, Kparker A, Niederberger CS. Depression and erectile dysfunction. Urol Clin North Am 2007;34:565–74.

52. Jankowski JT, Seftel AD, Strohl KP. Erectile dysfunction and sleep related disorders. J Urol 2008;179:837–41.

53. Rosen RC, Riley A, Wagner G, et al. The International Index of Erectile Function (IIEF): a multidimensional scale for assessment of erectile dysfunction. Urology 1997;49:822–30.

54. Rosen RC, Althof SE, Giuliano F. Research instruments for the diagnosis and treatment of patients with erectile dysfunction. Urology 2006;68(Suppl 3A):6–16.

55. Jackson G. The importance of risk factor reduction in erectile dysfunction. Curr Urol Rep 2007;8:463–6.

56. Hatzimouratidis K, Hatzichristou DG. Looking to the future for erectile dysfunction therapies. Drugs 2008;68:231–50.

57. Jang DJ, Lee MS, Shin BC, et al. Red ginseng for treating erectile dysfunction: a systematic review. Br J Clin Pharmacol 2008;4:444–50.

58. Kim TH, Jeon SH, Hahn EJ, et al. Effects of tissue-cultured mountain ginseng (Panax ginseng CA Meyer) extract on male patients with erectile dysfunction. Asian J Androl 2009;3:356–61.

59. Shamsa A, Hosseinzadeh H, Molaei M, et al. Evaluation of Crocus sativus L. (saffron) on male erectile dysfunction: a pilot study. Phytomedicine 2009;16(8): 690–3.

60. Zenico T, Cicero AF, Valmorri L, et al. Subjective effects of Lepidium meyenii (Maca) extract on well-being and sexual performances in patients with mild erectile dysfunction: a randomised, double-blind clinical trial. Andrologia 2009;41(2): 95–9.

61. Jeon JH, Shin S, Park D, et al. Fermentation filtrates of Rubus coreanus relax the corpus cavernosum and increase sperm count and motility. J Med Food 2008;3: 474–8.

62. Meyer JJ, Rakuambo NC, Hussein AA. Novel xanthones from Securidaca longepedunculata with activity against erectile dysfunction. J Ethnopharmacol 2008;3: 599–603.

63. Lee MS, Shin BC, Ernst E. Acupuncture for treating erectile dysfunction: a systematic review. BJU Int 2009;3:366–70.

Urinary Tract Infections

Janice A. Litza, MD*, John R. Brill, MD, MPH

KEYWORDS

- Urinary tract infection • Pyelonephritis
- Asymptomatic bacteriuria

Urinary tract infection (UTI) is the most common urological disorder among men and women, with most cases presenting to primary care physicians in the outpatient clinical setting.[1,2] UTIs represent 4% of all outpatient physician visits.[3] Of the total number of visits for UTI, 52% of patients present to primary care clinics, and 23% present to emergency departments.[4] UTIs are also the most common nosocomial infections of hospitalized patients. As men and women become older, UTI becomes more likely, and UTIs lead to more hospital-based care.[1,2]

A woman's lifetime risk of UTI is greater than 50%.[2] Women develop four times more urinary tract infections than men because of anatomic differences including a shorter urethra and because of normal vaginal flora that colonize the external urethra.[5,6] Infection in women most often results from perineal or periurethral bacteria that enter the urethra and ascend into the bladder, often in association with sexual activity, or due to mechanical instrumentation such as catheterization.[5,6]

ASYMPTOMATIC BACTERIURIA

Asymptomatic bacteriuria (ASB) is the presence of 100,000 microorganisms per milliliter of urine without clinical symptoms.[5] Usually no treatment is needed. Screening for ASB is not recommended for nonpregnant women,[6] elderly living in the community,[7] diabetic women,[8] institutionalized elderly,[9] or persons with spinal cord injuries.[9] However, screening with treatment of positive cultures is recommended for pregnant women in the first trimester.[5–7]

UNCOMPLICATED UTIS

An uncomplicated UTI is diagnosed in patients with cystitis symptoms who have normal urinary tract anatomy, no fever, no kidney disease, and no contributing medical

Department of Family Medicine, University of Wisconsin School of Medicine and Public Health, Milwaukee Academic Campus, 2801 West Kinnickinnic River Parkway, #250, Milwaukee, WI 53215, USA
* Corresponding author.
E-mail address: janice.litza@aurora.org

Prim Care Clin Office Pract 37 (2010) 491–507
doi:10.1016/j.pop.2010.04.001   **primarycare.theclinics.com**

problems such as diabetes, neurogenic bladder, or renal stones.[5,10,11] Characteristic symptoms of cystitis include dysuria, urgency, increased frequency, pyuria, and bacteriuria on urinalysis, and sometimes suprapubic pain, fullness, and hematuria.[5,6] No long-term adverse effects have been seen on renal function or increased mortality with acute uncomplicated UTI in the nonpregnant female population; therefore, treatment goals are aimed at symptom resolution.[10]

The differential diagnosis for uncomplicated UTI includes

Acute urethritis caused by sexually transmitted infections (STIs), often *Neisseria gonorrhea* or *Chlamydia trachomatis*.

Irritative voiding symptoms due to urethral syndrome, interstitial cystitis, recurrent UTI,[12] vaginitis, vulvovaginitis, or dysmenorrhea.[7]

Using Clinical Predictors

Helpful positive predictors include symptom onset with recent sexual intercourse, history of pyelonephritis, and resolution of symptoms within 48 hours of starting antibiotic treatment.[12] Negative predictors include nocturia more than twice per evening, and persistent symptoms between acute episodes; these patients should undergo work-up for other causes. Neutral predictors, neither favoring nor disfavoring the diagnosis of UTI, include hematuria and dyspareunia.[12] Patients with unsure pregnancy status should be tested,[7] as diagnostic criteria and treatment options differ.

Diagnostic Testing

Many studies and organizations refer to urine dipstick testing that is positive for leukocyte esterase or nitrite as confirmatory for uncomplicated UTI.[5–7] The European Association of Urology also recommends urine microscopy for white and red blood cells and nitrites.[9] In one study, the absence of four markers (blood, leukocyte esterase, nitrite, and protein) on urine dipstick at the point of care had a 98% negative predictive value, with sensitivity of 98.3% and specificity of 19.2%.[13] This conflicts with another study in which patients with clinical symptoms but negative urine dipstick symptomatically improved after taking antibiotics.[13] If treatment is driven by symptom reduction, use of empiric antibiotics for a 3-day course in low-risk patients with dysuria, frequency, and absence of vaginal symptoms can be recommended without use of dipstick, with 80% accuracy.[13,14]

Even with clinical predictors indicating greater than 90% probability of UTI, many physicians also order urine culture and sensitivities,[14] which add cost and laboratory workload and make little difference in the treatment of uncomplicated UTIs.[14,15] Urine culture is defined as positive for bacteriuria when there is isolation of no more than two microorganisms, each with at least 100,000 cfu/mL, from a clean voided midstream urine sample.[5,16] Changing this criterion to 1,000–10,000 cfu/mL would improve sensitivity to >90% without much loss of specificity,[5,9] and has been used by some practices.

Uropathogens

Escherichia coli remains the primary agent responsible for UTIs in both outpatient and inpatient settings.[5,6,17] Other common uropathogens are *Enterococcus faecalis*, *Enterobacter* species, *Staphylococcus saprophyticus*, *Klebsiella pneumoniae*, *Proteus mirabilis*, and *Pseudomonas* species.[5,6,10,18] Knowing local variations in sensitivity among the common uropathogens, in both inpatient and outpatient settings, can help physicians make the best treatment choices. First-line antibiotics may have better sensitivity rates in the outpatient setting compared with the inpatient setting.[18]

Treatment

Many studies have demonstrated that a 3-day antibiotic course is effective and cost-effective in 90% of uncomplicated UTIs.[2,5,6,19] A 1-day course is ineffective in most cases.[5,10] Treatment for longer than 3 days is reserved for complicated UTIs.[9,10] One source suggests symptomatic treatment only until culture results are available, to reduce unnecessary prescribing of antibiotics.[7]

Antibiotics for empiric treatment of uncomplicated UTI include

First-line antibiotic: trimethoprim/sulfamethoxazole (co-trimoxazole) in communities with resistance rates for *E coli* less than 20%.[5,7,9] Avoid in women who have been treated within 6 months, as they are more likely to have resistant organisms.[7,10]

Second-line antibiotics, or first-line in resistant communities: fluoroquinolones, such as ciprofloxacin, levofloxacin, norfloxacin, and ofloxacin. Their efficacy is comparable to co-trimoxazole, but increasing resistance rates have been noted.[10]

Alternates: third-generation cephalosporins, nitrofurantoin, fosfomycin.

The following should not be used unless indicated by individual patient culture sensitivities: first- or second-generation cephalosporins,[5,10] ampicillin,[5,10] and amoxicillin with clavulate.[5,6,10]

Follow-Up

Follow up is generally unnecessary for uncomplicated UTI unless there is treatment failure, or if clinical signs or symptoms suggest involvement of the upper urinary tract.[7] Cultures are indicated if symptoms persist after standard therapy,[6] or if symptoms recur 2 to 4 weeks after treatment.[7,9]

Use of Protocols for Uncomplicated UTIs

Empiric treatment based on suggested guidelines and protocols appears to be cost-effective, although some groups still advocate use of urine dipstick and culture to confirm diagnosis and allow accurate antimicrobial choices. Protocols that include nurse-directed triage and phone triage have not shown adverse clinical consequences.[18]

If the following criteria are met, then empiric antibiotics can be prescribed using a first-line agent for a 3-day course without further evaluation[7,18]:

Women younger than 55
No other comorbidities
Not postmenopausal
Not pregnant
No recent UTI
No vaginitis or cervicitis symptoms
Presence of increased urinary frequency
Presence of dysuria.

One outpatient family medicine study evaluated the use of standard guidelines using risk stratification and empiric therapy and found that use of electronic health record (EHR) templates increased compliance with protocols, reducing variability in use of urine dipstick, culture, and antibiotics.[18]

ACUTE PYELONEPHRITIS

Acute pyelonephritis is an infection of the kidney that starts either from ASB or from an ascending bladder infection.[6] Pyelonephritis can develop from an uncomplicated UTI; however, it is more commonly seen in the setting of obstruction, urinary tract malformations, urolithiasis, or pregnancy.[6] Typical symptoms include flank pain, chills, fever (>38°C), nausea or vomiting, and costovertebral angle tenderness. Common symptoms of cystitis also can be present, especially dysuria, increased frequency, and urgency.[5-7] Uncomplicated pyelonephritis can be treated as an outpatient with empiric therapy if only mild symptoms are present and the patient does not have significant nausea or vomiting to interfere with oral antibiotics.[10] Urine culture should be obtained at the initial evaluation. First-line antibiotic choices are the same as for uncomplicated UTIs, and the duration of therapy is typically 10 to 14 days. Hospitalization is appropriate if complicating factors cannot be ruled out, the patient clinically appears septic, or is unable to tolerate oral medication.[6,7] A clinical response is expected in 48 to 72 hours. If there is no improvement at that time, it is appropriate to evaluate for stones and obstruction.[5,6,9]

RECURRENT UTI

Recurrent UTI is defined as at least three episodes of symptomatic uncomplicated UTI with one or more documented positive cultures in 12 months,[6,12] without complicating factors. A relapse is infection with the same organism as the previous UTI.[5] A reinfection is when the initial UTI is treated, the patient becomes asymptomatic with a negative culture in between, and then develops symptoms again, or when the second infection is caused by a second organism.[5,6] American College of Obstetricians and Gynecologists (ACOG) data show reinfection occurs in 25% to 50% of women within the first year of an initial uncomplicated UTI, and recurrent UTI occurs in 3% to 5% of women.[5]

Patient education on the following behaviors has not been shown to reduce recurrent UTIs: wiping techniques, hygiene, postcoital voiding, douching, use of hot tubs, wearing of pantyhose, or timing of voiding.[6,7]

Age-based initial evaluation of recurrent UTI might include assessment for

Adolescent women (undiagnosed congenital abnormalities and onset of sexual activity)

Premenopausal women (frequent/recent sexual activity, diaphragm use, spermicide use, increasing parity, diabetes, obesity, sickle cell trait, and renal stones[5,7])

Postmenopausal women (tumors, obstructive problems, detrusor failure, genital infection,[9] vaginal atrophy, incontinence, incomplete bladder emptying, prolaps[5,7]).

After ruling out complicating factors and changing modifiable factors, the following are possible treatment regimens:

Antimicrobial prophylaxis with first-line agent (reduced dose daily[9]; after sexual intercourse[6,7,9]; three times a week for 6 months, after infection clearance is documented by a negative culture[7]).

Patient initiated treatment at an early symptom stage.[5,7,9,10] Patients can usually accurately self diagnose after the first infection.[7]

Food additive prophylaxis (Cranberry extract[6,9] inhibits adhesion of certain bacteria, decreasing subsequent infection.[19] Improvement is seen only in young and middle-aged women with recurrent UTI.[19] Further studies are needed to determine the optimal dosage and administration.[20] Cranberry extract is not indicated for treatment of UTI. Lactobacilli probiotics can restore the urogenital flora and decrease uropathogens.[21]).

Methenamine hippurate, a nonspecific antibacterial agent, may be effective for preventing UTI when no renal abnormalities are present. In one trial, it resulted in symptom reduction after 1 week of therapy.[22]

Local hormonal treatment in postmenopausal women.[10] In a Cochrane review, vaginal estrogens were more effective than placebo at preventing recurrent UTIs. Oral estrogens offered no benefit in reduction of recurrent UTI. More studies are needed to determine the best type of estrogen and most effective duration of therapy.[23]

MEN

Only 20% of UTIs occur in men. Male UTI rates increase dramatically with age, and most are complicated by prostate pathology.[1] Men at low risk with a first UTI may be treated using a 3-day course with a first-line agent.[14] Low-risk men are defined as under age of 45, with no prostatitis, urethritis, obstructive symptoms, or hematuria.[14] Urological evaluation is recommended in adolescents, men with febrile UTI, pyelonephritis, recurrent infections, or when complicating factors are suspected.[9] The European Association of Urology recommends a 7-day course with fluoroquinolones even in uncomplicated male UTI.[9] If fever is present, then a 2-week course of therapy is recommended, since prostatic involvement is common.[9] In contrast to uncomplicated UTI in women, a urine culture is recommended to confirm the diagnosis in all men. No further evaluation or imaging is needed if there is a positive culture along with resolution of symptoms in a man's first uncomplicated UTI. If symptoms persist or culture is negative, imaging with abdominal ultrasound is a reasonable next step.

NOSOCOMIAL UTIS

There has been a recent interest in prevention of catheter-associated UTI (CAUTI) in the hospital setting, since the Centers for Medicare and Medicaid Services (CMS) identified this as one of six unacceptable diagnoses for payment if UTI was not present on admission.[24,25] As of 2009, a CAUTI is one that occurs in a patient who had an indwelling urethral catheter at the time of or within 48 hours of the event.[26] A previous definition included those with a catheter within 7 days of the event.[16] CAUTIs account for 80% of nosocomial UTIs and 40% of all nosocomial infections.[24,26–29] Currently, the mechanism for infection is thought to be bacterial biofilm formation on the catheter; the longer the catheter is in place, the greater the risk of symptomatic CAUTI.[24,30–35]

The initial recommended strategy for patients who become symptomatic with a urinary catheter is to assess for catheter removal or replacement,[36] obtain urine and blood cultures,[36] begin treatment with first-line antibiotic agents based on local susceptibility patterns, and change to a specific antibiotic when sensitivities are available.[36] The source of urine for urine cultures should ideally be from a newly- placed catheter or urine obtained after removal.[37] Prevention of nosocomial UTIs involves using protocols for nursing, emergency rooms,[38] and physician order sets[39] to catheterize only for specific indications, removing the catheter as soon as possible, using sufficient lubricant with insertion, and inserting the smallest caliber catheter in a closed, gravity-dependent system.[36–38,40,41] Routine urinalysis and cultures are not recommended for patients who have been catheterized unless they develop symptoms suggestive of a UTI.[37] Likewise, treatment of ASB in this clinical situation is not recommended. The short-term use of silver- and antibiotic-coated catheters reduced UTI rate, but longer-term use of these catheters and maintenance of this reduction has yet to be assessed.[36,42,43] Application of topical antiseptics or antibiotics to the meatal opening is not currently recommended.[36,44,45] Currently, prophylactic antibiotics in patients with short-term catheters are not routinely recommended.[36] However, studies continue to show mixed results from various prophylactic regimens just before or immediately following catheter removal.[46,47]

PEDIATRIC PATIENTS

Infants and children diagnosed with UTIs more often present to emergency rooms than outpatient clinics.[48] In any setting, prompt identification, treatment, and follow-up of pediatric UTIs are key to preventing long-term complications.

When considering whether a UTI is the cause of unexplained fever in infants or children, physicians should assess pretest probability, using prevalence data by age, gender, race, and for male patients, circumcision status. A meta-analysis by Shaikh and colleagues[49] in 2008 showed that demographic and clinical characteristics are useful to help determine whether further testing is needed.[49] Cincinnati Children's Hospital Medical Center[50] and a recent review in *Journal of the American Medical Assocation*[51] have algorithms and worksheets for determining the pretest probability of a child having a UTI. The overall risk for all children with unexplained fever having a urinary tract infection is 7% to 9%.[52,53]

Initial Evaluation

If the pretest probability of UTI is less than 2%, observation with close follow-up in 24 hours can be considered.[51] If the pretest probability is greater than 2%, or if other risk factors are present, such as a history of UTI, temperature greater than 39°C, ill appearance, suprapubic tenderness, or fever greater than 24 hours, then testing and immediate treatment might be warranted.[51,54,55] The 2007 National Institute for Health and Clinical Excellence (NICE) guidelines suggest obtaining a clean urine specimen (bagged or midstream).[54] A negative dipstick is helpful in ruling out a UTI, while a test positive for leukocyte esterase, nitrite, or bacteriuria can guide treatment[51] and can help determine if catheterization or suprapubic aspiration is necessary.[54] Any positive urinalysis in children should be followed by a urine culture.[52] Imaging considerations are made based on risk factors, initial presentation, and response to treatment in the first 48hours. Hospitalization typically is recommended for infants younger than 1 year, ill-appearing children, and patients for whom follow-up might be difficult.[50,56,57]

Initial Antibiotic Treatment

Standard treatment for a first pediatric UTI includes a 7 to 14 day course of antibiotics,[50,51,54,58] selected based on local resistance patterns. The antibiotics most often used include parenteral ceftriaxone, cefotaxime, ampicillin, and gentamicin, and oral co-trimoxazole, cefixime, and cephalexin.[50,53,56] A Cochrane review in 2005 recommended a 3-day antibiotic course in well-appearing children over 3 months of age, but this does not appear to be widely accepted in the clinical protocols reviewed.[59,60]

Prophylactic Antibiotics

Recommendations for prophylactic antibiotics in children with renal scarring or vesicoureteral reflux have undergone significant changes.[50,53,54,58,61] Routine prophylaxis may not be indicated after an uncomplicated first UTI, or with absent/mild grade 1 to 3 vesicoureteral reflux.[55,61-64]

Imaging

The main goal of imaging is to evaluate for obstruction, pyelonephritis, previously undetected anomalies, vesicoureteral reflux, and renal scarring.[50,53,58] These findings may be important in deciding which children require antibiotic prophylaxis. Infants and children up to the age of 24 months with UTI have a 20% to 24% incidence of vesicoureteral reflux of all grades, with 8% to 9% showing other urinary tract abnormalities.[65] Imaging recommendations vary by institution, as more evidence-based, cost-effective, and patient-centered approaches are sought.

Imaging Studies

Renal ultrasound

This is helpful for anatomic variations, obstruction, pyelonephritis, and changes such as hydronephrosis that may suggest vesicoureteral reflux.

It is the least invasive, has no radiation exposure; therefore renal ultrasound is the most common initial test.[66,67]

Cystogram

The voiding cystourethrogram (VCUG) is the most invasive, requiring urethral catheterization and radiation exposure with fluoroscopy. It is used to detect pyelonephritis and to grade vesicoureteral reflux.

The radionuclide cystogram (RNC) is less invasive and less detailed compared with traditional VCUG. It requires radionuclide exposure.

Tc 99 m dimercaptosuccinic acid renal scanning

This is useful for detecting renal scarring and acute renal abnormalities. It can be used initially or as a follow-up study.[68]

Tc 99 m dimercaptosuccinic acid renal scanning (DMSA) involves intravenous injection and radiation exposure.[58]

The cost is higher cost and it requires radionuclide exposure.

Neonates and children with recurrent or atypical UTI (seriously ill, poor urine flow, abdominal or bladder mass on examination, elevated creatinine, septicemia, no response within 48 hours of antibiotics, or non-*E coli* infection) should have renal ultrasound during the acute infection and VCUG on follow-up, with possible DMSA.[53,54,58,69]

Imaging Guideline Highlights

The American Academy of Pediatrics 1999 guidelines highlight the following: 2 months to 2 years—renal ultrasound and either VCUG or RNC.[53]

NICE 2007 guidelines emphasize

Younger than 6 months with good response: renal ultrasound in 6 weeks, no further imaging[54]

6 months to 3 years with good response: no imaging

Greater than 3 years with good response: no imaging

Cincinnati Children's Hospital evidence-based guidelines from 2006 emphasize[50]

All males, females younger than 3 years, and females from age 3 to 7 years with
   fever of at least 38.5°C: ultrasound and cystogram
Females older than 3 years without fever: may not need imaging after first UTI.

Guidelines from the Albany Medical Center[58] include

All children younger than 5 years with febrile UTI: ultrasound and VCUG
All males with UTI: ultrasound and VCUG
Females younger than 2 years: ultrasound and VCUG
Females 2 to 3 years: ultrasound
Newborns with reflux: DMSA scan, possibly additional testing.

One additional tool is serum procalcitonin, used as an indicator of systemic upper
UTI.[58,70] It is potentially a less invasive clinical predictor of infants at low risk. Procalcitonin becomes elevated within 2 to 6 hours of initial significant bacterial infection.
Levels higher than 0.5 ng/mL are associated with renal parenchymal damage.[70] Newer
guidelines might include this marker if further studies confirm its usefulness.

IMMUNOSUPPRESSED PATIENTS

There is sparse literature on UTIs in immunosuppressed hosts, perhaps because
opportunistic infections are more likely to manifest in other organ systems.[71] Viruses
such as BK virus, adenovirus, and cytomegalovirus are a relatively commonly cause of
UTIs, particularly hemorrhagic cystitis, in the immunocompromised.[72] UTIs are
common in renal transplant patients, particularly in the first 3 months after transplantation.[73] An international guideline includes the following recommendations for
prevention and treatment of UTIs in renal transplant patients:

Treat infection in the recipient before transplantation.
Culture both the donor tissue sample and perfusate.
Use perioperative antibiotic prophylaxis.
Continue low-dose co-trimoxazole for 6 months.
Treat overt infection with a quinolone or co-trimoxazole for 10 to 14 days.[74]

PATIENTS WITH SPINAL CORD INJURY

Urologic complications are a primary source of morbidity and until recently were the
leading cause of death for the estimated 260,000 Americans living with spinal cord
injury (SCI).[75] Factors leading to UTIs in SCI patients are impaired voiding, stone
formation secondary to acute bone loss, and altered sensation and symptoms. Variables linked to development of UTI in spinal cord injured patients are prior history of
UTI, higher degree of functional impairment, and lack of exercise.[76] **Table 1** summarizes methods used to decrease the incidence of UTIs in SCI patients. For those using
intermittent catheterization, a Cochrane review concluded that various alternative
approaches are no better than clean technique with a simple catheter. Although
most guidelines recommend intermittent catheterization,[84] indwelling suprapubic
catheters may be preferred by patients and caregivers. A recent review by Sugimura
found a relatively low rate of infection or other complications with this approach.[85]
Darouiche observed that using an antimicrobial securing device (Stat-Lock TM) with
indwelling catheters reduced UTI rates.[86]
   Screening for UTIs in SCI patients is not recommended, as there is a high rate of
ASB and no demonstrable benefit to treatment without symptoms.[87] Observation
of a high rate of UTIs following bladder testing and manipulation suggests use of

Table 1
Strategies for reducing UTI in patients with spinal cord injury

Strategy	Subject Characteristics	Comparison	Effect	Comment
Hydrophilic catheter[77]	Self-intermittent catheterization	Noncoated catheters	20% reduction in total UTIs	Small sample (45 total)
Hydrophilic catheter[78]	123 male patients, > or = 16 y and SCI within 6 months	Noncoated catheters	18% reduction in percentage of patients without UTI	
Escherichia coli 83,972-coated catheters[79]	Intermittent Catheterization	Historical	62% achieved colonization with protective strain; these patients had 66% reduction in *E coli* UTIs	Small sample (13 subjects) historic controls, only *E coli* UTIs reported
Clean technique[80]	Tetraplegic patients requiring assisted intermittent catheterization	Sterile technique	No difference in number of UTIs or time to develop UTI	Small sample size (36 subjects)
Weekly oral cyclic antibiotic (WOCA)[81]	Clean intermittent catheterization, frequent UTIs	Historical controls	81% reduction in symptomatic UTI	Small sample size (38 subjects)
Cranberry tablets[82]	Documented neurogenic bladder	Placebo	70% relative reduction of UTIs	Small sample size (47 total)
Methenamine hippurate or cranberry tablets[83]	Neurogenic bladder, mostly community-dwelling	Placebo	No difference in UTI-free period	345 total subjects

Abbreviation: SCI, spinal cord injury.

antibiotic prophylaxis for SCI patients undergoing procedures.[88] A trial of a formal patient education program did not reduce UTI recurrence, but did enhance the SCI patients' sense of control.[89] UTIs may present as increased spasticity or autonomic dysreflexia in quadriplegic patients.[90] Treatment consists of 10 to 14 days of a fluoroquinolone antibiotic, guided by culture and sensitivity.

SENIORS

UTIs occur frequently in the elderly, and contribute significantly to morbidity and mortality. UTIs are a principal cause of falls in nursing home patients,[91] especially those with dementia.[92] UTIs frequently complicate acute medical conditions such as stroke.[93] A clear association exists between UTI and acute coronary syndrome, suggesting that systemic inflammation may even precipitate coronary ischemia.[94]

Several factors make the diagnosis of UTIs in the elderly challenging. ASB is highly prevalent. In a community-based study, increasing age, incontinence, and impaired mobility increased ASB prevalence; a woman over 80 with urinary incontinence and needing support to walk had a risk of nearly 50% of ASB.[95] Neither screening for ASB nor treatment of this condition in the elderly is recommended.[8,87] Diagnosis of UTI in nursing home residents is often difficult because of atypical symptoms. One study found the most useful signs and symptoms to be dysuria (relative risk [RR] = 1.58), change in character of urine (RR = 1.42), and change in mental status (RR = 1.38).[96] In patients with comorbidities, especially pulmonary disease, even diagnostic experts frequently cannot agree whether a patient has bacteriuria or a UTI.[97]

Several studies note the connection between impaired mobility and UTI development. Mobile nursing home patients had nearly a 70% less likelihood of being hospitalized for UTI than immobile counterparts, and maintaining or improving mobility reduced this risk by 39% to 76%.[98] Other strategies effective at reducing UTIs include avoiding catheterization and having a physician visit at the time of nursing home admission.[98] In older women with recurrent UTIs, daily cranberry extract was as effective as and safer than trimethoprim for prophylaxis.[99] Postmenopausal women with recurrent UTI treated with intravaginal estrogen have significantly reduced rates of recurrence.[9]

CAUTIs are a particular problem for the elderly. In 2004, Gokula found that less than half of urinary catheters placed in hospitalized seniors were indicated.[100] In addition to general guidelines for prevention of CAUTIs, recommendations for the elderly include

Avoid use of urinary catheters in nursing home residents for management of incontinence (category 1b)
Consider using external catheters (eg, condom catheters) as an alternative to indwelling urethral catheters in cooperative male patients without urinary retention or bladder outlet obstruction (category 2)

Appropriate indications for use of indwelling catheters in seniors include

To assist in healing of open sacral or perineal wounds in incontinent patients
To allow prolonged immobilization of potentially unstable thoracic or lumbar spine injuries or pelvic fractures
To improve comfort for end-of-life care.[84]

Recent studies have challenged the traditional notion that age alone constitutes a complicated UTI. Grover studied older women seen for UTI in a family practice center and concluded that treatment employed with co-trimoxazole and without the use of culture and sensitivity may be effective for appropriately selected older women.[101] A Cochrane review found that otherwise healthy elderly patients given longer than 3 days of antibiotics had significantly higher rates of adverse drug reactions, with no improvement in efficacy.[102] Thus, evidence suggests that the type and duration of treatment should be based on comorbidities and complications, not age.

DIABETIC PATIENTS

ASB is common in diabetic patients. Although diabetics with ASB have higher rates of developing symptomatic UTIs, there is no good evidence that antibiotic treatment of ASB reduces UTI rates, as recolonization occurs rapidly.[103] Nicolle states succinctly: "Bacteriuria is benign, and seldom permanently eradicable."[104] The United States Preventive Services Task Force does not recommend screening for ASB in diabetic patients.[8]

However, a UTI in a diabetic patient is considered a complicated UTI. Diabetic patients have more frequent and severe UTIs, and often have asymptomatic upper tract involvement. Insulin therapy and a history of prior cystitis are associated with a higher risk of UTI.[105] Well-controlled studies of optimal type and duration of therapy for UTIs in diabetes are lacking, but expert recommendations suggest a 10- to 14-day course of antibiotics with an antimicrobial agent that achieves high levels both in the urine and in urinary tract tissues.[77] Diabetics have a higher risk of recurrence than nondiabetics.[78] Funguria is also found more frequently in diabetics. It should not be routinely treated, but an indwelling catheter, if present, should be changed.[36]

REFERENCES

1. Griebling TL. Urologic diseases in America project: trends in resource use for urinary tract infections in men. J Urol 2005;173(4):1288–94.
2. Griebling TL. Urologic diseases in America project: trends in resource use for urinary tract infections in women. J Urol 2005;173(4):1281–7.
3. Hing E, Hall MJ, Xu J. National health statistics reports. National hospital ambulatory medical care survey: 2006 outpatient department summary. Division of Health Care Statistics; 2008.
4. Schappert SM, Rechtsteiner EA. National health statistics reports. Ambulatory medical care utilization estimates for 2006. Summary. Division of Health Care Statistics; 2006.
5. American College of Obstetricians and Gynecologists. ACOG Practice Bulletin No. 91: treatment of urinary tract infections in nonpregnant women. Obstet Gynecol 2008;111(3):785–94.
6. Sheffield JS, Cunningham FG. Urinary tract infection in women. Obstet Gynecol 2005;106(5 Pt 1):1085–92.
7. Car J. Urinary tract infections in women: diagnosis and management in primary care. BMJ 2006;332(7533):94–7.
8. Calogne N. Screening for asymptomatic bacteriuria in adults: U.S. Preventive Services Task Force reaffirmation recommendation statement. Ann Intern Med 2008;149(1):43–7.
9. Grabe M. Uncomplicated urinary tract infections in adults. In: Grabe M, Bishop MC, Bjerklund-Johansen TE, et al, editors. Guidelines on the management of urinary and male genital tract infections. Arnhem (The Netherlands): European Association of Urology (EAU); 2008. p. 11–40.
10. Wagenlehner FM, Weidner W, Naber KG. An update on uncomplicated urinary tract infections in women. Curr Opin Urol 2009;19(4):368–74.

11. De Alleaume L, Tweed EM, Bonacci R. Clinical inquiries. When are empiric antibiotics appropriate for urinary tract infection symptoms? J Fam Pract 2006; 55(4):338, 341–2.

12. Gopal M, Northington G, Arya L. Clinical symptoms predictive of recurrent urinary tract infections. Am J Obstet Gynecol 2007;197:74.e4.

13. Richards D, Toop L, Chambers S, et al. Response to antibiotics of women with symptoms of urinary tract infection but negative dipstick urine test results: double blind randomised controlled trial. BMJ 2005;331(7509):143.

14. Breen DP, Wanserski GR, Smith PC. Clinical inquiries. What is the recommended workup for a man with a first UTI? J Fam Pract 2007;56(8):657–9.

15. Patel HD, Livsey SA, Swann RA, et al. Can urine dipstick testing for urinary tract infection at point of care reduce laboratory workload? J Clin Pathol 2005;58(9): 951–4.

16. Horan TC, Andrus M, Dudeck MA. CDC/NHSN surveillance definition of health care-associated infection and criteria for specific types of infections in the acute care setting. Am J Infect Control 2008;36(5):309–32.

17. Guay DR. Contemporary management of uncomplicated urinary tract infections. Drugs 2008;68(9):1169–205.

18. Grover ML, Bracamonte JD, Kanodia AK, et al. Assessing adherence to evidence-based guidelines for the diagnosis and management of uncomplicated urinary tract infection. Mayo Clin Proc 2007;82(2):181–5.

19. Guay DR. Cranberry and urinary tract infections. Drugs 2009;69(7):775–807.

20. Jepson RG, Craig JC. Cranberries for preventing urinary tract infections. Cochrane Database Syst Rev 2008;1:CD001321.

21. Falagas ME, Betsi GI, Tokas T, et al. Probiotics for prevention of recurrent urinary tract infections in women: a review of the evidence from microbiological and clinical studies. Drugs 2006;66(9):1253–61.

22. Lee BB, Simpson JM, Craig JC, et al. Methenamine hippurate for preventing urinary tract infections. Cochrane Database Syst Rev 2007;(4):CD003265.

23. Perrotta C, Aznar M, Mejia R, et al. Oestrogens for preventing recurrent urinary tract infection in postmenopausal women. Cochrane Database Syst Rev 2008;2: CD005131.

24. Zhan C, Elixhauser A, Richards CL Jr, et al. Identification of hospital-acquired catheter-associated urinary tract infections from Medicare claims: sensitivity and positive predictive value. Med Care 2009;47(3):364–9.

25. National Healthcare Safety Network (NHSN). Catheter-Associated Urinary Tract Infection (CAUTI) Event. Available at: http://www.cdc.gov/nhsn/pdfs/pscManual/7pscCAUTIcurrent.pdf. Accessed February 16, 2010.

26. Nasr AM, ElBigawy AF, Abdelamid AE, et al. Evaluation of the use vs nonuse of urinary catheterization during cesarean delivery: a prospective, multicenter, randomized controlled trial. J Perinatol 2009;29(6):416–21.

27. Liang CC, Lee CL, Chang TC, et al. Postoperative urinary outcomes in catheterized and noncatheterized patients undergoing laparoscopic-assisted vaginal hysterectomy—a randomized controlled trial. Int Urogynecol J 2009;20(3): 295–300.

28. Onile TG, Kuti O, Orji EO, et al. A prospective randomized clinical trial of urethral catheter removal following elective cesarean delivery. Int J Gynaecol Obstet 2008;102(3):267–70.

29. Sekhavat L, Farajkhoda T, Davar R. The effect of early removal of indwelling urinary catheter on postoperative urinary complications in anterior colporrhaphy surgery. Aust N Z J Obstet Gynaecol 2008;48(3):348–52.

30. Trautner BW, Hull RA, Darouiche RO. Prevention of catheter-associated urinary tract infection. Curr Opin Infect Dis 2005;18(1):37–41.
31. Simpson C, Clark AP. Nosocomial UTI: are we treating the catheter or the patient? Clin Nurse Spec 2005;19(4):175–9.
32. Stickler DJ. Bacterial biofilms in patients with indwelling urinary catheters. Nat Clin Pract Urol 2008;5(11):598–608.
33. Graves N, Tong E, Morton AP, et al. Factors associated with health care-acquired urinary tract infection. Am J Infect Control 2007;35(6):387–92.
34. Grabe M, Bishop MC, Bjerklund-Johansen TE, et al. Catheter-associated UTIs. In: Grabe M, Bishop MC, Bjerklund-Johansen TE, et al, editors. Guidelines on the management of urinary and male genital tract infections. Arnhem (The Netherlands): European Association of Urology (EAU); 2008. p. 70–1.
35. Igawa Y, Wyndaele JJ, Nishizawa O. Catheterization: possible complications and their prevention and treatment. Int J Urol 2008;15(6):481–5.
36. Gokula RM, Smith MA, Hickner J. Emergency room staff education and use of a urinary catheter indication sheet improves appropriate use of foley catheters. Am J Infect Control 2007;35(9):589–93.
37. Topal J, Conklin S, Camp K, et al. Prevention of nosocomial catheter-associated urinary tract infections through computerized feedback to physicians and a nurse-directed protocol. Am J Med Qual 2005;20(3):121–6.
38. Parker D, Callan L, Harwood J, et al. Catheter-associated urinary tract infections: fact sheet. J Wound Ostomy Continence Nurs 2009;36(2):156–9.
39. Godfrey H, Fraczyk L. Preventing and managing catheter-associated urinary tract infections. Br J Community Nurs 2005;10(5):205–12.
40. Schumm K, Lam TB. Types of urethral catheters for management of short-term voiding problems in hospitalized adults: a short version Cochrane review. Neurourol Urodyn 2008;27(8):738–46.
41. Schumm K, Lam TB. Types of urethral catheters for management of short-term voiding problems in hospitalized adults. Cochrane Database Syst Rev 2008;2: CD004013.
42. Nasiriani K, Kalani Z, Farnia F, et al. Comparison of the effect of water vs. povidone-iodine solution for periurethral cleaning in women requiring an indwelling catheter prior to gynecologic surgery. Urol Nurs 2009;29(2):122–3.
43. Willson M, Wilde M, Webb ML, et al. Nursing interventions to reduce the risk of catheter-associated urinary tract infection: part 2: staff education, monitoring, and care techniques. J Wound Ostomy Continence Nurs 2009;36(2): 137–54.
44. Pfefferkorn U, Lea S, Moldenhauer J, et al. Antibiotic prophylaxis at urinary catheter removal prevents urinary tract infections: a prospective randomized trial. Ann Surg 2009;249(4):573–5.
45. Esposito S, Noviello S, Leone S, et al. A pilot study on prevention of catheter-related urinary tract infections with fluoroquinolones. J Chemother 2006;18(5): 494–501.
46. Freedman AL. Urologic diseases in North America Project: trends in resource utilization for urinary tract infections in children. J Urol 2005;173(3):949–54.
47. Shaikh N, Morone NE, Bost JE, et al. Prevalence of urinary tract infection in childhood: a meta-analysis. Pediatr Infect Dis J 2008;27(4):302–8.
48. UTI Guideline Team. Cincinnati Children's Hospital Medical Center: evidence-based care guideline for medical management of first urinary tract infection in children 12 years of age or less. Available at: http://www.cincinnatichildrens. org/svc/dept-div/health-policy/evbased/uti.htm. Accessed November 27, 2009.

49. Shaikh N, Morone NE, Lopez J, et al. Does this child have a urinary tract infection? JAMA 2007;298(24):2895–904.
50. Zorc JJ, Levine DA, Platt SL, et al. Clinical and demographic factors associated with urinary tract infection in young febrile infants. Pediatrics 2005; 116(3):644–8.
51. American Academy of Pediatrics Committee on Quality Improvement. Subcommittee on Urinary Tract Infection. Practice parameter: the diagnosis, treatment, and evaluation of the initial urinary tract infection in febrile infants and young children. Arlington Heights (IL): American Academy of Pediatrics; 1999.
52. Baumer JH, Jones RW. Urinary tract infection in children, National Institute for Health and Clinical Excellence. Arch Dis Child Educ Pract Ed 2007;92(6): 189–92.
53. Conway P, Cnaan A, Zaoutis T, et al. AHRQ site reference: recurrent urinary tract infections in children: risk factors and association with prophylactic antimicrobials. JAMA 2007;298(2):179–86.
54. Dore-Bergeron MJ, Gauthier M, Chevalier I, et al. Urinary tract infections in 1- to 3-month-old infants: ambulatory treatment with intravenous antibiotics. Pediatrics 2009;124(1):16–22.
55. Cohen AL, Rivara FP, Davis R, et al. Compliance with guidelines for the medical care of first urinary tract infections in infants: a population-based study. Pediatrics 2005;115(6):1474–8.
56. Bauer R, Kogan BA. New developments in the diagnosis and management of pediatric UTIs. Urol Clin North Am 2008;35(1):47–58.
57. Hodson EM, Willis NS, Craig JC. Antibiotics for acute pyelonephritis in children. Cochrane Database Syst Rev 2007;4:CD003772.
58. Bloomfield P, Hodson EM, Craig JC. Antibiotics for acute pyelonephritis in children. Cochrane Database Syst Rev 2003;(3):CD003772.
59. Montini G, Hewitt I. Urinary tract infections: to prophylaxis or not to prophylaxis? Pediatr Nephrol 2009;24(9):1605–9.
60. Gaspari RJ, Dickson E, Karlowsky J, et al. Multidrug resistance in pediatric urinary tract infections. Microb Drug Resist Mechanisms Epidemiol Dis 2006; 12(2):126–9.
61. Kotoula A, Gardikis S, Tsalkidis A, et al. Procalcitonin for the early prediction of renal parenchymal involvement in children with UTI: preliminary results. Int Urol Nephrol 2009;41(2):393–9.
62. Montini G, Rigon L, Zucchetta P, et al. Prophylaxis after first febrile urinary tract infection in children? A multicenter, randomized, controlled, noninferiority trial. Pediatrics 2008;122(5):1064–71.
63. Kanellopoulos TA, Salakos C, Spiliopoulou I, et al. First urinary tract infection in neonates, infants and young children: a comparative study. Pediatr Nephrol 2006;21(8):1131–7.
64. Muller L, Preda I, Jacobsson B, et al. Ultrasonography as predictor of permanent renal damage in infants with urinary tract infection. Acta Paediatr 2009; 98(7):1156–61.
65. Brader P, Riccabona M, Schwarz T, et al. Value of comprehensive renal ultrasound in children with acute urinary tract infection for assessment of renal involvement: comparison with DMSA scintigraphy and final diagnosis. Eur Radiol 2008;18(12):2981–9.
66. Preda I, Jodal U, Sixt R, et al. Normal dimercaptosuccinic acid scintigraphy makes voiding cystourethrography unnecessary after urinary tract infection. J Pediatr 2007;151(6):581–4.e1.

67. Hsieh MH, Madden-Fuentes RJ, Roth DR. Urologic diagnoses among infants hospitalized for urinary tract infection. Urology 2009;74(1):100–3.

68. Hellerstein S. Acute urinary tract infection—evaluation and treatment. Curr Opin Pediatr 2006;18(2):134–8.

69. Frank U, Daschner FD, Schulgen G, et al. Incidence and epidemiology of nosocomial infections in patients infected with human immunodeficiency virus. Clin Infect Dis 1997;25(2):318–20.

70. Paduch DA. Viral lower urinary tract infections. Curr Urol Rep 2007;8(4):324–35.

71. Tolkoff-Rubin NE, Rubin RH. Urinary tract infection in the immunocompromised host. Lessons from kidney transplantation and the AIDS epidemic. Infect Dis Clin North Am 1997;11(3):707–17.

72. Grabe M. UTIs in renal insufficiency, transplant recipients, diabetes mellitus and immunosuppression. In: Grabe M, Bishop MC, Bjerklund-Johansen TE, et al, editors. Guidelines on the management of urinary and male genital tract infections. Arnhem (The Netherlands): European Association of Urology (EAU); 2008. p. 52–63.

73. Chen Y. National Spinal Cord Injury Statistical Center. Available at: https://www.nscisc.uab.edu/public_content/facts_figures_2009.aspx. Accessed November 23, 2009.

74. Kroll T, Neri MT, Ho PS. Secondary conditions in spinal cord injury: results from a prospective survey. Disabil Rehabil 2007;29(15):1229–37.

75. Gould CV, Umscheid CA, Agarwal RK. Guideline for prevention of catheter-associated urinary tract infections. Available at: http://www.cdc.gov/ncidod/dhqp/dpac_uti_pc.html. 2009. Accessed November 11, 2009.

76. Sugimura T, Arnold E, English S, et al. Chronic suprapubic catheterization in the management of patients with spinal cord injuries: analysis of upper and lower urinary tract complications. BJU Int 2008;101(11):1396–400.

77. Cardenas DD, Hoffman JM. Hydrophilic catheters versus noncoated catheters for reducing the incidence of urinary tract infections: a randomized controlled trial. Arch Phys Med Rehabil 2009;90(10):1668–71.

78. De Ridder DJ, Everaert K, Fernandez LG, et al. Intermittent catheterisation with hydrophilic-coated catheters (SpeediCath) reduces the risk of clinical urinary tract infection in spinal cord injured patients: a prospective randomised parallel comparative trial. Eur Urol 2005;48(6):991–5.

79. Prasad A, Cevallos ME, Riosa S, et al. A bacterial interference strategy for prevention of UTI in persons practicing intermittent catheterization. Spinal Cord 2009;47(7):565–9.

80. Moore KN, Burt J, Voaklander DC. Intermittent catheterization in the rehabilitation setting: a comparison of clean and sterile technique. Clin Rehabil 2006; 20(6):461–8.

81. Salomon J, Denys P, Merle C, et al. Prevention of urinary tract infection in spinal cord-injured patients: safety and efficacy of a weekly oral cyclic antibiotic (WOCA) programme with a 2 year follow-up–an observational prospective study. J Antimicrob Chemother 2006;57(4):784–8.

82. Hess MJ, Hess PE, Sullivan MR, et al. Evaluation of cranberry tablets for the prevention of urinary tract infections in spinal cord injured patients with neurogenic bladder. Spinal Cord 2008;46(9):622–6.

83. Lee BB, Haran MJ, Hunt LM, et al. Spinal-injured neuropathic bladder antisepsis (SINBA) trial. Spinal Cord 2007;45(8):542–50.

84. Darouiche RO, Goetz L, Kaldis T, et al. Impact of StatLock securing device on symptomatic catheter-related urinary tract infection: a prospective, randomized, multicenter clinical trial. Am J Infect Control 2006;34(9):555–60.

85. Nicolle LE, Bradley S, Colgan R, et al. Infectious Diseases Society of America guidelines for the diagnosis and treatment of asymptomatic bacteriuria in adults. Clin Infect Dis 2005;40:643.

86. Pannek J, Nehiba M. Morbidity of urodynamic testing in patients with spinal cord injury: is antibiotic prophylaxis necessary? Spinal Cord 2007;45(12): 771–4.

87. Cardenas DD, Hoffman JM, Kelly E, et al. Impact of a urinary tract infection educational program in persons with spinal cord injury. J Spinal Cord Med 2004;27(1):47–54.

88. DeMaio J. Urinary tract infection, complicated. Available at: http://hopkins-abxguide. org/diagnosis/genitourinary/urinary_tract_infection__complicated__uti_.html. Accessed November 23, 2009.

89. Rhoads J, Clayman A, Nelson S. The relationship of urinary tract infections and falls in a nursing home. Director 2007;15(1):22–6.

90. Eriksson S, Strandberg S, Gustafson Y, et al. Circumstances surrounding falls in patients with dementia in a psychogeriatric ward. Arch Gerontol Geriatr 2009; 49(1):80–7.

91. Stott DJ, Falconer A, Miller H, et al. Urinary tract infection after stroke. QJM 2009;102(4):243–9.

92. Sims JB, de Lemos JA, Maewal P, et al. Urinary tract infection in patients with acute coronary syndrome: a potential systemic inflammatory connection. Am Heart J 2005;149(6):1062–5.

93. Rodhe N, Molstad S, Englund L, et al. Asymptomatic bacteriuria in a population of elderly residents living in a community setting: prevalence, characteristics and associated factors. Fam Pract 2006;23(3):303–7.

94. Juthani-Mehta M, Quagliarello V, Perrelli E, et al. Clinical features to identify urinary tract infection in nursing home residents: a cohort study. J Am Geriatr Soc 2009;57(6):963–70.

95. Gau JT, Shibeshi MR, Lu IJ, et al. Interexpert agreement on diagnosis of bacteriuria and urinary tract infection in hospitalized older adults. J Am Osteopath Assoc 2009;109(4):220–6.

96. Rogers MA, Fries BE, Kaufman SR, et al. Mobility and other predictors of hospitalization for urinary tract infection: a retrospective cohort study. BMC Geriatr 2008;8:31.

97. McMurdo ME, Argo I, Phillips G, et al. Cranberry or trimethoprim for the prevention of recurrent urinary tract infections? A randomized controlled trial in older women. J Antimicrob Chemother 2009;63(2):389–95.

98. Gokula RR, Hickner JA, Smith MA. Inappropriate use of urinary catheters in elderly patients at a midwestern community teaching hospital. Am J Infect Control 2004;32(4):196–9.

99. Grover ML, Bracamonte JD, Kanodia AK, et al. Urinary tract infection in women over the age of 65: is age alone a marker of complication? J Am Board Fam Med 2009;22(3):266–71.

100. Lutters M, Vogt-Ferrier NB. Antibiotic duration for treating uncomplicated, symptomatic lower urinary tract infections in elderly women. Cochrane Database Syst Rev 2008;3:CD001535.

101. Harding GK, Zhanel GG, Nicolle LE, et al. Antimicrobial treatment in diabetic women with asymptomatic bacteriuria. N Engl J Med 2002;347:1576.

102. Nicolle LE, Zhanel GG, Harding GK. Microbiological outcomes in women with diabetes and untreated asymptomatic bacteriuria. World J Urol 2006;24(1): 61–5.

103. Jackson SL, Boyko EJ, Scholes D, et al. Predictors of urinary tract infection after menopause: a prospective study. Am J Med 2004;117(12):903–11.
104. Hoepelman AI, Meiland R, Geerlings SE. Pathogenesis and management of bacterial urinary tract infections in adult patients with diabetes mellitus. Int J Antimicrob Agents 2003;22(Suppl 2):35–43.
105. Schneeberger C, Stolk RP, Devries JH, et al. Differences in the pattern of antibiotic prescription profile and recurrence rate for possible urinary tract infections in women with and without diabetes. Diabetes Care 2008;31(7):1380–5.

Sexually Transmitted Infections in Men

John R. Brill, MD, MPH

KEYWORDS

- Sexually transmitted infection • Gonorrhea
- Chlamydia • Urethritis • Herpes

A wide variety of bacterial, viral, and ectoparasitic infections are spread through sexual contact. The Centers for Disease Control and Prevention (CDC) estimates that in the United States 19 million new sexually transmitted infections (STIs) are acquired each year, costing $14.7 billion, and half of these are in persons 15 to 24 years old.[1,2] STIs are a major cause of morbidity including systemic and reproductive complications, a major cause of mortality in young people, and a leading cause of quality-adjusted life years lost.[1] Although STIs exist in every demographic, clinicians working with urban underserved populations need to be particularly vigilant. Nearly all STIs disproportionately strike minority populations, and there are particular concentrations of gonorrhea and syphilis in cities. Primary care clinicians frequently are the point of first contact for men with STIs, given the highly variable manifestations of these disorders. Primary care clinicians are also ideally suited for establishing rapport and confidence, obtaining a thorough history of sexual exposures, seeking examination and laboratory findings to corroborate the history, and appropriately treating for the most likely infections.

STI EVALUATION

The STI evaluation requires sensitivity, trust, alertness to co-infections, and an understanding of local epidemiology. A thorough sexual history should be obtained as shown in **Box 1**. Clinicians should recognize that some persons may be unwilling to fully disclose these sensitive items.

The examination should include all sites of sexual exposure, noting the patient's general condition and presence of any rashes. Clinicians should examine the genital area for inguinal adenopathy and pubic hair infestations. The penis should be inspected for lesions and the urethra gently milked to express discharge. The urethral meatus may be exposed by placing fingers on either side to identify occult discharge, erythema, or ulcers. Any discharge seen should be collected for gonorrhea and

No external funding.
Department of Family Medicine, University of Wisconsin School of Medicine and Public Health, Milwaukee Academic Campus, 2801 West Kinnickinnic Parkway #250, Milwaukee, WI 53215, USA
E-mail address: john.brill.md@aurora.org

Prim Care Clin Office Pract 37 (2010) 509–525
doi:10.1016/j.pop.2010.04.003
0095-4543/10/$ – see front matter © 2010 Published by Elsevier Inc. **primarycare.theclinics.com**

Box 1
Elements of a sexual history

Symptom duration, frequency, severity

Associated symptoms, including fever, weight loss, malaise, rash

History of STIs

Prior treatments or home remedies used

Gender of sexual partner(s)

Sites of exposure, including whether receptive or insertive, at each site

Frequency of condom use

History of having sex under the influence of alcohol or drugs

From French P. BASHH 2006 National Guidelines—consultations requiring sexual history taking. Int J STD AIDS 18(1):17–22, 2007; Jeffries 4th WL. Sociodemographic, sexual, and HIV and other sexually transmitted disease risk profiles of nonhomosexual-identified men who have sex with men. Am J Public Health 2009;99(6):1042–5.

---

chlamydia testing. Ulcers present may be swabbed for herpes simplex virus testing and dark field examination for syphilis, if available. The scrotum should be elevated to expose the perineal area. Each testis and epididymal region should be palpated for tenderness or swelling. If sexually exposed or symptomatic, the anus should be inspected and samples for gonorrhea and chlamydia collected. The oropharynx should be examined for exudates, and a sample for gonorrhea collected if sexually exposed or symptomatic.

URETHRITIS

Men with an STI most commonly present with symptoms of urethral inflammation, including discharge, dysuria, or urethral itching or tingling. Urethritis can be caused by STIs as well as noninfectious irritants. In most cases, no organism is definitively identified.

A man with any one of the following findings can be diagnosed with urethritis: mucopurulent penile discharge, a positive leukocyte esterase test on first-void urine, or at least 10 white blood cells (WBCs) per high-power field on microscopy of a first-void urine sediment.[3] For men with symptoms of urethral irritation but lacking these diagnostic criteria, treatment should generally be reserved until test results are available. Exceptions include high-risk patients whose return seems doubtful.

Urethritis has traditionally been classified as gonococcal or nongonococcal urethritis (NGU); however, the replacement of Gram stain testing of urethral discharge with combined laboratory testing for both gonococcal and chlamydial infections makes this distinction less important. In addition, about 20% of men with gonococcal urethritis are also co-infected with *Chlamydia* or another organism.[4]

Neisseria gonorrhoeae infects an estimated 700,000 US residents each year.[5] Gonococcal urethritis tends to present with a more copious and purulent discharge than NGU,[4] and asymptomatic infections are unusual in men. In the United States, gonorrhea is heavily concentrated in urban areas. African American male adolescents have a 40 times higher incidence than white male adolescents.[6] Appropriate treatment can relieve symptoms, prevent complications such as prostatitis and epididymitis, reduce subsequent infertility, decrease transmission of other STIs, and prevent pelvic inflammatory disease (PID) and its sequelae in female partners.[7]

Chlamydia trachomatis is the most common pathogen identified in NGU. The CDC estimates that there are 3 cases of chlamydia for every case of gonorrhea in the United States.[8] In contrast to gonorrhea, up to 90% of chlamydia infections in men are asymptomatic. A recent large study found a slight increase in prostatitis and a fourfold risk of epididymitis following chlamydial infection, but no increase in subsequent male infertility.[9] Again, a major goal of chlamydia treatment in men is to prevent PID in female partners.

Diagnosis of both gonorrhea and chlamydia is now primarily by nucleic acid amplification tests (NAATs). NAATs offer some advantages over culture, including higher sensitivity (up to 97%), equal specificity (99%), noninvasive collection (urine), and a single test for both organisms.[10] Recent literature has demonstrated the potential effectiveness of rapid NAAT testing and patient-collected specimens for more immediate and convenient diagnosis.[11,12]

Extragenital chlamydial and gonococcal infections are usually asymptomatic. Because of this, the CDC has recommended periodic screening for asymptomatic men who have sex with men (MSM) and for high-risk individuals, as shown in **Box 2**. Although NAATs are far more sensitive than culture, the Food and Drug Administration (FDA) has not approved them for rectal or pharyngeal diagnosis.[13]

Mycoplasma genitalium is becoming increasingly recognized as a cause of NGU.[14] In men, an infection with this atypical bacterium may be more symptomatic than an infection with chlamydia.[15] Diagnostic tests for *Mycoplasma* and the related *Ureaplasma* species are not readily available at this time, but DNA assays with up to 97% sensitivity have been developed.[16] To date, evidence is lacking that these organisms cause long-term complications.[17]

Several other infectious agents can cause NGU. Trichomonas should be suspected in endemic areas, in patients with purulent discharge, and when usual treatments have failed.[18] Adenovirus and herpes simplex virus have been associated with insertive oral sex in MSM.[19] Enteric bacteria have been linked to insertive anal sex.[3]

Unless test results are available when urethritis is diagnosed, antibiotics to treat both chlamydia and gonorrhea should be prescribed. A management algorithm and recommended regimens are shown in **Fig. 1**. Evaluation for other STIs is strongly recommended.[20]

For *Chlamydia urethritis*, the enhanced compliance of single-dose azithromycin makes it generally preferred to doxycycline, unless cost concerns predominate.[21]

Box 2
CDC recommended annual screenings for men who have sex with men

Do a urethral swab or urine DNA test for gonorrhea and chlamydia in men who have had insertive intercourse during the preceding year;

Test for rectal infection with gonorrhea and chlamydia in men who have had receptive anal intercourse during the preceding year;

Do a DNA swab or culture for pharyngeal infection with gonorrhea in men who have had receptive oral intercourse during the preceding year; testing for oropharyngeal chlamydia infection is not recommended

From Centers for Disease Control and Prevention. Sexually transmitted disease treatment guideline 2006. Available at: http://www.cdc.gov/std/treatment/2006/specialpops. htm#specialpops4. Accessed September 30, 2009.

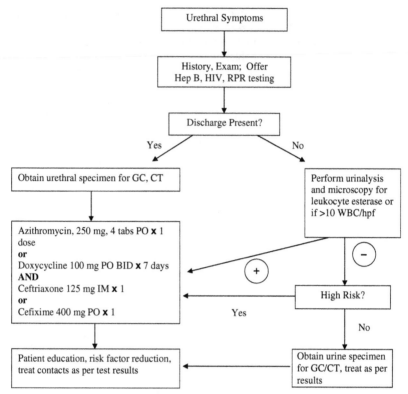

Fig. 1. Management of men with urethral symptoms.

Azithromycin is also the treatment of choice for both *Mycoplasma* and *Ureaplasma* species,[22] and results in symptom clearance for most men whose tests are negative for all known pathogens.[23] Increasing gonorrheal resistance to fluoroquinolones means ciprofloxacin and ofloxacin are no longer recommended for empiric treatment. If a fluoroquinolone is inadvertently used,[24] it may be effective, but a test of cure would be recommended. Extragenital gonorrhea and chlamydia infections are treated the same as genital infections, except that cefixime is not recommended for oropharyngeal gonorrhea. Men presenting with urethritis should be educated regarding medication instructions, testing for other STIs, risk factor reduction, and partner notification, as shown in **Box 3**.

GENITAL ULCERS

Several STIs may present with genital ulceration, with herpes and syphilis being the most common in the United States. However, a variety of other infectious and noninfectious etiologies for genital ulcers exist, and in some cases patients may have multiple co-infections.[25] The history and examination are frequently inaccurate, so all patients with genital ulcers should be offered syphilis and herpes testing. See **Table 1** for additional information about infections that can cause genital ulcers.

Herpes simplex virus (HSV) infections are widespread in the United States, with an estimated 50 million persons having herpes genital infections, most of whom are undiagnosed.[26] Women with new-onset herpes most commonly complain of genital pain,

---

Box 3
Patient education for urethritis

Avoid sex for 1 week after starting the antibiotics and until after your sexual partners have been treated.

Finish all your pills, even if you feel okay, unless your doctor tells you to stop.

If no infection is found, your doctor may advise you to avoid other things that can cause irritation of the urethra:

Spicy foods

Perfumed soaps, body washes, lotions, or lubricants

Caffeinated beverages (coffee, soda)

Overly vigorous or frequent masturbation or intercourse

Your doctor will advise you to drink enough water so that your urine is clear most of the time.

If your symptoms do not improve within 1 week after finishing treatment, please contact your doctor.

Safer sex practices may be advised to help prevent urethritis. These include

Using condoms correctly with sex every time,

Not exchanging money or drugs for sex,

Not having sex after drinking alcohol or taking drugs, and

Limiting the number of your sex partners.

From Centers for Disease Control and Prevention. Sexually transmitted disease treatment guideline 2006. Available at: http://www.cdc.gov/STD/treatment/2006/urethritis-and-cervicitis.htm. Accessed October 30, 2009.

---

whereas men more commonly complain of lesions.[27] However, most already suspect they have herpes. HSV infection can be diagnosed clinically, by direct testing of lesions, or by serology. Clinical diagnosis, however, is frequently incorrect, largely because of atypical presentations.[28] Previously HSV-1 was linked to oral lesions and HSV-2 to genital lesions, but the incidence of new HSV-1 genital infections has surpassed that of HSV-2.[26] HSV-1 causes fewer and less severe genital recurrences than HSV-2.

The CDC suggests confirmatory testing and typing, given the diagnostic pitfalls and difference in prognosis between the 2 types.[26] This can be done either by culture or by polymerase chain reaction (PCR). Both methods require viral shedding, which declines during recurrent outbreaks and with increased duration of an outbreak. Most published literature suggests that culture remains the recommended method for diagnosis in the United States[29]; however, most commercial laboratories prefer PCR, because it is at least 3 times more sensitive than culture[30] and less labor intensive (Dr Stephanie Koplin, Aurora Health Care laboratories, personal communication, 2009). PCR is not yet FDA approved for cutaneous lesions.

When lesions are not present, antibody tests can be used to look for evidence of herpes infection. Serologic tests for antibodies to HSV-1 do not distinguish between a new HSV-1 genital infection and a previously acquired oral infection.[31] HSV-2 appears to be always genitally acquired, and new point-of-care tests have been developed for this type, with sensitivity of 80% to 98% (rising with time since infection) and specificity of greater than 95%.[32] HSV-2 testing may be helpful in those with other STIs and for those exposed to genital herpes so patients can be counseled about

Table 1
Disorders causing genital ulcers

Disorder	Etiology	Distinguishing Features	Diagnosis and Management
Syphilis	Treponema pallidum	Painless, usually solitary.	Dark field microscopy if available, RPR/VDRL; bicillin 2.4 million units IM
HSV	Herpes Simplex Virus types 1 or 2	Painful, usually multiple, last¯ 10 days.	Consider viral culture or PCR, see Table 2
Chancroid	Haemophilus ducreyi	Painful genital ulcer and tender suppurative inguinal adenopathy	No commercially available test. Azithromycin 1 g orally × 1 OR Ceftriaxone 250 mg IM × 1 OR Ciprofloxacin 500 mg orally twice a day for 3 days
Donovaniasis (not endemic to the United States)	Klebsiella granulomatis	Painless, progressive beefy-red, ulcerative lesions, no lymphadenopathy.	Donovan bodies on tissue biopsy. Doxycycline 100 mg orally twice a day for at least 3 weeks and until all lesions have healed
Lymphogranuleum venereum (LGV)	Chlamydia trachomatis serovars L1, L2, or L3	Transient ulcer, tender inguinal lymphadenopathy, typically unilateral	CT culture, PCR[a] Doxycycline 100 mg orally twice a day for 21 days
Bite wound	Human mouth flora	Can be deep, painful	Amoxicillin-clavulanic acid
Neurodermatitis, irritant, chemical	Noninfectious	Recurrent, negative evaluation	Antipruritics, Eliminate offending agent, psychological therapy

Abbreviations: CT, chlamydia trachomatis; IM, intramuscularly; VDRL, Venereal Disease Research Laboratory; RPR, rapid plasma reagin.
[a] PCR is not FDA approved for skin lesions and does not distinguish serovars.
Data from Refs.[78–80]

ways to decrease transmission.[33] Unfortunately, evidence of protective behavioral change after diagnosis of HSV-2 is lacking.[34]

When HSV is diagnosed, education should focus on treatment options and reduction of transmission. Patients with a new diagnosis of HSV infection frequently experience significant morbidity, loss of functioning, and anxiety.[35] Antiviral agents can be used episodically or daily, as shown in **Table 2**. Both strategies benefit patient quality of life. Episodic treatment, begun at the first sign of recurrence, can speed ulcer healing and decrease symptom severity.[31] Daily suppressive therapy has a greater impact on measures of disease frequency and burden, but with increased cost.[36] Factors favoring daily suppressive antiviral therapy in men are primary infection within the past year, history of frequent outbreaks, HIV positivity, and presence of HSV Type 2.[31] Because HSV-2 has been demonstrated to shed frequently, for short intervals, and without symptoms,[37] suppressive antiviral treatment may reduce transmission more than episodic treatment, but neither is infallible. A recent expert review suggests the use of once-daily suppressive therapy with valacyclovir for the first year after diagnosis.[38–40] A meta-analysis found this regimen had a relative risk for recurrent outbreak of 0.53, with the number needed to treat (NNT) of 2.15 patients to prevent 1 outbreak annually.[41]

For patients infected with both HSV-2 and HIV, HSV suppressive therapy reduces HIV expression by up to 55%, particularly in those whose CD4 counts are higher than 500.[36] Unfortunately, suppressive therapy has not been shown to decrease acquisition of HIV in HSV-2 positive patients.[41]

Consistent condom use reduces HSV transmission by 30%.[42] In one recent study in Uganda, adult circumcision reduced the rate of seroconversion to HSV-2 positivity by 25% over a 2-year period.[43] Ultimately, however, we currently have no way to cure genital HSV, nor any fail-safe means of preventing transmission among sexual partners.

Table 2
Antiviral treatment for genital herpes simplex virus

Agent	First Outbreak Regimens	Episodic Treatment	Suppressive Therapy; Cost/Month	Notes
Acyclovir	400 mg orally 3 times a day for 7–10 days OR 200 mg orally 5 times a day for 7–10 days	400 mg orally 3 times a day for 5 days OR 800 mg orally twice a day for 5 days OR 800 mg orally 3 times a day for 2 days	400 mg orally 2 to 3 times a day; $115.80 (generic), $251.40 (Zovirax)	Topical therapy not recommended.
Famcyclovir	250 mg orally 3 times a day for 7–10 days	125 mg orally twice daily for 5 days OR 1000 mg orally twice daily for 1 day	250 mg orally twice a day; $318.00 (Famvir)	
Valacyclovir	1 g orally twice a day for 7–10 days	500 mg orally twice a day for 3 days OR 1.0 g orally once a day for 5 days	500 mg to 1.0 g orally once a day; $177.00 (Valtrex)	

Data from Drugs for non-HIV viral infections. Treat Guidel Med Lett 2007;59:59–70.

Syphilis is a highly infectious STI caused by the spirochete *Treponema pallidum*. The disease is characterized by stages, with little change in classification over the past century. The primary stage is marked by development of a painless ulcer, the chancre, at the site of sexual exposure. The chancre usually develops 2 to 3 weeks after contact (range 9–90 days) and will spontaneously resolve in 5 to 6 weeks (range 3–10 weeks), whereupon one-third of untreated patients will develop secondary syphilis.[44] This stage is marked by changes in mucous membranes, hair, and skin, including the classic symmetric maculopapular rash on palms and soles, as well as systemic symptoms, such as fever, lymphadenopathy, and malaise. Untreated, the disease can remain latent for years, progressing in about 15% of patients to tertiary syphilis, and causing severe damage to numerous systems, including brain, nerves, eyes, heart, and joints.

In the United States, approximately 100,000 cases of primary and secondary syphilis are diagnosed each year; however, this is less than 1% of the estimated 12 million new cases worldwide.[45] Syphilis is most prevalent among men, MSM, ethnic minorities, and regionally in the coastal and southeast areas of the United States. It is reported 7 times more frequently in African Americans than whites.[46] A strong association exists between syphilis and HIV, with each conferring a three- to fivefold increased risk of discovering the other.[47]

Diagnosis of syphilis in the primary care setting is generally serologic, using a screening nontreponemal assay Venereal Disease Research Laboratory, rapid plasma reagin (VDRL, RPR) followed by a confirmatory treponemal pallidum hemagglutination test, fluorescent treponemal antibody-absorption (TPHA, FTA-Abs). All assays may be negative in the early days of primary syphilis, so suspicious lesions should be treated presumptively, and serology followed over time.[45]

Treatment of syphilis is designed to relieve symptoms, halt progression to tertiary stages, decrease transmission of other STIs, and prevent perinatal transmission. Penicillin is curative for early syphilis, and *Treponema pallidum* has remained remarkably sensitive to the antibiotic. Patients whose syphilis is known to be acquired in the past year can be treated with a single dose of 2.4 million units of benzathine penicillin; those whose infection is of longer or unknown duration require 3 doses 1 week apart. A fourfold drop in the RPR or VRDL titer is considered evidence of adequate treatment.[48]

MALE ACCESSORY GLAND INFECTIONS

Male accessory gland infections (MAGIs) affect the prostate, epididymis, seminal vesicles, and ductus deferens. Sexually acquired MAGIs are generally caused by the same organisms as urethritis, and laboratory studies should be obtained as for urethritis. Depending on the severity of the illness, complete blood count (CBC) and blood cultures may be useful.[49]

PROCTITIS

Proctitis may be caused by STIs, autoimmune disorders, radiation treatment, irritants or chemicals, or nonsexually acquired infections. Proctitis manifests as rectal bleeding (73%), pain (62%), discharge (58%), and blood in the stool (54%).[50] Gonorrhea, chlamydia, herpes, *Trichomonas vaginalis, Mycoplasma genitalium*, and syphilis can cause proctitis; mixed infections are common, and frequently the cause is not identified.[51] Over the past decade, lymphogranuloma venereum (LGV), caused by certain *Chlamydia trachomatis* serovars, has reemerged as a cause of proctitis, particularly in MSM who are HIV positive.[52] Empiric treatment with doxycycline and ceftriaxone generally leads to rapid improvement.[50]

Table 3
Treatment options for genital warts

Treatment	Mechanism	How Administered; Efficacy	Advantages	Disadvantages
No treatment	Natural immunity	N/A; 0%–50%. Smoking cessation enhances cure.	Low cost; high incidence of spontaneous resolution	Anxiety, embarrassment, negative effect on relationships
Imiquimod 5% cream (Aldara)	Immunomodulator	Patient applied to lesions 3 times per week for up to 16 weeks; 37%–54% cure, woman cured > men.	No systemic effects, may decrease future recurrence	Mild local irritation, cost
Podophyllotoxin (Podophyllin 0.5% gel or cream)	Antimitotic agent	Patient applied twice a day × 3 days, then 4 days off, repeat cycle up to 4 weeks; 45%–77% cure	No systemic effects	Local inflammation
Sinecatechin 15% ointment (Veregen)	Green tea extract; mechanism not clearly elucidated	Patient applied 3 times per day for up to 16 weeks ; 54%–65% cure, women cured > men	May decrease future recurrence	Local irritation, cost, 3 x/day application
Cryotherapy with liquid nitrogen	Destroys affected tissues	Provider applied × 1, repeat every 1–2 weeks as necessary; 71%–79% cure	Inexpensive; works best for discrete lesions. May be used on mucous membranes	Painful, limited use for multiple or diffuse lesions
Surgical excision	Direct removal	Provider; 35%–72% cure	Inexpensive; works best for discrete lesions	Requires local anesthetic; scarring possible
Electrodessication	Destroys affected tissues	Provider applied, 57%–94% cure	Inexpensive; works best for large warts	Requires local anesthetic; scarring possible
CO_2 laser	Destroys affected tissues	Provider applied, 82%–100% cure	Useful for intra urethral warts	Cost, requires local anesthetic; scarring possible. Laser plume may spread HPV.
Podophyllin 10%–25%	Antimitotic agent	Provider applied; 20%–77% success	Inexpensive	External lesions only; serious systemic effects reported after mucosal use.
Trichloroacetic acid, Bichloroacetic acid	Destroys affected tissues	Provider applied 3 times per week for up to 4 weeks; 63%–70% cure	Inexpensive product	Pain, ulceration; can be difficult to limit application to wart only
Interferon	Immunomodulator	Intralesional or interlesional injection; 34%–52% cure	Can be used as adjuvant or second-line agent for refractory cases	Painful; flu-like symptoms; cost

Data from Refs.[54,81–83]

Table 4
US Preventive Services Task Force screening recommendations for STIs

Disease	Recommendation	Screening Method	Rationale
Chlamydia	Screen all sexually active nonpregnant young women aged 24 and younger (A), older nonpregnant women at increased risk (A), all pregnant women aged 24 and younger (B), and older pregnant women who are at increased risk (B). Evidence insufficient to recommend screening for men (I).	Blood or cervical or urethral chlamydia fluid by Nucleic Acid Amplification Test	CT is common and has significant morbidity for women, especially during pregnancy. There is little evidence that screening men prevents morbidity. Low-risk patients may be harmed by false-positive tests.
Gonorrhea	Screen all sexually active women at increased risk (B). Insufficient evidence to recommend screening low-risk pregnant women or high-risk men (I). Do not screen men or nonpregnant lower risk women (D).	Blood or cervical or urethral fluid by Nucleic Acid Amplification Test	Women with asymptomatic GC have high morbidity, especially during pregnancy; however, it is less common than CT. Men are usually symptomatic. Low-risk patients may be harmed by false-positive tests.
Hepatitis B virus	Screen pregnant women at their first prenatal visit (A). Do not screen others (D).	Blood for HBsAg	Universal prenatal screening substantially reduces prenatal transmission. Low prevalence and high spontaneous resolution limit general benefit.

Human immunodeficiency virus (HIV)	Blood, ELISA + Western blot	Screen pregnant women, and all adolescents and adults at increased risk (A). No recommendation either for or against screening of lower-risk persons (C).	Universal prenatal screening substantially reduces prenatal transmission. Screening and early intervention lead to improved health. Although false positives are rare, low prevalence and potential harms of screening limit general benefit.
Syphilis	Blood, RPR or VDRL + treponemal test	Screen all pregnant women and persons at increased risk (A). Do not screen others (D).	Universal screening of pregnant women decreases congenital syphilis. Screening tests can accurately detect syphilis, which is easily cured. Low prevalence and potential harms of screening preclude general use.
Herpes Simplex Virus	Serology	Do not screen pregnant women (D) or other asymptomatic persons (D).	Screening asymptomatic pregnant women does not reduce transmission to newborns. Screening others can identify exposed persons but there is no evidence of improved outcomes.

Abbreviations: ELISA, enzyme-linked immunosorbent assay; HBsAg, hepatitis B surface antigen; RPR, rapid plasma reagin, VDRL; Veneral Disease Research Laboratory.
Data from US Preventive Services Task Force. Clinical recommendations. Available at: http://www.ahrq.gov/CLINIC/uspstfix.htm#Recommendations. Accessed November 13, 2009.

GENITAL PAPULES

The most common STIs presenting as genital papules are genital warts and molluscum contagiosum. Genital warts are caused by the human papilloma virus (HPV). Genital warts must be distinguished from variants of normal anatomy such as pearly penile papules,[53] other infections (such as molluscum, or the accuminata lata lesions of syphilis), and premalignant and malignant lesions including Bowenoid papulosis and squamous cell cancer.[54] It is estimated that more than $200 million per year is spent on genital warts in the United States.[55] An estimated 5.6% of sexually active US adults between the ages of 18 and 59 years have been diagnosed by a medical provider with genital warts.[56] A recent study of 240 heterosexually active male US college students demonstrated a cumulative incidence of new infection of any genital HPV type of 62.4% over a 24-month period.[57] Risk factors significantly associated with HPV colonization include smoking and a higher lifetime number of female sex partners.[58]

Treatment of genital warts in men is primarily geared toward removal of the lesions themselves, because treatment has not been shown to decrease recurrence, decrease the development of cervical cancer in female partners, or prevent perinatal transmission.[54] Treatment options are shown in **Table 3**. In general, patient-applied therapies have become preferred.[54] Although no randomized trials have been conducted, clinicians should discuss anal Pap smear for dysplastic changes in patients who receive anal intercourse, especially if they are HIV positive.[59]

Molluscum contagiosum in adults is primarily sexually acquired. The viral infection is recognized clinically by painless, flesh-colored, centrally umbilicated papules. Although self-limited, spontaneous resolution may take months to years. Treatment options are similar to those of warts, although most methods are more successful with molluscum.[60] A recent clinical inquiry found no treatment to be specifically favored, but verified high success and satisfaction rates with the patient-applied therapies.[61]

ECTOPARASITES

Ectoparasitic infections, including scabies and pubic lice, typically present with itching and excoriation. A hypersensitivity rash, or pediculid, may mimic a viral exanthem.[62] These infestations are often seen as co-infections with other STIs, and are more frequent in MSM.[63] Primary treatment is topically administered 1% permethrin, with malathion used for treatment failures. Treatment of intimate contacts and environmental decontamination measures can help to prevent recurrence.[64]

BLOOD-BORNE STIS

Hepatitis B and HIV are chronic viral infections that in the United States are chiefly acquired through sexual contact. These infections are diagnosed primarily through laboratory identification of asymptomatic persons. Sexual transmission of hepatitis C is rare, but can occur when a genital ulcer from another STI makes blood contact more likely.

Worldwide, about 360 million people are chronically infected with the hepatitis B virus (HBV).[65] Over the past 2 decades, the United States has seen significant declines in hepatitis B, with incidence falling 81% to the lowest rate ever recorded (1.6 cases per 100,000 population in 2006). This success seems primarily attributable to childhood immunization, as rates declined the greatest amount for children younger than 15 years.[66] Nonetheless, the Hepatitis B Foundation estimates that 1 in 20 Americans has been infected with HBV, and 1 million are chronically infected.[67] Those at greatest risk for HBV positivity are those with multiple heterosexual partners (39%), MSM (24%), the foreign born,[68] and injection drug users.

HBV is most commonly diagnosed by laboratory studies in the subclinical state (70%), with elevations of transaminases (alanine aminotransferase [ALT] > aspartate aminotransferase [AST]), confirmed by HBV serology. Most symptomatic patients present with jaundice, nausea, weight loss, or right upper quadrant pain. Fortunately, progression of HBV to hepatic failure or hepatocellular cancer is unusual for sexually acquired infections; more than 95% of HBV thus acquired will spontaneously resolve.[69] Persistent elevation of serum ALT for more than 6 months indicates progression to chronic hepatitis.[70]

Antiviral treatment should be considered for all patients diagnosed with chronic HBV.[71] High viral load seems to be the best indicator of developing cirrhosis or hepatocellular carcinoma,[72] with risk beginning at 300 copies/mL. An international guideline recommends a threshold of 2000 copies/mL for initiating therapy.[73]

Primary care physicians have been involved in the care of HIV-infected patients for the past 3 decades. Although screening recommendations differ, there is a consensus that all persons with another STI and all pregnant women should be screened.[74] Primary care physicians should also be familiar with recommendations for occupational or sexual exposure.[75] Vigilance should be maintained for the acute retroviral syndrome that occurs in the first few weeks of HIV infection, before antibody test results become positive. Symptoms include fever, malaise, lymphadenopathy, and skin rash. Such patients can be highly contagious and should be advised to stop risky behaviors.[76]

Although a full discussion of HIV treatment is beyond the scope of this article, the following 4 general principles apply[77]:

1. Appropriate combination treatment with highly active antiretroviral therapy (HAART), prolongs health and extends life.
2. Specific medications are selected based on resistance testing.
3. Therapy is lifelong.
4. Cost, drug interactions, side effects, and pill burden can be problematic.

SCREENING FOR STIS

The US Preventive Services Task Force primarily recommends screening for STIs in high-risk persons, young women, and at the first prenatal visit. Specific recommendations are shown in **Table 4**.

REFERENCES

1. CDC. Trends in reportable sexually transmitted diseases in the United States, 2007. Atlanta (GA): U.S. Department of Health and Human Services; 2008. Available at: http://www.cdc.gov/std/stats07/trends.htm. Accessed October 11, 2010.
2. Chesson HW, Blandford JM, Gift TL, et al. The estimated direct medical cost of sexually transmitted diseases among American youth, 2000. Perspect Sex Reprod Health 2004;36(1):11–9.
3. Centers for Disease Control and Prevention. Sexually transmitted disease treatment guideline 2006. Available at: http://www.cdc.gov/STD/treatment/2006/urethritis-and-cervicitis.htm. Accessed October 30, 2009.
4. Shahmanesh M, Moi H, Lassau F, et al. 2009 European Guideline on the Management of Male Non-gonococcal Urethritis. Int J STD AIDS 2009;20:458–64.

5. Centers for Disease Control and Prevention. Gonorrhea fact sheet. Available at: http://www.cdc.gov/std/gonorrhea/stdfact-gonorrhea.htm. Accessed October 11, 2010.

6. Centers for Disease Control and Prevention. Sexually Transmitted Disease Surveillance. Table 21b Gonorrhea — Rates per 100,000 population by race/ethnicity, age group and sex: United States, 2004–2008. Available at: http://www.cdc.gov/std/stats08/tables/21b.htm. Accessed February 14, 2010.

7. Vickerman P, Peeling RW, Watts C, et al. Detection of gonococcal infection: pros and cons of a rapid test. Mol Diagn 2005;9(4):175–9.

8. Centers for Disease Control and Prevention, Division of STD Prevention. Sexually transmitted diseases in the United States, 2008 National Surveillance Data for Chlamydia, Gonorrhea, and Syphilis. Available at: http://www.cdc.gov/std/stats08/trends.htm. Accessed February 14, 2010.

9. Trei JS, Canas LC, Gould PL. Reproductive tract complications associated with *Chlamydia trachomatis* infection in US Air Force males within 4 years of testing. Sex Transm Dis 2008;35(9):827–33.

10. Gaydos CA, Ferrero DV, Papp J. Laboratory aspects of screening men for *Chlamydia trachomatis* in the new millennium. Sex Transm Dis 2008;35(11 Suppl): S45–50.

11. van der Helm JJ, Hoebe CJ, van Rooijen MS, et al. High performance and acceptability of self-collected rectal swabs for diagnosis of *Chlamydia trachomatis* and *Neisseria gonorrhoeae* in men who have sex with men and women. Sex Transm Dis 2009;36(8):493–7.

12. Nadala EC, Goh BT, Magbanua JP, et al. Performance evaluation of a new rapid urine test for chlamydia in men: prospective cohort study. BMJ 2009;339:b2655.

13. Renault CA, Hall C, Kent CK. Use of NAATs for STD diagnosis of GC and CT in non-FDA-cleared anatomic specimens. MLO Med Lab Obs 2006;38(7):10–24.

14. Totten PA, Schwartz MA, Sjostrom KE, et al. Association of *Mycoplasma genitalium* with nongonococcal urethritis in heterosexual men. J Infect Dis 2003; 187(9):1506.

15. Moi H, Reinton N, Moghaddam A. Mycoplasma genitalium is associated with symptomatic and asymptomatic non-gonococcal urethritis in men. Sex Transm Infect 2009;85(1):15–8.

16. Edberg A, Jurstrand M, Johansson E, et al. A comparative study of three different PCR assays for detection of *Mycoplasma genitalium* in urogenital specimens from men and women. J Med Microbiol 2008;57:304–9.

17. Short VL, Totten PA, Ness RB, et al. Clinical presentation of *Mycoplasma genitalium* infection versus *Neisseria gonorrhoeae* infection among women with pelvic inflammatory disease. Clin Infect Dis 2009;48(1):41–7.

18. Schwebke JR, Hook EW III. High rates of *Trichomonas vaginalis* among men attending a sexually transmitted diseases clinic: implications for screening and urethritis management. J Infect Dis 2003;188:465–8.

19. Bradshaw CS, Tabrizi SN, Read TR, et al. Etiologies of nongonococcal urethritis: bacteria, viruses, and the association with orogenital exposure. J Infect Dis 2006; 193:336.

20. Patel M, Corboy JE, Hitchcock K, et al. Clinical inquiries. What other STI testing should we do for a patient with chlamydia? J Fam Pract 2007;56(1):64–6.

21. Campos-Outcalt D. Sexually transmitted disease: easier screening tests, single-dose therapies. J Fam Pract 2003;52(12):965–9.

22. Jernberg E, Moghaddam A, Moi H. Azithromycin and moxifloxacin for microbiological cure of *Mycoplasma genitalium* infection: an open study. Int J STD AIDS 2008;19:676–9.

23. Maeda S, Yasuda M, Ito S, et al. Azithromycin treatment for nongonococcal urethritis negative for *Chlamydia trachomatis, Mycoplasma genitalium, Mycoplasma hominis, Ureaplasma parvum*, and *Ureaplasma urealyticum*. Int J Urol 2009;16(2):215–6.

24. Centers for Disease Control and Prevention (CDC). Update to CDC's sexually transmitted diseases treatment guidelines, 2006: fluoroquinolones no longer recommended for treatment of gonococcal infections. MMWR Morb Mortal Wkly Rep 2007;56(14):332–6.

25. Samuel M, Aderogba K, Dutt N, et al. A hat trick of ulcerating pathogens in a single genital lesion. Int J STD AIDS 2007;18(1):65–6.

26. Centers for Disease Control and Prevention. Sexually transmitted disease treatment guideline 2006. Available at: http://www.cdc.gov/std/treatment/2006/genital-ulcers.htm#genulc3. Accessed October 30, 2009.

27. Richards J, Krantz E, Selke S, et al. Healthcare seeking and sexual behavior among patients with symptomatic newly acquired genital herpes. Sex Transm Dis 2008;35(12):1015–21.

28. Sen P, Barton SE. Genital herpes and its management. BMJ 2007;334(7602): 1048–52.

29. Sullivan M, Sams R, Jamieson B, et al. Clinical inquiries. What is the best test to detect herpes in skin lesions? J Fam Pract 2006;55(4):346–8.

30. Strick LB, Wald A. Diagnostics for herpes simplex virus: is PCR the new gold standard? Mol Diagn Ther 2006;10(1):17–28.

31. Clinical Effectiveness Group. 2007 national guideline for the management of genital herpes. London (UK): British Association for Sexual Health and HIV (BASHH) 2007. Available at: http://www.guideline.gov. Accessed October 30, 2009.

32. Philip SS, Ahrens K, Shayevich C, et al. Evaluation of a new point-of-care serologic assay for herpes simplex virus type 2 infection. Clin Infect Dis 2008; 47(10):e79–82.

33. Heintzman J, Rugge B, Judkins DZ, et al. Clinical inquiries. What's the best test for HSV-2 after exposure? J Fam Pract 2007;56(3):221–2.

34. Crosby RA, Head S, DiClemente RJ, et al. Do protective behaviors follow the experience of testing positive for herpes simplex type 2? Sex Transm Dis 2008; 35(9):787–90.

35. Bickford J, Barton SE, Mandalia S. Chronic genital herpes and disclosure. The influence of stigma. Int J STD AIDS 2007;18(9):589–92.

36. Fife KH, Almekinder J, Ofner S. A comparison of one year of episodic or suppressive treatment of recurrent genital herpes with valacyclovir. Sex Transm Dis 2007; 34(5):297–301.

37. Mark KE, Wald A, Magaret AS, et al. Rapidly cleared episodes of herpes simplex virus reactivation in immunocompetent adults. J Infect Dis 2008;198(8):1141–9.

38. Martinez V, Caumes E, Chosidow O. Treatment to prevent recurrent genital herpes. Curr Opin Infect Dis 2008;21(1):42–8.

39. Baeten JM, Strick LB, Lucchetti AM, et al. Herpes simplex virus (HSV)-suppressive therapy decreases plasma and genital HIV-1 levels in HSV-2/HIV-1 coinfected women: a randomized, placebo-controlled, cross-over trial. J Infect Dis 2008;198(12):1804–8.

40. Celum C, Wald A, Hughes J, et al. Effect of acyclovir on HIV-1 acquisition in herpes simplex virus 2 seropositive women and men who have sex with men: a randomised, double-blind, placebo-controlled trial. Lancet 2008;371(9630): 2109–19.

41. Lebrun-Vignes B, Bouzamondo A, Dupuy A, et al. A meta-analysis to assess the efficacy of oral antiviral treatment to prevent genital herpes outbreaks. J Am Acad Dermatol 2007;57(2):238–46.
42. Martin ET, Krantz E, Gottlieb SL, et al. A pooled analysis of the effect of condoms in preventing HSV-2 acquisition. Arch Intern Med 2009;169(13):1233–40.
43. Tobian AA, Serwadda D, Quinn TC, et al. Male circumcision for the prevention of HSV-2 and HPV infections and syphilis. N Engl J Med 2009;360(13):1298–309.
44. French P. Syphilis. BMJ 2007;334(7585):143–7.
45. Centers for Disease Control and Prevention. Sexually transmitted disease treatment guideline 2006. Available at: http://www.cdc.gov/std/treatment/2006/genital-ulcers.htm#genulc6. Accessed October 30, 2009.
46. Heffelfinger JD, Swint EB, Berman SM, et al. Trends in primary and secondary syphilis among men who have sex with men in the United States. Am J Public Health 2007;97(6):1076–83.
47. Fleming DT, Wasserheit JN. From epidemiological synergy to public health policy and practice: the contribution of other sexually transmitted diseases to sexual transmission of HIV infection. Sex Transm Infect 1999;75:3–17.
48. Zetola NM, Engelman J, Jensen TP, et al. Syphilis in the United States: an update for clinicians with an emphasis on HIV coinfection. Mayo Clin Proc 2007;82(9):1091–102.
49. Krause W. Male accessory gland infection. Andrologia 2008;40:113–6.
50. Davis TW, Goldstone SE. Sexually transmitted infections as a cause of proctitis in men who have sex with men. Dis Colon Rectum 2009;52(3):507–12.
51. Francis SC, Kent CK, Klausner JD, et al. Prevalence of rectal Trichomonas vaginalis and Mycoplasma genitalium in male patients at the San Francisco STD clinic, 2005–2006. Sex Transm Dis 2008;35(9):797–800.
52. White JA. Manifestations and management of lymphogranuloma venereum. Curr Opin Infect Dis 2009;22(1):57–66.
53. Monroe JR. Does this man have genital warts? Pearly penile papules. JAAPA 2009;22(2):16.
54. Mayeaux EJ Jr, Dunton C. Modern management of external genital warts. J Low Genit Tract Dis 2008;12(3):185–92.
55. Markowitz LE, Dunne EF, Saraiya M, et al. Quadrivalent human papillomavirus vaccine: recommendations of the Advisory Committee on Immunization Practices (ACIP). MMWR Recomm Rep 2007;56(RR–2):1–24.
56. Dinh TH, Sternberg M, Dunne EF, et al. Genital warts among 18- to 59-year-olds in the United States, National Health and Nutrition Examination Survey, 1999–2004. Sex Transm Dis 2008;35(4):357–60.
57. Partridge JM, Hughes JP, Feng Q, et al. Genital human papillomavirus infection in men: incidence and risk factors in a cohort of university students. J Infect Dis 2007;196(8):1128–36.
58. Nielson CM, Harris RB, Dunne EF, et al. Risk factors for anogenital human papillomavirus infection in men. J Infect Dis 2007;196(8):1137–45.
59. Chiao EY, Giordano TP, Palefsky JM, et al. Screening HIV-infected individuals for anal cancer precursor lesions: a systematic review. Clin Infect Dis 2006;43(2):223–33.
60. Guirguis-Blake J. Interventions for molluscum contagiosum. Am Fam Physician 2006;74(9):1504.
61. Brown MR, Paulson CP, Henry SL. Treatment for anogenital molluscum contagiosum. Am Fam Physician 2009;80(8):864.
62. Ko CJ, Elston DM. Pediculosis. J Am Acad Dermatol 2004;50(1):1–12.

63. Varela JA, Otero L, Espinosa E, et al. *Phthirus pubis* in a sexually transmitted diseases unit: a study of 14 years. Sex Transm Dis 2003;30(4):292–6.
64. Flinders DC, De Schweinitz P. Pediculosis and scabies. Am Fam Physician 2004; 69(2):341–8.
65. Chen DS. Hepatitis B vaccination: the key toward elimination and eradication of hepatitis B. J Hepatol 2009;50(4):805–16.
66. Wasley AU, Grytdal S, Gallagher K, et al. Surveillance for acute viral hepatitis—United States, 2006. MMWR Surveill Summ 2008;57(2):1–24.
67. Hepatitis B foundation. Available at: http://www.hepb.org/hepb/statistics.htm. Accessed November 11, 2009.
68. Tran TT. Understanding cultural barriers in hepatitis B virus infection. Cleve Clin J Med 2009;76(Suppl 3):S10–3.
69. Shi YH, Shi CH. Molecular characteristics and stages of chronic hepatitis B virus infection. World J Gastroenterol 2009;15(25):3099–105.
70. Carey WD. The prevalence and natural history of hepatitis B in the 21st century. Cleve Clin J Med 2009;76(Suppl 3):S2–5.
71. Gish RG. Hepatitis B treatment: current best practices, avoiding resistance. Cleve Clin J Med 2009;76(Suppl 3):S14–9 [0891–1150] yr.
72. Iloeje UH, Yang HI, Su J, et al. The Risk Evaluation of Viral Load Elevation and Associated Liver Disease/Cancer-in HBV (the REVEAL-HBV) Study Group. Predicting cirrhosis risk based on the level of circulating hepatitis B viral load. Gastroenterology 2006;130:678–86.
73. European Association for the Study of the Liver. EASL clinical practice guidelines: management of chronic hepatitis B. J Hepatol 2009;50:227–42.
74. Campos-Outcalt D. Time to revise your HIV testing routine. J Fam Pract 2007; 56(4):283–4.
75. Cohen MS, Gay C, Kashuba AD, et al. Narrative review: antiretroviral therapy to prevent the sexual transmission of HIV-1. Ann Intern Med 2007;146(8):591–601.
76. Centers for Disease Control and Prevention. Sexually transmitted disease treatment guideline 2006. Available at: http://www.cdc.gov/std/treatment/2006/hiv. htm. Accessed October 30, 2009.
77. Romanelli F, Matheny SC. HIV infection: the role of primary care. Am Fam Physician 2009;80(9):946–95.
78. Feily A, Namazi MR, Saboktakin M, et al. Self-inflicted non-healing genital ulcer: a rare form of factitious disorder. Acta Dermatovenerol Alp Panonica Adriat 2009; 18(2):83–5.
79. Rosen T, Vandergriff T, Harting M. Antibiotic use in sexually transmissible diseases. Dermatol Clin 2009;27(1):49–61.
80. Center for Disease Control and Prevention. Sexually transmitted disease treatment guideline 2006. Management of patients who have genital ulcers. Available at: http://www.cdc.gov/std/treatment/2006/genital-ulcers.htm#genulc1. Accessed September 30, 2009.
81. Cook K, Brownell I. Treatments for genital warts. J Drugs Dermatol 2008;7(8): 801–7.
82. Schneider C, Segre T. Green tea: potential health benefits. Am Fam Physician 2009;79(7):591–4.
83. Kodner CM, Nasraty S. Management of genital warts. Am Fam Physician 2004; 70:2335–42.

Urologic Chronic Pelvic Pain Syndrome

Viviana Martinez-Bianchi, MD*, Brian H. Halstater, MD

KEYWORDS
- Interstitial cystitis • Bladder pain syndrome • Dysuria
- Urgency • Urologic chronic pelvic pain syndrome

DYSURIA

Dysuria is urination that is painful or uncomfortable. It is often associated with increased urinary frequency, abnormally frequent urination, *or urgency*, an abrupt, strong, often overwhelming need to urinate. The most common cause of dysuria is urethral or bladder inflammation, often because of infection. Patients with acute dysuria have symptoms of short duration, usually a few days, often associated with frequency and urgency. Most of these patients have an infection. **Table 1** shows the causes of dysuria in four categories: gynecologic, urological, inflammatory, and miscellaneous. Chronic dysuria is defined as pain with urination that has been continuous or recurrent for at least 6 months. It is closely tied to chronic pelvic pain syndrome in women, and prostatodynia (chronic prostate pain) in men. Associated symptoms include allodynia (nonpainful stimuli are perceived as painful) and hyperalgesia (painful stimuli are perceived as more painful than expected). Chronic dysuria is associated with changes in the central nervous system (CNS) that may maintain the perception of pain in the absence of acute injury.[1] The various causes of chronic dysuria are shown in **Table 2**.

PAINFUL BLADDER SYNDROME AND INTERSTITIAL CYSTITIS

Painful bladder syndrome (PBS) is a chronic disease of unknown etiology. PBS presents with chronic pelvic pain, nocturia, increased urinary frequency, and urgency.[2] The International Continence Society (ICS) defines PBS as "the complaint of suprapubic pain related to bladder filling, accompanied by other symptoms such as increased daytime and night-time frequency, in the absence of proven urinary infection or other obvious pathology."[3] The European Society for the Study of Bladder Pain Syndrome/Interstitial Cystitis calls the disease bladder pain syndrome (BPS), including a history of more than 6 months of pelvic pain, pressure, or discomfort perceived to be related

Duke Family Medicine Residency Program, Division of Family Medicine, Department of Community and Family Medicine, Duke University, DUMC 3886, Durham, NC 27710, USA
* Corresponding author.
E-mail address: marti213@mc.duke.edu

Prim Care Clin Office Pract 37 (2010) 527–546
doi:10.1016/j.pop.2010.05.002
0095-4543/10/$ – see front matter © 2010 Elsevier Inc. All rights reserved.

primarycare.theclinics.com

Table 1 Acute causes of dysuria	

Urologic	Balanitis
	Bladder neck obstruction
	Carcinoma or carcinoma in situ
	Epididymitis/orchitis
	Infectious urethritis (common etiologies include *Chlamydia*,
	    gonorrhea, ureaplasma urealyticum, *Candida*, *Mycoplasma*,
	    and herpes simplex)
	Pyelonephritis
	Radiation urethritis
	Urethral caruncle
	Urethral diverticulum
	Urethral stricture
	Urethral trauma
	Urinary retention
	Urinary tract infections
	Urolithiasis (in bladder, urethra or lower ureters)

Gynecologic	Cancer of the cervix, uterus, and ovaries Bartholin adenitis or abscess Cervicitis (similar organisms as infectious urethritis) Pelvic inflammatory disease Vulvovaginitis Urinary retention
Inflammatory Conditions	Rheumatologic disorders: Spondyloarthropathies, reactive arthritis, Behçet syndrome
Skin Conditions	Dermatitis Contact irritants: contraceptive foams, douches, diaphragm
Psychiatric	Obsessive washing
Drug Side Effects	Amoxicillin, cyclophosphamides, aspirin, nonsteroidal anti- inflammatory agents, allopurinol.
Miscellaneous	Foreign bodies in bladder, penis, vagina

to the urinary bladder, accompanied by at least one other urinary symptom, such as persistent urge to void or urinary frequency.[1]

One common subset of PBS is interstitial cystitis (IC). IC traditionally is defined as a chronic sterile inflammatory disease of the bladder, with either glomerulations or a classic Hunner ulcer found on cystoscopy. IC is more common in women, with a median age at onset of 40 years. In recent years, the diagnostic approach to IC has become more dependent on symptoms and less reliant on cystoscopic evaluation and biopsy.[2-5]

PROSTATODYNIA

There appears to be a significant overlap between the symptoms experienced by women diagnosed with PBS (with or without IC) and those of men with chronic prostatitis/chronic pelvic pain syndrome (CPPS). Active trigger points in internal and external pelvic regions that consistently reproduce specific patterns of referred pain in both men with CPPS and women with PBS have been identified.[6,7] Up to 70% of men with symptoms of nonbacterial prostatitis and prostatodynia have glomerulations and submucosal hemorrhages when undergoing bladder distention under anesthesia, raising the possibility that some cases of prostatitis may actually be IC.[8]

Table 2
Differential diagnosis of chronic dysuria

Urological	Chronic prostatitis/prostate pain syndrome/UCPPS (urologic chronic pelvic pain syndrome)
	Epididymo-orchitis
	Interstitial cystitis/bladder pain syndrome/UCPPS
	Overactive bladder
	Postvasectomy pain syndrome
	Scrotal pain syndrome
	Urethral diverticulum
	Urethritis/urethral pain syndrome
Neoplastic	Renal cell tumors, bladder, prostate, vagina, vulvar, cervical and penile cancers
Inflammatory Conditions	Spondyloarthropathies
	Autoimmune disorders
Gynecologic	Atrophic vaginitis
	Cancer of the cervix, ovaries, uterus, vagina
	Endometriosis
	Generalized vaginal pain syndrome
	Vulvodynia
Anorectal	Proctitis
	Anal fissure
	Hemorrhoids
Neuromuscular	Pudendal neuropathy/pudendal neuralgia
	Sacral spinal cord pathology
Psychogenic Conditions	Somatization disorder
	Major depression
	Stress disorders, post-traumatic stress disorder
	Anxiety
Drug Side Effects	Cyclophosphamides, aspirin, nonsteroidal anti-inflammatory agents, allopurinol

The National Institute of Diabetes and Digestive and Kidney Diseases (NIDDK) classification of prostatitis has replaced the older terms nonbacterial prostatitis and prostatodynia with category 3 chronic prostatitis/chronic pelvic pain syndrome (CP/CPPS, or simply CPPS). Just as with IC, these patients have pelvic and genital pain, often associated with urinary and sexual symptoms, but no history of documented urinary tract infection (UTI). Given the overlap of symptoms, the NIDDK has proposed that Urologic Chronic Pelvic Pain Syndromes (UCPPS) be used as an umbrella term for CPPS and IC.[9]

PREVALENCE

The true prevalence of PBS is not known. In a population-based study of patients in primary care, the prevalence of PBS was between 0.45% and 12.6%.[10] A population-based study in Finland concluded that IC affects 0.3% to 0.68% of women.[11] Another study in the Pacific Northwest concluded that the prevalence of IC symptoms was between 6.2% and 11.2% in women, and 2.3% and 4.6% in men.[12]

PATHOPHYSIOLOGY

PBS appears to have a multifactorial etiology.[3] Some of the mechanisms cited include: immunologic mechanisms, uroepithelial dysfunction, mast cell activation, and neural inflammation. These mechanisms may be associated with the development of myo-fascial trigger points. Psychological factors can perpetuate these symptoms, with subsequent worsening and establishment of a chronic syndrome.[13]

UTIs may trigger PBS in some patients. In a retrospective study of 314 women with recent-onset PBS, 18% to 36% of them had evidence of a UTI at the onset of symp-toms.[14] However, neither bacterial nor viral DNA is found in bladder biopsies of patients with PBS/IC, making chronic infection an unlikely cause for this syndrome.[15]

Some IC patients have increased bladder epithelial permeability, where the bladder glycosaminoglycan layer is damaged or defective,[16] exposing nerves to irritants within the bladder. Mast cells may be involved in the neurogenic inflammation observed in patients with IC, which leads to urinary frequency and detrusor overactivity. Increases in nerve growth factor have been detected in women with IC and men with prostatitis.[17]

The pain associated with PBS appears to involve an alteration in bladder sensory physiology, such that bladder-afferent neurons respond in an exaggerated manner to normally innocuous stimuli (allodynia).[18] A small study of subjects with IC showed generalized hypersensitivity to deep tissue stimulation with lower thresholds, and tolerance of bladder, muscle, and ischemic stimulation compared with healthy subjects. In the same study, subjects with IC had more catastrophizing, a perception of decreased health, more somatic complaints, and increased vigilance to sensations.[19]

Patients with PBS often have myofascial trigger points, with tension and tenderness of the pelvic floor musculature on physical examination. It is not known, however, whether these musculoskeletal abnormalities are a consequence of the lower urinary tract symptoms, or are a primary disorder that gives rise to secondary urinary symp-toms.[20] Irritable bowel syndrome, IC, and other chronic pelvic pain (CPP) disorders often occur concomitantly, possibly because of neural cross-talk via the convergence of pelvic afferents.[21] This may occur at the level of the dorsal root ganglia, spinal cord, or brain.[22]

PATIENT PRESENTATION

A detailed history is extremely important in this clinical syndrome, because multiple etiologies need to be ruled out. Characteristics of the pain, location, radiation, timing, associated voiding symptoms (frequency, urgency), sexual history, sexual functioning, and comorbid conditions need to be discussed in detail with the patient.

In general, PBS patients report pain in the following locations: 83% suprapubic, 36% urethral, 21% genital, and 29% nongenitourinary. Many patients will report pain that changes locations and occurs in multiple sites.[7] Irritative voiding symptoms (urgency, increased frequency, nocturia, dysuria) and dyspareunia are common, and 84% to 90% of patients with PBS report worsening of pain with bladder filling.[3,23] Burning and pain during urination occurs in 69% of patients. Pain may be described as aching, throbbing, tender, and piercing. Most women note that pain is worsened by touching, tampons, and intercourse. Some have worsening with urination or while riding in a car,[7] and some women report a pain flare at the time of the menstrual cycle.[24]

CLINICAL SYMPTOM SCALES

Several validated questionnaires are used to distinguish PBS from other urinary tract pathologies, although none is specific enough to be used as the sole diagnostic indicator. These tools also can be used to monitor the treatment efficacy of those who have already been diagnosed.[25]

For women, these include

- The O'Leary-Sant IC Symptom Index (ICSI) and IC Problem Index (ICPI) measure urinary and pain symptoms and assess how problematic symptoms are for patients with IC.[26]
- The Pain, Urgency, Frequency Symptom Scale (PUF, **Fig. 1**) collects symptoms and bother information in women. A PUF score of 13 or greater should prompt the physician to further evaluate the patient for IC.[27]

PELVIC PAIN and URGENCY/FREQUENCY PATIENT SYMPTOM SCALE

Please circle the answer that best describes how you feel for each question.

		0	1	2	3	4	SYMPTOM SCORE	BOTHER SCORE
1	How many times do you go to the bathroom during the day?	3-6	7-10	11-14	15-19	20+		
2	a. How many times do you go to the bathroom at night?	0	1	2	3	4+		
	b. If you get up at night to go to the bathroom, does it bother you?	Never Bothers	Occasionally	Usually	Always			
3	a. Do you now or have you ever had pain or symptoms during or after sexual intercourse?	Never	Occasionally	Usually	Always			
	b. Has pain or urgency ever made you avoid sexual intercourse?	Never	Occasionally	Usually	Always			
4	Do you have pain associated with your bladder or in your pelvis (vagina, labia, lower abdomen, urethra, perineum, testes, or scrotum)?	Never	Occasionally	Usually	Always			
5	a. If you have pain, is it usually		Mild	Moderate	Severe			
	b. Does your pain bother you?	Never	Occasionally	Usually	Always			
6	Do you still have urgency after going to the bathroom?	Never	Occasionally	Usually	Always			
7	a. If you have urgency, is it usually		Mild	Moderate	Severe			
	b. Does your urgency bother you?	Never	Occasionally	Usually	Always			
8	Are you sexually active? Yes____ No____							

SYMPTOM SCORE = (1, 2a, 3a, 4, 5a, 6, 7a)	
BOTHER SCORE = (2b, 3b, 5b, 7b)	
TOTAL SCORE (Symptom Score + Bother Score) =	

© 2000 C. Lowell Parsons, M.D

Total score ranges from 1 to 35.
A total score of 10-14 = 74% likelihood of positive PST; 15-19 = 76%; 20 or above = 91% likelihood of positive PST.

Revised 11/17/2003   © 2000 C. Lowell Parsons, M.D. Reprinted with permission.

Fig. 1. Pelvic pain and urgency/frequency patient symptom scale. (*Courtesy of* C. Lowell Parsons, MD; with permission.)

For men, these include

- The National Institutes of Health (NIH) Chronic Prostatitis Symptom Index (CPSI), which allows quantification of the pain, voiding symptoms, and quality of life in men (**Fig. 2**).[28]

NIH-Chronic Prostatitis Symptom Index (NIH-CPSI)

Pain or Discomfort

1. In the last week, have you experienced any pain or discomfort in the following areas?

		Yes	No
a.	Area between rectum and testicles (perineum)	$\square_1$	$\square_0$
b.	Testicles	$\square_1$	$\square_0$
c.	Tip of the penis (not related to urination)	$\square_1$	$\square_0$
d.	Below your waist, in your pubic or bladder area	$\square_1$	$\square_0$

2. In the last week, have you experienced:

		Yes	No
a.	Pain or burning during urination?	$\square_1$	$\square_0$
b.	Pain or discomfort during or after sexual climax (ejaculation)?	$\square_1$	$\square_0$

3. How often have you had pain or discomfort in any of these areas over the last week?

$\square_0$ Never
$\square_1$ Rarely
$\square_2$ Sometimes
$\square_3$ Often
$\square_4$ Usually
$\square_5$ Always

4. Which number best describes your AVERAGE pain or discomfort on the days that you had it, over the last week?

$\square$	$\square$	$\square$	$\square$	$\square$	$\square$	$\square$	$\square$	$\square$	$\square$	$\square$
0	1	2	3	4	5	6	7	8	9	10

NO PAIN   PAIN AS BAD AS YOU CAN IMAGINE

Urination

5. How often have you had a sensation of not emptying your bladder completely after you finished urinating, over the last week?

$\square_0$ Not at all
$\square_1$ Less than 1 time in 5
$\square_2$ Less than half the time
$\square_3$ About half the time
$\square_4$ More than half the time
$\square_5$ Almost always

6. How often have you had to urinate again less than two hours after you finished urinating, over the last week?

$\square_0$ Not at all
$\square_1$ Less than 1 time in 5
$\square_2$ Less than half the time
$\square_3$ About half the time
$\square_4$ More than half the time
$\square_5$ Almost always

Impact of Symptoms

7. How much have your symptoms kept you from doing the kinds of things you would usually do, over the last week?

$\square_0$ None
$\square_1$ Only a little
$\square_2$ Some
$\square_3$ A lot

8. How much did you think about your symptoms, over the last week?

$\square_0$ None
$\square_1$ Only a little
$\square_2$ Some
$\square_3$ A lot

Quality of Life

9. If you were to spend the rest of your life with your symptoms just the way they have been during the last week, how would you feel about that?

$\square_0$ Delighted
$\square_1$ Pleased
$\square_2$ Mostly satisfied
$\square_3$ Mixed (about equally satisfied and dissatisfied)
$\square_4$ Mostly dissatisfied
$\square_5$ Unhappy
$\square_6$ Terrible

Scoring the NIH-Chronic Prostatitis Symptom Index Domains

Pain: Total of items 1a, 1b, 1c,1d, 2a, 2b, 3, and 4 = _____

Urinary Symptoms: Total of items 5 and 6 = _____

Quality of Life Impact: Total of items 7, 8, and 9 = _____

Fig. 2. NIH-Chronic Prostatitis Symptom Index (NIH-CPSI). (*From* Litwin MS, McNaughton-Collins M, Fowler FJ Jr, et al. The National Institutes of Health chronic prostatitis symptom index: development and validation of a new outcome measure. J Urol 1999;162:369–75.)

PAST MEDICAL HISTORY

The past medical history should be obtained, including the following:[13,29]

- UTI history
- Sexually transmitted disease (STD) history
- History of bladder problems or known urological diseases
- Voiding dysfunction in childhood, including enuresis, urgency, increased frequency, or recurrent UTIs
- Sexual history
- Previous pelvic surgery or radiation
- Presence of allergies (systemic or dermatologic)
- Presence of autoimmune diseases
- History of cardiovascular conditions
- History of neurologic conditions
- Concomitant chronic syndromes (irritable bowel syndrome, fibromyalgia, migraine headaches, vulvodynia, chronic fatigue syndrome, low back pain)
- Psychiatric history, including depression, anxiety, obsessive–compulsive disorder, maladaptive coping, and social support.

RISK ASSESSMENT

Women tend to have a higher risk of PBS than men, with a female-to-male risk ratio of approximately 9:1.[30] Several recent studies and reviews have looked at the correlation between PBS and other chronic conditions. In a study published in 2009 by Warren and colleagues, 11 antecedent syndromes were diagnosed more often in those with PBS, the most common being fibromyalgia-chronic widespread pain, chronic fatigue syndrome, sicca syndrome, and irritable bowel syndrome. Other less commonly associated syndromes include migraine headaches, depression, and allergies.[31] Several studies have reported an association between IC and sexual, physical, and emotional abuse.[32]

Familial occurrence of PBS is suggested by a study that found that adult female first-degree relatives of patients with IC may have a prevalence of IC 17 times that found in the general population. A greater concordance of IC among monozygotic than dizygotic twins also has been described.[3] Another group of researchers found an autosomal-dominant link in a cohort of families.[33]

SEXUAL FACTORS

Vulvodynia and dyspareunia are common among women with PBS.[34] Anticipation of pain with intercourse causes anxiety, and patients may try to avoid intimacy, putting strain on their romantic relationships. Depression also can occur as a result of the chronic pain, the impact the pain is having on the patient's life, or from shame and guilt due to current or past sexual experiences. There can be a connection with post-traumatic stress disorder (PTSD), leading to avoidance, hyperarousal, or re-experiencing difficult past encounters.[35] In a study of 122 vulvodynia patients, most (84%) had a positive Potassium Sensitivity Test, and 80% had urgency or increased frequency, leading the authors to conclude that the etiology of the patients' pain was in the bladder (IC), and that vulvodynia in many patients was likely referred pain from the urinary bladder.[36]

In obtaining a sexual history, questions should be clear and direct:[37,38]

- Many people with IC or painful bladder syndrome experience difficulty with sexual functioning. Is this a problem for you?
- Does the sexual problem happen all the time?
- How long have you had the sexual problem?
- Does the problem occur with masturbation?
- Do you have problems when your partner attempts penetration?
- Does the problem happen with specific activities?
- How does the problem affect your relationship?
- Could you point out where it hurts on this diagram of the genitalia?
- How does this sexual problem affect you?
- How is your partner affected by the sexual problem?
- Does the sexual problem cause you to withdraw from your partner?
- Does the problem cause you to refrain from sexual activity, including masturbation?
- What tests have you already had in the evaluation of your sexual health concern?
- What treatments have you already received, and what are the outcomes of the various treatments?

NUTRITION

PBS symptoms are influenced by food and beverages in 90% of patients. The most frequently reported bothersome items were caffeinated drinks, tea, carbonated and alcoholic beverages, fruits (tomatoes, grapefruit, lemons, oranges, pineapple) and juices (grapefruit, cranberry, orange, pineapple), artificial sweeteners, and spicy foods containing tomato products or hot pepper. Three quarters of patients in one study reported that larger meals caused more bladder symptoms than smaller meals. Some had symptom relief following the ingestion of alkalizing agents, such as calcium glycerophosphate (Prelief) or sodium bicarbonate (baking soda).[39]

MENTAL HEALTH

Depression and panic disorder are significantly more common in men and women with pelvic pain conditions. Patients with PBS also report worse quality of life in regard to mental health. They report significant sleep dysfunction, depression, anxiety, and stress compared with asymptomatic controls. Patients with PBS do more catastrophic thinking, have greater sexual dysfunction, and perceive lower social support than controls. These levels of stress and anxiety appear related to patient symptom severity.[40,41] Helpful questionnaires[42] include the Patient Health Questionnaire (PHQ-9) (**Fig. 3**),[43] which assesses depression and anxiety, and the Pain Catastrophizing Scale (PCS),[44] which measures negative thoughts associated with pain.

PHYSICAL EXAMINATION

The physical examination should include:

- Abdominal examination for scars, hernias, areas of tenderness, masses, or organomegaly

PATIENT HEALTH QUESTIONNAIRE (PHQ-9)

NAME:_____   DATE:_____

Over the last *2 weeks,* how often have you been
bothered by any of the following problems?
(use "✓" to indicate your answer)

	Not at all	Several days	More than half the days	Nearly every day
1. Little interest or pleasure in doing things	0	1	2	3
2. Feeling down, depressed, or hopeless	0	1	2	3
3. Trouble falling or staying asleep, or sleeping too much	0	1	2	3
4. Feeling tired or having little energy	0	1	2	3
5. Poor appetite or overeating	0	1	2	3
6. Feeling bad about yourself—or that you are a failure or have let yourself or your family down	0	1	2	3
7. Trouble concentrating on things, such as reading the newspaper or watching television	0	1	2	3
8. Moving or speaking so slowly that other people could have noticed. Or the opposite — being so figety or restless that you have been moving around a lot more than usual	0	1	2	3
9. Thoughts that you would be better off dead, or of hurting yourself	0	1	2	3

add columns _____ + _____ + _____

(Healthcare professional: For interpretation of TOTAL,   TOTAL: _____
please refer to accompanying scoring card).

10. If you checked off *any problems,* how *difficult* have these problems made it for you to do your work, take care of things at home, or get along with other people?	Not difficult at all _____ Somewhat difficult _____ Very difficult _____ Extremely difficult _____

Fig. 3. Patient Health Questionnaire (PHQ-9). (*Courtesy of* Pfizer, Inc, New York, New York. Copyright © Pfizer, Inc.; all rights reserved.)

- Musculoskeletal examination for kyphosis and abduction and adduction of the hips
- Skin examination for rashes or lesions
- Neurologic examination for motor strength and areas of increased or decreased sensation.

PHQ-9 Patient Depression Questionnaire

For initial diagnosis:

1. Patient completes PHQ-9 Quick Depression Assessment.
2. If there are at least 4 ✓s in the shaded section (including Questions #1 and #2), consider a depressive disorder. Add score to determine severity.

Consider Major Depressive Disorder
- if there are at least 5 ✓s in the shaded section (one of which corresponds to Question #1 or #2)

Consider Other Depressive Disorder
- if there are 2-4 ✓s in the shaded section (one of which corresponds to Question #1 or #2)

Note: Since the questionnaire relies on patient self-report, all responses should be verified by the clinician, and a definitive diagnosis is made on clinical grounds taking into account how well the patient understood the questionnaire, as well as other relevant information from the patient.
Diagnoses of Major Depressive Disorder or Other Depressive Disorder also require impairment of social, occupational, or other important areas of functioning (Question #10) and ruling out normal bereavement, a history of a Manic Episode (Bipolar Disorder), and a physical disorder, medication, or other drug as the biological cause of the depressive symptoms.

To monitor severity over time for newly diagnosed patients or patients in current treatment for depression:

1. Patients may complete questionnaires at baseline and at regular intervals (eg, every 2 weeks) at home and bring them in at their next appointment for scoring or they may complete the questionnaire during each scheduled appointment.
2. Add up ✓s by column. For every ✓: Several days = 1 More than half the days = 2 Nearly every day = 3
3. Add together column scores to get a TOTAL score.
4. Refer to the accompanying **PHQ-9 Scoring Box** to interpret the TOTAL score.
5. Results may be included in patient files to assist you in setting up a treatment goal, determining degree of response, as well as guiding treatment intervention.

Scoring: add up all checked boxes on PHQ-9

For every ✓ Not at all = 0; Several days = 1;
More than half the days = 2; Nearly every day = 3

Interpretation of Total Score

Total Score	Depression Severity
1-4	Minimal depression
5-9	Mild depression
10-14	Moderate depression
15-19	Moderately severe depression
20-27	Severe depression

Fig. 3. *(continued)*

Pelvic examination in women needs to be detailed, mapping areas of tenderness and grading the degree of tenderness:[29]

- Inspect vulva and introitus for areas of irritation, ulceration, desquamation, and signs of endometriosis or herpes.
- Palpate for tenderness of vestibular glands or vulvar skin.
- Look for vaginal spasms or tenderness during insertion and opening of speculum. Inspect for vaginal discharge, vaginal wall irritation. Check vaginal fornices for endometriosis.
- Inspect cervix for ulcerations or discharge.

- Do bimanual examination and palpate the whole pelvic floor musculature. Evaluate for tightness, tenderness, taut bands, or pain radiation that duplicates symptoms, particularly in the muscles and connective tissue lateral to the urethra.[45]

Genitourinary examination in men also needs to be detailed and may include a pelvic examination in lithotomy position:

- Inspect for lesions, asymmetry, and skin changes.
- Do a digital rectal examination (DRE) to evaluate for prostate changes and tenderness of prostate or anorectal area. Examine the muscles lateral to the prostate and in the urogenital diaphragm. Palpate for trigger points in the perineal body.[45] Palpate for tenderness of the bladder, prostate, levator, and adductor muscles of the pelvic floor.
- Palpate scrotal contents for tenderness or masses in the testis or epididymus.
- Inspect penis for meatal discharge, penile lesions, and balanitis.
- Measure postvoid residual urine with ultrasound.[46]

LABORATORY AND OTHER TESTING
Voiding Diary

Patients should keep a 3-day voiding diary, recording volumes of intake and output, as well as voiding times and sensation at voiding.

Urine Analysis, Culture, Cytology

- Urinalysis for blood, glucose, nitrites, and leukocyte esterase should be performed. If hematuria is present, further testing may be necessary to exclude other disease processes with which IC can be mistaken, including neoplasia.[47]
- The midstream urine culture for women and the two-glass test for men (urine cultures of initial stream before prostatic massage, and midstream after massage) should be performed to rule out infection.[42] If sterile pyuria is identified, an acid fast bacilli smear and culture to rule out tuberculosis (TB) should be performed in high-risk populations.
- Urine cytology is recommended on all patients. In a large study of patients diagnosed with IC, 1% actually had transitional cell carcinoma.[48]

Cystoscopy

The role of cystoscopy in diagnosing IC has become controversial. Although PBS is now considered a clinical syndrome, until recently cystoscopy was regarded as an essential diagnostic tool, and cystoscopy and hydrodistension under anesthesia were the gold standards for the diagnosis and initial treatment of IC.[3] To be diagnosed with IC, patients previously needed to have either glomerulations on cystoscopic examination or classic Hunner ulcer, and either pain associated with the bladder or urinary urgency. Some authors still advocate that a cystoscopic examination for glomerulations should be done after distention of the bladder under anesthesia to 80 to 100 cm H_2O for 1 to 2 minutes,[3] looking for glomerulations, suburothelial hemorrhages, or ulceration. Any suspicious lesion should be biopsied.[46,47] In Europe, biopsy findings that are accepted as positive signs of BPS are inflammatory infiltrates, granulation tissue, detrusor mastocytosis, or intrafascicular fibrosis.[49]

Urodynamics

A full cystometrogram may need to be performed to define the patient's bladder sensation, capacity, and compliance, and to rule out detrusor overactivity, significant hypocompliance, or bladder outlet obstruction.[46] A small study comparing overactive bladder (OAB) patients with those diagnosed with PBS showed that the urodynamic characteristics of the patients with PBS were significantly different from those of the patients with OAB. The PBS/IC group showed a greater premature filling sensation and decreased bladder capacity compared to the OAB group and were able to handle smaller urine volumes. 70% patients with OAB had involuntary detrusor contraction while IDC was not observed in the PBS/IC group.[50]

Potassium Sensitivity Test

In individuals with a healthy bladder, less than 3% will experience symptoms of urgency or pain in response to intravesical potassium; when they do, their reactions are mild. However, about 80% of patients with IC have a positive potassium sensitivity test. Their dysfunctional bladder epithelium allows potassium to diffuse into the bladder muscularis layer, causing an irritating effect that depolarizes nerve and muscle and leads to tissue injury. The potassium sensitivity test is considered positive if the patient assigns a grade of 2 or higher on either the urgency or the pain scales.[51]

TREATMENT

Only two treatments are currently approved by the US Food and Drug Administration for treating IC: oral pentosan polysulfate and intravesical dimethyl sulfoxide (DMSO), but many other treatments have been used. Treatment for patients with PBS should be addressed individually, based on the patient's most significant symptom(s). Often, patients will need a multisystem, multidisciplinary approach. The mnemonic UPOINT[40] can be helpful in individualizing therapy:

   Urinary symptoms
   Psychosocial dysfunction
   Organ-specific findings
   Infection
   Neurologic dysfunction
   Tenderness of muscles.

Oral Medications

1. Amitriptyline 25 to 100 mg by mouth at bedtime appears to be safe and effective in the treatment of IC, resulting in a 64% response rate[52] and decreasing pain and urgency intensity. Patients need to be counseled about anticholinergic adverse effects, with mouth dryness being the most common. Dose should be increased gradually, and the lowest effective dose should be used.[53]
2. Pentosan polysulfate sodium (PPS) 300 mg by mouth three times daily has been shown to improve quality of life in some patients.[54] Studies (supported by the manufacturer) concluded that initiation of PPS treatment within 6 months of establishing the diagnosis of IC may be associated with greater improvement.[55]
3. Cyclosporine A 1.5 mg/kg twice daily was shown to be more effective than PPS but caused more adverse effects.[56]
4. Cimetidine 400 mg twice daily was shown to be slightly better than placebo in a small study.[57]

5. L-arginine 500 mg three times daily was found to show some improvement in pain and urgency in a subset of patients with bladder capacity of 800 mL or larger.[58]
6. Hydroxyzine 25 to 75 mg at bedtime has been used alone or combined with PPS, but studies have not shown that it provides significant benefit.[59]
7. Prednisone, dosed at 25 mg daily for 1 to 2 months, then tapered to the minimum required for relief of symptoms, can be used for patients with severe ulcerative IC.[60]
8. Muscle relaxants can be used to address the cycle of tight muscles and hypertonic muscular states of the pelvic floor. Myorelaxant drugs such as metaxolone and cyclobenzaprine generally have been shown to be beneficial for myofascial pain. Tizanidine can be beneficial for muscle spasticity and secondarily for myofascial pain.[61]
9. Pregabalin has been beneficial for patients with a significant myofascial pain disorder as well as neuropathic symptoms, such as burning.[62]
10. Montelukast 10 mg daily, evaluated in a pilot study published in 2001, showed some promise in the treatment of IC, but further clinical trials have yet not confirmed the initial findings.[62]
11. Duloxetine, a 5-HT and NA reuptake inhibitor with low activity on dopamine reuptake, showed no favorable therapeutic results in the treatment of PBS patients.[63]

It is important to note that 67% of 104 patients in a recent study have reported that some oral medications made their symptoms worse, including antibiotics, aspirin, ibuprofen, and decongestants.[39]

Intravesical Medications

A recent Cochrane review of the effectiveness of six intravesical treatments for PBS/IC (resiniferatoxin, dimethyl sulfoxide [DMSO], Bacillus Calmette-Guerin [BCG] intravesical immunotherapy, pentosan polysulfate, oxybutynin, and alkalinization of urine pH) concluded that the evidence behind the use of most intravesical preparations is limited.[64]

1. DMSO is a readily absorbed solvent that is a byproduct of the wood pulp industry. It is the only agent approved in the United States for intravesical treatment of IC. Its pharmacologic properties include rapid membrane penetration, enhanced drug absorption, anti-inflammatory action, analgesic action, collagen dissolution, muscle relaxation, and mast cell histamine release. It appears to desensitize nociceptive pathways in the urinary tract. Its most common adverse effect is a garlic-like odor in the patient's breath. It is administered intravesically, 50 mL of 50% DMSO with 10 mg of triamcinolone, 40,000 units of heparin, and 44 mEq of sodium bicarbonate.[3]
2. Heparin appears to act by mimicking the activity of the bladder's own mucopolysaccharide lining and has anti-inflammatory effects. Administration of 10,000 U of heparin in sterile water, either alone or with DMSO, at varying intervals, provided good results according to observational studies. A solution of 40,000 U heparin, 2% lidocaine, and 3 mL 8.4% sodium bicarbonate, administered intravesically used three times a week for 2 weeks, can provide relief of voiding symptoms, pain, and dyspareunia in patients with IC.[65] The symptom relief appears to last beyond the duration of the local anesthetic activity of lidocaine, suggesting a suppression of neurologic upregulation.[66]
3. Alkalinized lidocaine (200 mg lidocaine, alkalinized with 8.4% sodium bicarbonate solution to a final volume of 10 mL), instilled intravesically five times a week in 99 women, resulted in moderate to marked improvement.[67]

4. Sodium hyaluronate (a phosphate-buffered saline solution with 40 mg sodium hyaluronate weekly) provided 85% of patients with improvement in voiding symptoms and pain, and 55% remained with no pain or minimal bladder symptoms after therapy; 34% continued to monthly therapy.[3]
5. Chondroitin sulfate instilled weekly for 20 weeks, then monthly for 3 months, improved urinary symptoms.
6. Pentosan polysulfate, 300 mg twice weekly in 50 mL of normal saline intravesically, has shown modest response.[3]
7. Intravesical BCG immunotherapy appeared promising in some studies,[68] but other studies found that the benefits of BCG were minimal, or argued against routine use of BCG immunotherapy in IC patients, even if it had an acceptable safety profile.[69,70]
8. Resiniferatoxin, a capsaicin analog and vanilloid receptor agonist, is being considered as a new intravesical strategy for IC. Further studies are pending.[71]

Topical Medications

Lubricants and moisturizers (eg, Astroglide, Replens, and Femglide) can improve orgasmic function in patients with complaints of vaginal dryness and dyspareunia, without any long-term safety concerns.[72] Patients who are trying to conceive should be made aware of their effect on decreasing sperm motility.[72] Plain petrolatum (Vaseline) will benefit some patients.[73] Topical anesthetics can be used immediately before intercourse to relieve pain.[72,73] Lidocaine ointment 5% or lidocaine jelly 2% can be applied as required for symptoms and 30 minutes before sexual activity. Male sexual partners may experience penile numbness and should avoid oral contact.[73] Estrogen vaginal cream can be helpful for postmenopausal women who have dyspareunia related to atrophy.[74] A very small study of Zestra (a lubricating oil with herbal ingredients) showed it can improve sexual experience in women due to increasing blood flow to the genital area when applied directly to the mons pubis in patients with IC. The effects can last 45 minutes.[75]

Herbal Therapy

Oral herbal preparations have been used as a treatment alternative for patients with PBS. A pilot study used the herbs cornus, gardenia, curculigo, rhubarb, psoralea, and rehmannia in a tea twice a day for 6 days a week for 3 months, then once a day. Of the 25 patients studied, 61% had a significant decrease in pain at 4 weeks, and an additional 22% had a significant response at 3 months. More research is needed in this area.[76]

Physical Therapy

A randomized multicenter pilot trial showed benefit of manual therapy in treatment of urologic chronic pelvic pain syndrome.[20] Pelvic floor manual therapy for decreasing pelvic floor hypertonicity can effectively ameliorate the symptoms of the urgency/frequency syndrome and IC in 70% to 80% of patients.[45]

Psychosocial Therapy

Psychotherapy with a certified psychologist, psychiatrist, or social worker can be beneficial. Interventions aimed at increasing adaptive coping, such as guided imagery, appear to positively impact the female experience with IC.[77] Relaxation techniques, diaphragmatic breathing, progressive muscle relaxation, exercise, self-visualization, and self-hypnosis have been shown to be effective in reducing stress.[76] National support groups are also available, including the Interstitial Cystitis Association and the Interstitial Cystitis Network.

Sexual Therapy

Sexual functioning has been identified as a strong predictor of physical quality of life and as the only strong predictor of mental quality of life in patients with severe IC.[78] Patients can be taught self-care strategies, such as emptying the bladder before and after sex, avoiding prolonged intercourse, minimizing pressure on the urethra, engaging in outercourse, cleansing after sexual activity, and taking pain killers or anti-spasmotics before engaging in sexual activity. Patients also should discuss with their partner their goals for expressing intimacy. Therapists can evaluate the patient's level of knowledge and help patients redefine normal and adequate sexual functioning with this condition. Treatment can start with nonintercourse exercises, where patients use film, erotic reading, and self-stimulation to learn what they can tolerate. Therapy can reintroduce sexual thought into patients' lives and help them feel sensual and sexual again. Sexuality in the IC patient is best managed by decreasing pain and by using a sex therapist to identify and treat desire, arousal, and orgasmic disorders.[76]

Dietary Modifications

Surveys have reported that dietary modifications are the fourth most common therapy patients choose. There are no controlled studies in regards to diet, but a reasonable approach is to have the patient implement a diet that for 2 or 3 months eliminates all the proposed beverages and foods that exacerbate PBS symptoms, and then add them back in one at a time.[79]

Other Treatments

1. Sacral neuromodulation is effective in the treatment of refractory urgency and increased frequency caused by PBS.[80]
2. Laser ablation of Hunner ulcers in a small study was reported to provide symptomatic relief for patients with PBS/IC previously refractory to medical treatment. The reduction in pain lasted for over a year, but half of the patients experienced relapse and had to be re-treated.[81] Cystectomy with urinary diversion and bladder augmentation is considered to be a last-resort treatment option reserved for severe cases when all other approaches have failed.[82]
3. Local anesthetics, such as Lidocaine or Marcaine 1 to 3 mL without epinephrine can be injected into trigger point areas in the pelvis. Typically a series of three to five injections is used, with increasing sustained relief after each injection.[60]
4. Botulinum toxin type A (Botox) 80 U (20 U/mL) injected into puborectalis and pubococcygeus muscles under conscious sedation was no more effective than placebo in improving quality of life or reducing pain.[83]
5. Bladder training can extend the voiding interval by inhibiting the urge to urinate, and it has been successful in some patients. Progressive increases in the voiding interval by 15 to 30 minutes every 3 to 4 weeks can result in a decrease in frequency, nocturia, and urgency.[76]

CARING FOR THE PATIENT WITH PBS

Quality-of-life studies suggest that PBS patients are six times more likely than individuals in the general population to cut down on work time due to health problems, but only half as likely to do so as patients with arthritis.[3] Several illnesses are associated with PBS: migraine, asthma, fibromyalgia, incontinence, chronic fatigue syndrome, and vulvodynia.[84] The combination of any of these illnesses can be challenging to manage and control. Women with PBS report global deficits in quality of life compared with healthy controls, and they experience greater depressive symptoms.[85]

The quality of life of patients with PBS is affected by chronic pain, sexual dysfunction, and difficulty sleeping, and most patients need a multisystem, multidisciplinary approach. The primary care physician, as the leader of a patient-centered medical home, can offer the strongest support to patients by enlisting appropriate members of the team to aid patients in their self-management. A patient-centered team may include the primary care physician, urologist, counselor, physical therapist, pharmacist, nutritionist, social worker, and sexual therapist. The team needs to be ready to help patients who present for the management of IC flares.[86]

PBS is recognized as a serious medical condition associated with significant disability. Because many of the modalities used to treat this syndrome can provide only inadequate or short-term relief, continuous support of these patients is paramount. A team-based approach that can offer the patient all the modalities mentioned is necessary to decrease anxiety, depression, and recurrence of problems.

REFERENCES

1. van de Merwe J, Nordling J, Bouchelouche P, et al. Diagnostic criteria, classification, and nomenclature for painful bladder syndrome/interstitial cystitis: an ESSIC. Eur Urol 2008;53:60–7.
2. Bogart LM, Berry SH, Clemens JQ. Symptoms of interstitial cystitis, painful bladder syndrome and similar diseases in women: a systematic review. J Urol 2007;177(2):450–6.
3. Hanno PM. Painful bladder syndrome/interstitial cystitis and related disorders. In: Wein AJ, editor. Campbell-Walsh urology. 9th edition. Philadelphia: Saunders; 2007. p. 330–70.
4. Hanno PM, Landis JR, Mathews-Cook Y, et al. The diagnosis of interstitial cuystitis revisited: lessons learned from the NIH Interstitial Cistitis Database Study. J Urol 1999;161(2):553–7.
5. Sant GR, Hanno PM. Interstitial cystitis: current issues and controversies in diagnosis. Urology 2001;6(1):82–8.
6. Anderson RU, Sawyer T, Wise D, et al. Painful myofascial trigger points and pain sites in men with chronic prostatitis/chronic pelvic pain syndrome. J Urol 2009; 182(6):2753–8.
7. Warren JW, Langenberg P, Greenberg P, et al. Sites of pain from interstitial cystitis/painful bladder syndrome. J Urol 2008;180(4):1373–7.
8. Hanno PM. Interstitial cystitis—epidemiology, diagnostic criteria, clinical markers. Rev Urol 2002;4(Suppl 1):S3–8.
9. Abrams P, Baranowski A, Berger R, et al. A new classification is needed for pelvic pain syndromes—are existing terminologies of spurious diagnostic authority bad for patients? J Urol 2006;175(6):1989–90.
10. Rosenberg M, Hazzard M. Prevalence of Interstitial cystitis symptoms in women: a population based study in the primary care office. J Urol 2005;174(6):2231–4.
11. Leppilahti, Sairanen J, Tammela TL, et al, for the Finnish Interstitial Cystitis-Pelvic Pain Syndome Study Group. Prevalence of clinically confirmed interstitial cystitis in women: a population based study in Finland. J Urol 2005;174(2):407–801.
12. Clemens J, Meenan R, O'Keeffe-Rosetti M, et al. Prevalence of prostatitis-like symptoms in a managed care population. J Urol 2005;176(2):576–80.

13. Doggweiler-Wiygul R. Urologic myofascial pain syndromes. Curr Pain Headache Rep 2004;8:445–51.
14. Warren JW, Brown V, Jacobs S, et al. Urinary tract infection and inflammation at onset of interstitial cystitis/painful bladder syndrome. Urology 2008;71(6):1085–90.
15. Al-Hadithi HN, Williams H, Hart CA, et al. Absence of bacterial and viral DNA in bladder biopsies from patients with interstitial cystitis/chronic pelvic pain syndrome. J Urol 2005;174(1):151–4.
16. Hurst RE, Rhodes SW, Adamson PB, et al. Functional and structural characteristics of the glycosaminoglycans of the bladder luminal surface. J Urol 1987; 138(1):433–7.
17. Dupont MC, Spitsbergen JM, Kim KB, et al. Histological and neurotrophic changes triggered by varying models of bladder inflammation. J Urol 2001; 166(3):1111–8.
18. Mukerji G, Yiangou Y, Agarwal SK, et al. Transient receptor potential vanilloid receptor subtype 1 in painful bladder syndrome and its correlation with pain. J Urol 2006;176(2):797–801.
19. Ness TJ, Powell-Boone T, Cannon R, et al. Psychophysical evidence of hypersensitivity in subjects with interstitial cystitis. J Urol 2005;173(6):1983–7.
20. Fitzgerald MP, Anderson RU, Potts J, et al, for the Urological Pelvic Pain Collaborative Research Network. Randomized multicenter feasibility trial of myofascial physical therapy for the treatment of urological chronic pelvic pain syndromes. J Urol 2009;182(2):570–80.
21. Pezzone MA, Liang R, Fraser MO. A model of neural cross-talk and irritation in the pelvis: implications for the overlap of chronic pelvic pain disorders. Gastroenterology 2005;128(7):1953–64.
22. Noronha R, Akbarali H, Malykhina A, et al. Changes in urinary bladder smooth muscle function in response to colonic inflammation. Am J Physiol Renal Physiol 2007;293(5):1461–7.
23. FitzGerald MP, Brensinger C, Brubaker L, et al. What is the pain of interstitial cystitis like? Int Urogynecol J Pelvic Floor Dysfunct 2006;17(1):69–72.
24. Powell-Boone T, Ness TJ, Cannon R, et al. Menstrual cycle affects bladder pain sensation in subjects with interstitial cystitis. J Urol 2005;174(5):1832–6.
25. Kushner L, Moldwin RM. Efficiency of questionnaires used to screen for interstitial cystitis. J Urol 2006;176(2):587–92.
26. O'Leary MP, Sant GR, Fowler FJ, et al. The interstitial cystitis symptom index and problem index. Urology 1997;49(Suppl 5A):58–63.
27. Parsons CL, Dell J, Stanford EJ, et al. Increased prevalence of interstitial cystitis: previously unrecognized urologic and gynecologic cases identified using a new symptom questionnaire and intravesical potassium sensitivity. Urology 2002;60(4):573–8.
28. Litwin MS, McNaughton-Collins M, Fowler FJ Jr, et al. The National Institutes of Health chronic prostatitis symptom index: development and validation of a new outcome measure. Chronic Prostatitis Collaborative Research Network. J Urol 1999;162(2):369–75.
29. Nordling J, Anjum F, Bade J, et al. Primary evaluation of patients suspected of having interstitial cystitis (IC). Eur Urol 2004;45(5):535–682.
30. Clemens JQ, Joyce GF, Wise M, et al. Interstitial cystitis and painful bladder syndrome. In: Litwin MS, Saigal CS, editors. Urologic diseases in America. US Department of Health and Human Services, Public Health Service, National Institutes of Health, National Institute of Diabetes and Digestive and Kidney Diseases. Washington, DC: US Government Printing Office; 2007. p. 125–54 NIH Publication # 07-5512.

31. Warren JW, Howard FM, Cross RK, et al. Antecedent nonbladder syndromes in case–control study of interstitial cystitis/painful bladder syndrome. Urology 2009;73(1):52–7.
32. Peters KM, Kalinowski SE, Carrico DJ, et al. Fact or fiction—is abuse prevalent in patients with interstitial cystitis? Results from a community survey and clinic population. J Urol 2007;178(3 Pt 1):891–5.
33. Dimitrakov J, Guthrie D. Genetics and phenotyping of urological chronic pelvic pain syndrome. J Urol 2009;181(4):1550–7.
34. Gardella B, Porru D, Ferdeghini F, et al. Insight into urogynecologic features of women with interstitial cystitis/painful bladder syndrome. Eur Urol 2008;54(5): 1145–51.
35. Peters KM, Carrico DJ, Diokno AC. Characterization of a clinical cohort of 87 women with interstitial cystitis/painful bladder syndrome. Urology 2008;71(4):634–40.
36. Kahn BS, Tatro C, Parsons CL, et al. Prevalence of interstitial cystitis in vulvodynia patients detected by bladder potassium sensitivity. J Sex Med 2010;7: 996–1002.
37. Ohl L. Essentials of female sexual dysfunction from a sex therapy perspective. Urol Nurs 2007;27(1):57–63.
38. Goldstein I. Urologic management of women with sexual health concerns. In: Wein AJ, editor. Wein: Campbell-Walsh urology. Philadelphia: Saunders; 2007. Chapter 28.
39. Shorter B, Lesser M, Moldwin RM, et al. Effect of comestibles on symptoms of interstitial cystitis. J Urol 2007;178(1):145–52.
40. Nickel JC, Tripp DA, Pontari M, et al. Psychosocial phenotyping in women with interstitial cystitis/painful bladder syndrome: a case-control study. J Urol 2010; 183(1):167–72.
41. Nickel JC, Payne CK, Forrest J, et al. The relationship among symptoms, sleep disturbances and quality of life in patients with interstitial cystitis. J Urol 2009; 181(6):2555–61.
42. Shoskes DA, Nickel JC, Rackley RR, et al. Clinical phenotyping in chronic prostatitis/chronic pelvic pain syndrome: a phenotypic classification of UCPPS. Prostate Cancer Prostatic Dis 2009;12:177–83.
43. Kroenke K, Spitzer RL, Williams JB. The PHQ-9: validity of a brief depression severity measure. J Gen Intern Med 2001;16(9):606–13.
44. Sullivan MJL, Bishop S, Pivik J, et al. The pain catastrophizing scale: development and validation. Psychol Assess 1995;7(4):524–32.
45. Weiss JM. Pelvic floor myofascial trigger points: manual therapy for interstitial cystitis and the urgency-frequency syndrome. J Urol 2001;166(6):2226–31.
46. Irwin P, Samsudin A. Reinvestigation of patients with a diagnosis of interstitial cystitis: common things are sometimes common. J Urol 2005;174(2): 584–7.
47. Neal DE. Interstitial cystitis: evaluation and related conditions. J Urol 2009;181(6): 2414–5.
48. Tissot WD, Diokno AC, Peters KM. A referral center's experience with transitional cell carcinoma misdiagnosed as interstitial cystitis. J Urol 2004;172(2): 478–80.
49. Wein A. Primary evaluation of patients suspected of having interstitial cystitis (IC). J Urol 2004;172(6):2494–5.
50. Kim SH, Kim TB, Kim SW, et al. Urodynamic findings of the painful bladder syndrome/interstitial cystitis: a comparison with idiopathic overactive bladder. J Urol 2009;181(6):2550–4.

51. Parsons CL, Bullen M, Kahn BS, et al. Gynecologic presentation of interstitial cystitis as detected by intravesical potassium sensitivity. Obstet Gynecol 2001; 98(1):127–32.
52. van Ophoven A, Hertle L. Long term results of amitripyline treatment for interstitial cystitis. J Urol 2005;174(5):1837–40.
53. van Ophoven A, Pokupic S, Heinecke A, et al. A prospective, randomized, placebo controlled, double-blind study of amitriptyline for the treatment of interstitial cystitis. J Urol 2004;172(2):533–6.
54. Nickel JC, Barkin J, Forrest J, et al, for the Elmiron Study Group. Randomized, double-blind, dose-ranging study of pentosan polysulfate sodium for interstitial cystitis. Urology 2005;65(4):654–8.
55. Nickel JC, Kaufman DM, Zhang HF, et al. Time to initiation of pentosan polysulfate sodium treatment after interstitial cystitis diagnosis: effect on symptom improvement. Urology 2008;71(1):57–61.
56. Sairanen J, Tammela TL, Leppilahti M, et al. Cyclosporine A and pentosan polysulfate sodium for the treatment of interstitial cystitis: a randomized comparative study. J Urol 2005;174(6):2235–8.
57. Thilagarajah R, Witherow RO, Walker MM. Oral cimetidine gives effective symptom relief in painful bladder disease: a prospective, randomized, double-blind placebo-controlled trial. BJU Int 2001;87(3):207–12.
58. Korting GE, Smith SD, Wheeler MA, et al. A randomized double-blind trial of oral L-arginine for treatment of interstitial cystitis. J Urol 1999;161(2):558–65.
59. Sant GR, Propert KJ, Hanno PM, et al. A pilot clinical trial of oral pentosan polysulfate and oral hydroxyzine in patients with interstitial cystitis. The Interstitial Cystitis Clinical Trials Group. J Urol 2003;170(3):810–5.
60. Soucy F, Grégoire M. Efficacy of prednisone for severe refractory ulcerative interstitial cystitis. J Urol 2005;173(3):841–3.
61. Butrick CW. Pelvic floor hypertonic disorders: identification and management. Obstet Gynecol Clin North Am 2009;36(3):707–22.
62. Bouchelouche K, Nordling J, Hald T, et al. The cysteinyl leukotriene D4 receptor antagonist montelukast for the treatment of interstitial cystitis. J Urol 2001;166(5):1734–7.
63. van Ophoven A, Hertle L. The dual serotonin and noradrenaline reuptake inhibitor duloxetine for the treatment of interstitial cystitis: results of an observational study. J Urol 2007;177(2):552–5.
64. Dawson TE, Jamison J. Intravesical treatments for painful bladder syndrome/interstitial cystitis. Cochrane Database Syst Rev 2007;4:CD006113.
65. Welk BK, Teichman JM. Dyspareunia response in patients with interstitial cystitis treated with intravesical lidocaine, bicarbonate, and heparin. Urology 2008;71(1): 67–70.
66. Parsons CL. Successful down-regulation of bladder sensory nerves with combination of heparin and alkalinized lidocaine in patients with interstitial cystitis. Urology 2005;65(1):45–8.
67. Nickel JC, Moldwin R, Lee S, et al. Intravesical alkalinized lidocaine (PSD597) offers sustained relief from symptoms of interstitial cystitis and painful bladder syndrome. BJU Int 2009;103(7):910–8.
68. Mayer R, Propert KJ, Peters KM, et al. A randomized controlled trial of intravesical bacillus Calmette-Guerin for treatment refractory interstitial cystitis. The Interstitial cystitis CLinical trials Group. J Urol 2005;173:1186–91.
69. Propert KJ, Mayer R, Nickel JC, et al. Follow-up of patients with interstitial cystitis responsive to treatment with intravesical bacillus calmette-guerin or placebo. J Urol 2008;179.

70. Mayer R, Propert KJ, Peters KM, et al. A randomized controlled trial of intravesical bacillus calmette-guerin for treatment refractory interstitial cystitis. J Urol 2005; 173(4):1186–91.
71. Lazzeri M, Beneforti P, Spinelli M, et al. Intravesical resiniferatoxin for the treatment of hypersensitive disorder: a randomized placebo controlled study. J Urol 2000;164(3 Pt 1):676–9.
72. Anderson L, Lewis SE, McClure N. The effects of coital lubricants on sperm motility in vitro. Hum Reprod 1998;13:3351–6.
73. Haefner HK, Collins ME, Davis GD, et al. The vulvodynia guideline. J Low Genit Tract Dis 2005;9(1):40–51.
74. Clayton A, Hamilton D. Female sexual dysfunction. Psychiatr Clin North Am 2010; 33(2):323–38.
75. Ferguson DM, Steidle CP, Singh GS, et al. Randomized, placebo-controlled, double-blind, crossover design trial of the efficacy and safety of "Zestra for Women" in women with and without female sexual arousal disorder. J Sex Marital Ther 2003;29(Suppl 1):33–44.
76. Whitmore KE. Complementary and alternative therapies as treatment approaches for interstitial cystitis. Rev Urol 2002;4(Suppl 1):S28–35.
77. Rothrock NE, Lutgendorf SK, Kreder KJ. Coping strategies in patients with interstitial cystitis: relationships with quality of life and depression. J Urol 2003;169(1): 233–6.
78. Nickel JC, Tripp D, Teal V, et al, for the Interstitial Cystitis Collaborative Trials Group. Sexual function is a determinant of poor quality of life for women with treatment refractory interstitial cystitis. J Urol 2007;177(5):1832–6.
79. Rovner E, Propert KJ, Brensinger C, et al. Treatments used in women with interstitial cystitis: the interstitial cystitis data base (ICDB) study experience. The Interstitial Cystitis Data Base Study Group. Urology 2000;56(6):940–5.
80. Powell CR, Kreder KJ. Long-term outcomes of urgency–frequency syndrome due to painful bladder syndrome treated with sacral neuromodulation and analysis of failures. J Urol 2010;183(1):173–6.
81. Rofeim O, Hom D, Freid RM, et al. Use of the neodymium: YAG laser for interstitial cystitis: a prospective study. J Urol 2001;166(1):134–6.
82. Webster DC, Brennan T. Interstitial cystitis. Arch Gynecol Obstet 2007;275(4): 223–9.
83. Abbott JA, Jarvis SK, Lyons SD, et al. Botulinum toxin type A for chronic pain and pelvic floor spasm in women: a randomized controlled trial. Obstet Gynecol 2006; 108(4):915–23.
84. Marinkovic SP, Moldwin R, Gillen LM, et al. The management of interstitial cystitis or painful bladder syndrome in women. BMJ 2009;339:b2707.
85. Rothrock NE, Lutgendorf SK, Hoffman A, et al. Depressive symptoms and quality of life in patients with interstitial cystitis. J Urol 2002;167(4):1763–7.
86. Forrest JB, Dell JR. Successful management of interstitial cystitis in clinical practice. Urology 2007;69(Suppl 4):82–6.

Prostatitis: Acute and Chronic

Kalyanakrishnan Ramakrishnan, MD*,
Robert C. Salinas, MD, CAQ Geriatrics

KEYWORDS

- Prostatitis • Acute prostatitis • Acute bacterial prostatitis
- Chronic prostatitis • Evaluation and treatment of prostatitis
- Urological infections

Prostatitis is one of the most common urological infections afflicting adult men and has recently been divided into 4 different categories based on the National Institutes of Health (NIH) consensus classification.[1] This category system includes category I (acute bacterial prostatitis), category II (chronic bacterial prostatitis), category III chronic nonbacterial prostatitis and pelvic pain syndrome, including inflammatory and noninflammatory types (CP/CPPS), and category IV (asymptomatic inflammatory prostatitis). **Table 1** shows the frequencies of the various types of prostatitis as well as the symptoms and physical examination findings characteristic of each type. Bacterial prostatitis is also classified as acute or chronic based on the duration of symptoms, with chronic cases having symptoms persisting for at least 3 months.[2] Acute and chronic bacterial prostatitis affects less than 5% of men with prostatitis.[3] Most patients with prostatitis are found to have either nonbacterial prostatitis or prostatodynia.[4]

One survey of 5000 primary care doctors and 545 urologists estimated the prevalence of prostatitis to be about 9.7%.[5] The cumulative incidence of recurrence is much higher (20%–50%), increasing in the older age groups.[5] A more recent population-based study involving men 25 to 80 years old indicated that nearly 1 in 9 men reported experiencing prostatitis-like symptoms.[6] The incidence of acute prostatitis peaks between 20 and 40 years of age and then peaks again after 60 years. Patients with symptoms of prostatitis seem to be at increased risk for recurrent episodes. One retrospective analysis of 968 patients with acute prostatitis showed the mean age at presentation of acute bacterial prostatitis to be 53.3 years. In this study, 15% reported having had previous episodes, another 10% had recently undergone lower urinary tract procedures (mostly prostate biopsy or urethral catheterization), and 13.6% had undergone urologic surgery.[7] Chronic prostatitis is more common after the middle of the fifth decade.[4]

Department of Family and Preventive Medicine, University of Oklahoma Health Sciences Center, Oklahoma City, OK 73104, USA
* Corresponding author.
E-mail address: kramakrishnan@ouhsc.edu

Prim Care Clin Office Pract 37 (2010) 547–563
doi:10.1016/j.pop.2010.04.007
0095-4543/10/$ – see front matter © 2010 Elsevier Inc. All rights reserved.

Table 1
NIH Consensus definition and classification of prostatitis[1]

Type	Description	Legend
I	Acute bacterial prostatitis (2%–5%)	Acute infection of the prostate gland characterized by local and systemic symptoms (dysuria, frequency, suprapubic/pelvic/perineal pain, fevers, chills, malaise); uropathogen identified; responds to antibiotics
II	Chronic bacterial prostatitis (2%–5%)	Chronic infection of prostate characterized by episodic dysuria, frequency, and suprapubic/pelvic/perineal pain); no systemic symptoms, uropathogen identified; responds to antibiotics, asymptomatic between infections
III	Chronic abacterial prostatitis/ Chronic pelvic pain syndrome (90%–95%)	No demonstrable infection. Causes local symptoms (pelvic pain, urinary symptoms, ejaculatory dysfunction); usually no identifiable uropathogen or infection; treatment often unsuccessful. The National Institutes of Health Chronic Prostatitis Symptom Index (NIH-CPSI) used to quantify severity
A	Inflammatory CPPS	White blood cells in semen, expressed prostatic secretions or urine obtained after prostate massage
B	Noninflammatory CPPS	No white blood cells in these body fluids
IV	Asymptomatic inflammatory prostatitis	No subjective symptoms; white blood cells in prostate secretions or in prostate tissue found incidentally during evaluation for other disorders

Data from Krieger JN, Nyberg L Jr, Nickel JC. NIH consensus definition and classification of prostatitis JAMA 1999;282(3):236–7.

From 1990 to 1994, prostatitis accounted for almost 2 million outpatient visits per year in the United States.[8] Race and ethnicity do not affect the incidence. Unemployment, lower education, and annual income of less than $50,000 are associated with more severe episodes of CPPS and more disability.[9] An estimated $84,452,000 was spent on treating prostatitis in 2000.[10] Men with CP/CPPS experienced considerable impairment in health-related quality of life (HRQOL), worse than patients in the most severe subgroups of diabetes mellitus and congestive heart failure.[11] Men with benign prostatic hypertrophy have an 8-fold greater risk of prostatitis. Other risk factors include lower urinary tract infection, a history of sexually transmitted disease, and stress.[12] Prostatitis also poses an international health problem, with epidemiologic studies suggesting a worldwide prevalence of more than 10%.[12]

Acute bacterial prostatitis in most patients probably originates from ascending urethral infections, and probably results from the reflux of infected urine into the ejaculatory and prostatic ducts that empty into the posterior urethra (intraprostatic urinary reflux). Ascending urethral infection may follow sexual intercourse or cystourethral instrumentation, such as bladder catherization.[13] Most infections occur in the periphery of the gland. Rarer causes include direct inoculation of infection into the prostate gland (such as during prostate biopsies), direct or lymphatic spread from the rectum, and hematogenous spread.[13] Acute bacterial prostatitis develops in 0.5% of patients after initial prostate biopsy and 4.7% of patients after re-biopsy, despite preprocedural prophylactic antibiotic administration.[14] However, the incidence of bacteremia is as high as 44% in patients undergoing transrectal biopsy of the prostate without preprocedural antibiotics. Factors that increase the likelihood of infectious inoculation of the prostate are the presence of an indwelling catheter and documented bacteriuria at the time of biopsy.[15,16] Common risk factors for bacterial prostatitis are enumerated in **Table 2**. The etiology and pathogenesis of chronic bacterial prostatitis, NIH category II (recurrent infection of the prostate), may involve several mechanisms, including high voiding pressures due to bladder neck obstruction, detrusor sphincter dyssynergia, pelvic floor muscle dysfunction, chronic urethral stricture, dysfunctional voiding, intraprostatic ductal reflux, alongside autoimmune and neuromuscular mechanisms.[17]

The most frequent organism causing acute prostatitis is *Escherichia coli* (87.5%), followed by *Pseudomonas, Proteus, Klebsiella*, and polymicrobial infections, as shown in **Table 3**.[7] Rarer organisms worthy of mention include *Streptococcus, Anaerobes, Ureaplasma, Mycoplasma genitalium, Trichomonas vaginalis, Chlamydia trachomatis*, and *Candida*. Pseudomonas and mixed infections are thought to be more common (20 and 9.5 times, respectively) after lower urinary tract manipulations.[7] Enterococci account for 5% to 10% of documented acute infections. *Neisseria gonorrhoeae* should be suspected in sexually active men younger than 35 years.[13] In patients

Table 2
Risk factors and pathogenesis of acute and chronic bacterial prostatitis

Acute Prostatitis	Chronic Prostatitis
Intraprostatic urine reflux	Lower urinary tract infection
Unprotected intercourse	Anatomic/physiologic lower
Phimosis, urethral stricture	urinary tract obstruction
Lower urinary tract infection	Voiding dysfunction
including epididymitis	Pelvic floor muscle dysfunction
Benign prostatic hypertrophy	Intraprostatic reflux of urate and
Indwelling urethral catheter	creatinine
Cystourethral instrumentation	Immune response
Prostate biopsies	Form of reflex sympathetic
Proctitis	dystrophy
	Benign prostatic hypertrophy

Data from Rhee JJ, Piesman M, Costabile RA. Acute bacterial prostatitis and prostatic abscess. Emedicine 2008. http://emedicine.medscape.com/article/439968. Accessed Sep. 5, 2009; Lobel B, Rodriguez A. Chronic prostatitis: what we know, what we do not know, and what we should do! World J Urol 2003;21(2):57–63.

Table 3
Bacteriology in acute and chronic bacterial prostatitis

Common Organisms	Uncommon Organisms
Escherichia coli	Neisseria gonorrhoeae[a]
Pseudomonas[c]	Ureaplasma urealyticum[b]
Proteus	Mycoplasma genitalium[b]
Klebsiella	Trichomonas vaginalis[a]
Streptococcus	Chlamydia trachomatis[a]
Enterococcus	Mycobacterium tuberculosis[c]
Staphylococcus aureus	Serratia[c]
Polymicrobial infections++	Salmonella[c]
	Fungi[c] (Candida, Histoplasma, Aspergillus, Cryptococcus)

[a] More common in younger sexually active men.
[b] Usually seen in immunosuppressed individuals.
[c] More common after transurethral procedures, including bladder drainage.
   Data from Millan-Rodriguez F, Palou J, Bujons-tour A, et al. Acute bacterial prostatitis: two different sub-categories according to a previous manipulation of the lower urinary tract. World J Urol 2006;24(1):45–50; Benway BM, Moon TD. Bacterial prostatitis. Urol Clin N Am 2008;35(1):23–32; Etienne M, Chavanet P, Sibert L, et al. Acute bacterial prostatitis: heterogeneity in diagnostic criteria and management. Retrospective multicentric analysis of 371 patients diagnosed with acute prostatitis. BMC Infect Dis 2008;30;8–12.

with immune deficiencies including human immune deficiency viral syndrome (HIV), pathogens such as Mycobacterium tuberculosis, Serratia, Salmonella, and fungi (Candida, Histoplasma, Aspergillus, Cryptococcus) have been found.[18] The most common pathogens isolated in chronic prostatitis include E coli (over 80%), followed by Klebsiella, Pseudomonas, and Proteus. In one study, 27% of patients with chronic prostatitis were noted to have a urethral infection or colonization by Chlamydia.[19]

The ability of certain bacteria to adhere to uroepithelial cells through specific fimbriae and adhesins is thought to be critical for the initiation of prostatic infection. Virulence factors play important roles in the pathogenesis of acute prostatitis due to the common organism E coli. E coli strains causing prostatitis are more pathogenic than other strains, and have a greater degree of biofilm formation.[20]

Acute bacterial prostatitis is characterized by localized suprapubic or rectal pain, systemic symptoms (chills, fever, malaise, nausea, vomiting), and lower urinary tract symptoms (dysuria, frequency, urgency). Fever and dysuria are the most common presenting complaints and occur in more than three-fourths of patients, whereas pelvic pain and chills are identified in less than half the patients.[21] Hematuria is seen in 17% to 20% of patients.[7,21] Other systemic complaints may include generalized aches and pains, anorexia, lethargy, and acute mental status changes, especially in elderly patients. Bladder neck spasm may result in urinary retention and is seen in around one-fifth of patients. A history of urinary tract infection is noted in over a third of patients (37%), and 40% also report a prior history of prostatitis.[21] Patients may also present with gram-negative bacteremia and sepsis, characterized by acute mental status changes, high fevers and chills, diaphoresis, and hypotension due to cardiovascular compromise.

On examination, lower abdominal tenderness and a distended bladder may be present. A thickened and tender unilateral or bilateral epididymis and perianal spasm may be detected. An enlarged tender prostate is characteristic, and is seen in more than 90% of patients.[7] Rectal examination should be performed gently, and prostatic massage is not advised in acute prostatitis, as it may precipitate bacteremia or frank sepsis.

A common presentation of NIH category II chronic bacterial prostatitis is one of recurrent lower urinary tract infections responding to appropriate antibiotics. The infections typically recur with the same pathogen.[22] Pain (lower abdominal, perineal, testicular, scrotal, rectal, back) and lower urinary tract symptoms (dysuria, frequency, hesitancy, weak urinary stream) are the most common symptoms in patients with chronic prostatitis. Other features are painful ejaculation, change in color of semen, retarded ejaculation, and erectile dysfunction. Miscellaneous symptoms include depression, anxiety, and fatigue.[17] The NIH chronic prostatitis symptom index (NIH-CPSI, shown in **Table 4**) is a measure of the presence and intensity of symptoms in chronic prostatitis and their impact on quality of life. This index is useful in diagnosis, progression, and assessment of the effects of various treatment measures. It is easily self-administered and highly discriminative.[23]

In immunocompetent patients with acute prostatitis, a complete blood count shows a leukocytosis with an increased number of immature neutrophils (a "left shift"). Dipstick urinalysis may detect proteinuria, pyuria, and hematuria. A complete urinalysis, including Gram stain and culture, can help to identify the offending organism. A combination of the leukocyte esterase and nitrite tests (both tests positive) has a sensitivity of 68% to 88%; in the presence of a contributory history and examination it is also sufficiently specific to rule in infection.[24]

Table 4
NIH Chronic Prostatitis Symptom Index (NIH-CPSI) (maximum score = 38)

Symptom		Patient Response, Score
Pain/Discomfort	Perineal pain	Yes 1; No 0
	Penile pain (unrelated to urination)	Yes 1; No 0
	Testicular pain	Yes 1; No 0
	Hypogastric pain	Yes 1; No 0
	Dysuria, burning micturition	Yes 1; No 0
	Painful ejaculation	Yes 1; No 0
Average pain intensity over past week over any of these areas (0–10)		No pain 0; worst pain 10
Urination	Sense of incomplete emptying (0–5 based on frequency)	Never 0; <1 in 5 1; <half the time 2; half the time 3; >half the time 4; almost always 5
	Needing to urinate again within 2 h (0–5 based on frequency)	As above
Impact of symptoms	Preventing routine activities over past week (0–3, based on frequency)	Never 0; a little 1; some 2; a lot 3
	Thought of symptoms (0–3 based on frequency)	As above
Quality of life	Patient perception of quality of life if symptoms persisted for rest of life (0–6 based on level of satisfaction)	Delighted 0; pleased 1; satisfied 2; neither satisfied/dissatisfied 3; dissatisfied 4; unhappy 5; terrible 6.

Data from Litwin MS, McNaughton-Collins M, Fowler FJ Jr, et al. The National Institutes of Health chronic prostatitis symptom index: development and validation of a new outcome measure. Chronic Prostatitis Collaborative Research Network. J Urol 1999;162(2):369–75.

Gram stain analysis of urine can help guide the choice of initial antibiotic therapy. Urine microscopy usually shows numerous red and white blood cells, and the presence of greater than 5 to 10 white cells per high-power field is highly suggestive of a urinary infection. Gram stain of urethral swabs, culture of urethral secretions, and DNA amplification tests are all useful in detecting Gonococci and Chlamydia. Expressed prostatic secretions will contain many leukocytes and macrophages. Blood cultures may be positive but are generally indicated only in immunosuppressed patients, if a hematogenous source is suspected, or if complications occur. In one retrospective study of 338 patients with upper urinary tract infection, only one blood culture grew a uropathogen not found on urine culture.[25] Altered renal or hepatic function can occur due to sepsis, as well as from back pressure following prostate enlargement. Serum C-reactive protein is usually elevated. Prostate-specific antigen (PSA) levels are elevated in most patients with acute bacterial prostatitis because inflammation disrupts the prostatic ducts and causes leakage of PSA. PSA levels normalize when infection resolves following antibiotic treatment.[26] PSA testing has little clinical value in acute prostatitis, and if elevated, should be repeated 30 to 60 days after adequate treatment. Transrectal ultrasonography (TRUS) and computed tomography (CT) are useful in excluding abscess formation. However, nearly 50% of patients have sonographically demonstrable lesions in peripheral lobules of the prostate, most of which resolve or shrink after treatment.[27] Ultrasound is useful in documenting residual urine and confirming urinary retention. Imaging studies are also indicated when clinical and other laboratory results are equivocal, or when no improvement is observed within 36 hours after institution of medical therapy.[22] Indium-111–labeled leukocyte imaging can be useful in diagnosing acute prostatitis and monitoring treatment response.[28] Prostate biopsy should not be performed in acute prostatitis because it may precipitate gram-negative sepsis.

Urinalysis and urine culture are useful in diagnosis and treatment of chronic prostatitis. The urine specimen should include midstream pre-massage and post-massage specimens known as the 2-glass test.[29] In the 4-glass test, as described by Meares and Stamey, first voided urine (VB1), midstream urine (VB2), urine after prostatic massage (VB3), and expressed prostatic secretions (EPS) are collected and used to localize the site of infection. The initial 10 mL of voided urine represents urethral source; the standard midstream specimen localizes vesical infection. The last 2 specimens directly examine prostatic secretions. A direct comparison of the sensitivities of the standard 4-glass test with the 2-glass test found the 2-glass test to be 96% to 98% as accurate as the 4-glass test, with the VB3 specimen failing to predict positive EPS specimens in only a small number of patients (sensitivity 92%, specificity 98%).[30] Semen cultures are more sensitive than EPS (97% vs 82.4%) in diagnosing chronic bacterial prostatitis.[31] Urodynamic studies are useful in patients with predominantly voiding symptoms, and can be used to supplement office evaluations of uroflow and post-void residual urine volumes. These tests can help to diagnose prostatic obstruction, primary bladder neck obstruction, dysfunctional voiding, urethral obstruction, and detrusor-sphincter dyssynergia.[32] Cystoscopy is recommended in any patient with a history of hematuria or abnormal urine cytology. Cystoscopy should also be considered in elderly patients with irritative or obstructive voiding symptoms, which are potential manifestations of bladder cancer in this age group.

An abscess involving the prostate gland is uncommon but can be a potentially serious complication of acute prostatitis. Risk factors include long-term urinary catheterization, recent urethral manipulation, hepatic cirrhosis, diabetes mellitus, renal failure, and other immunosuppressed states, including HIV/AIDS.[18,33] The pathogenesis and clinical features of prostate abscess are similar to those of acute bacterial prostatitis. *E coli* and *Staphylococcus* are the most common pathogens. Rarer pathogens, including *Mycobacterium tuberculosis*, *Actinomyces*, and *Bacteroides fragilis*, may be seen in immunosuppressed patients.[18] Left untreated an abscess may enlarge, spreading beyond the prostate to involve the bladder and the perirectal space, forming a pelvic abscess. Abscesses appear as hypoechoic areas with increased blood flow on TRUS.[33] TRUS is the imaging modality of choice due to its high sensitivity, cost-effectiveness, and diagnostic and treatment potential. CT is useful in delineating widespread infections or when findings on TRUS are equivocal. Recommended treatment consists of hospitalization, intravenous broad-spectrum antibiotics, and pain relief. Percutaneous or transrectal ultrasound-guided perineal drainage is minimally invasive and effective.[34,35] In large abscesses, temporary urinary diversion through suprapubic cystostomy or nephrostomy is often required.

Evaluation of prostatitis should commence with a history and examination (**Box 1**). Questions should address the presence or absence of lower urinary tract symptoms, sexual history including erectile and ejaculatory dysfunction, history of sexually transmitted diseases or urethritis, other coexisting medical problems such as diabetes

---

Box 1
Evaluation of acute and chronic prostatitis

Acute prostatitis

   History: Lower urinary tract symptoms, sexual history, history of sexually transmitted diseases/urethritis, coexisting medical problems, history of prior inguinal or pelvic surgery

   Physical examination: Abdominal, genital, perineal, and gentle digital rectal examination

   Complete blood count, urinalysis, and urine culture

   Blood culture: If immunosuppressed patient, suspected hematogenous source, or complications such as sepsis, abscess formation

   Transrectal ultrasonography (TRUS): Useful in diagnosis of prostatitis and abscess, abscess drainage

   Computed tomography (CT): Useful in diagnosis and drainage of prostatic/pelvic abscess, ruling out other pelvic pathology mimicking prostatitis

   Labeled leukocyte studies (Indium-111, Gallium-67): Useful in diagnosing acute prostatitis and complications, monitoring treatment response

Chronic prostatitis

   History of recurrent lower urinary tract infections, duration of symptoms longer than 3 months

   Abdominal, genital, perineal, and rectal examination

   NIH-CPSI scoring: Assesses impact of symptoms on patient's quality of life

   Urinalysis and culture, urine cytology

   Prostate-specific antigen monitoring, and biopsy if risk for prostate cancer

   Measurement of post-void residual urine

   Lower urinary tract bacterial localization (2-glass or 4-glass) test

   Semen analysis and semen culture: If foul-smelling semen or infertile patient

   Imaging studies or other invasive investigations (cystoscopy, urodynamics) should be based on pathology suspected on initial investigations

mellitus and neurologic disorders, and history of prior inguinal or pelvic surgery.[32] Physical examination should include an abdominal, genital, perineal, and a gentle digital rectal examination. Urinalysis and urine culture should be performed on all patients.[32] Patients suspected of having acute prostatitis do not require further evaluation, and treatment can be started unless complications such as abscess formation are suspected. Chronic prostatitis should be suspected when there is a history of recurrent infections and duration of symptoms lasting longer than 3 months. The impact of the symptoms on the patient's quality of life should be documented using an instrument such as the NIH-CPSI. Prostate cancer should be excluded by serial PSA measurements, or with biopsy in patients considered to be at risk. PSA levels, if elevated, should be repeated following a few weeks of antibiotic treatment to ensure normalization.[36] Additional evaluation should focus on identifying the responsible organism and underlying pathology, and may be performed either before or during treatment. This evaluation may include post-void residual urine measurements to identify incomplete emptying, measuring urine flow rates to identify bladder outlet obstruction or decreased detrusor contractility, urine cytology to detect malignancy, and lower urinary tract bacterial localization tests (2-glass or 4-glass test). Semen analysis and culture are useful in patients complaining of foul-smelling semen or fertility problems. The decision to perform imaging studies or other invasive investigations (cystoscopy, urodynamics) should be based on pathology suspected on initial investigations.[32]

Antimicrobial treatment in patients with severe acute bacterial prostatitis or associated systemic sepsis should be initiated immediately after obtaining urine and blood cultures (**Fig. 1**). Patients may require hospital admission until systemic features of the illness are controlled, analgesia and voiding are satisfactory, and sepsis and complications are ruled out. Bladder drainage, if necessary, should be suprapubic to reduce the risk of prostatic abscess and septicemia.[37] Parenteral administration of a fluoroquinolone, an aminoglycoside with or without ampicillin, or an extended-spectrum cephalosporin with or without an aminoglycoside is recommended until fever and other signs and symptoms of infection subside (**Table 5**).[38] Aminoglycosides should be avoided in patients with preexisting renal disease. Oral antibiotics are commenced as soon as patients become afebrile, have improved clinically, and can tolerate oral hydration and medications. A fluoroquinolone or other antibiotic, based on culture reports, should be continued for at least 4 weeks. In less severe cases, a shorter duration of treatment (2–4 weeks) with a fluoroquinolone may be sufficient.[38,39] Resistance to fluoroquinolones among the common uropathogens remains very low (1%–3%).[40] Fluoroquinolones are generally well absorbed from the gastrointestinal tract and have excellent prostate penetration, favorable pharmacokinetic properties, good safety profile, and a broad-spectrum of antibacterial activity against gram-negative pathogens, including *Pseudomonas*.[38] Levofloxacin is also effective against gram-positive pathogens, and chlamydia and mycoplasma infections. In selected patient populations with moderate to severe urinary tract infections, intravenous and oral fluoroquinolones give equivalent clinical outcomes.[41] Fluoroquinolones have some disadvantages (phototoxicity, drug interactions, rash, jaundice, tendonitis and tendon rupture, peripheral neuropathy, central nervous system effects), and patients need to be monitored during prolonged treatment.

In the absence of fever and severe lower urinary tract symptoms, immediate antibacterial therapy is not routinely indicated in chronic prostatitis. Investigations to rule out other underlying causes should be initiated (within 1–2 weeks) and once determined or excluded, all patients (both culture-positive and culture-negative) should

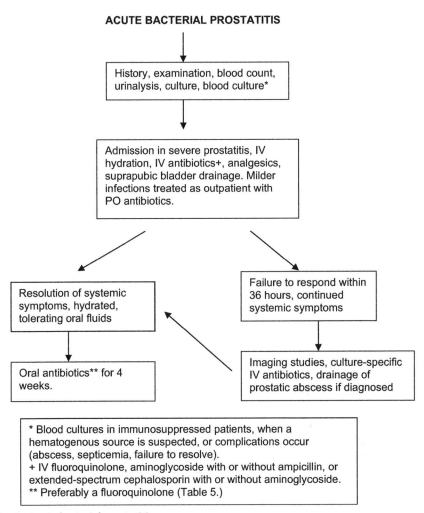

ACUTE BACTERIAL PROSTATITIS

History, examination, blood count, urinalysis, culture, blood culture*

Admission in severe prostatitis, IV hydration, IV antibiotics+, analgesics, suprapubic bladder drainage. Milder infections treated as outpatient with PO antibiotics.

Resolution of systemic symptoms, hydrated, tolerating oral fluids

Failure to respond within 36 hours, continued systemic symptoms

Oral antibiotics** for 4 weeks.

Imaging studies, culture-specific IV antibiotics, drainage of prostatic abscess if diagnosed

* Blood cultures in immunosuppressed patients, when a hematogenous source is suspected, or complications occur (abscess, septicemia, failure to resolve).
+ IV fluoroquinolone, aminoglycoside with or without ampicillin, or extended-spectrum cephalosporin with or without aminoglycoside.
** Preferably a fluoroquinolone (Table 5.)

Fig. 1. Acute bacterial prostatitis.

receive antibiotics, the choice of which will be influenced by the culture results (see **Table 2**). Antibiotics should be administered for an initial 2 weeks after diagnosis (**Fig. 2**). If cultures (urine, EPS, semen) are positive, or the patient notices significant clinical improvement, a total treatment period of 4 to 6 weeks is recommended.[36] In culture-negative prostatitis, antibiotics should be discontinued after 2 weeks in the absence of clinical improvement.[36] In chronic prostatitis and inflammatory CPPS (NIH types II and IIIA), the drugs of choice are high doses of oral fluoroquinolones that concentrate well in the urine, such as ciprofloxacin or levofloxacin. Other options include trimethoprim-sulfamethoxazole (Bactrim), tetracyclines, and macrolides. Bactrim has good penetration into prostatic tissue, may be administered orally or parenterally, is inexpensive, and is active against most common urologic pathogens (except *Pseudomonas* and some enterococci) (see **Table 5**). The tetracyclines share many of the advantages of Bactrim (inexpensive, available orally) and are active against chlamydia and mycoplasma. However, tetracyclines are contraindicated in hepatic or

Table 5
Antibiotic choices in acute and chronic bacterial prostatitis

Medication	Dosage and Administration (Parenteral, Oral)	Side Effects
Levofloxacin	250–750 mg daily IV or PO	GI effects, phototoxicity, drug interactions, rash, jaundice, tendonitis and tendon rupture, peripheral neuropathy, central nervous system effects
Ciprofloxacin	250–750 mg BID 400 mg IV BID	GI effects, headache, rash, photosensitivity
Ceftriaxone	1–2 g IV or IM daily	Phlebitis, rash, diarrhea, elevated liver enzymes
Cefotaxime	1–2 g every 8–12 h	As above
Gentamicin	3–5 mg/kg IV daily	GI effects, ototoxicity, nephrotoxicity, numbness, tingling, weakness, confusion, headache, drug interactions
Trimethoprim-sulfamethoxazole	8–10 mg/kg of trimethoprim IV every 12 h 160/800 mg PO every 12 h	GI effects, allergic reaction, erythema multiforme, weakness, insomnia
Ampicillin	1–2 g IV every 4–6 h 500 mg PO every 6 h	GI side effects, rash
Doxycycline	100 mg IV BID 100 mg PO BID	GI effects, *Clostridium difficile* colitis, photosensitivity, drug interactions, headache, allergic reactions
Clarithromycin	250–500 mg PO BID	GI effects, cholestatic jaundice, *C difficile* colitis, seizures
Azithromycin	250–500 mg daily	GI effects, headache, rash

Abbreviations: BID, twice a day; GI, gastrointestinal; IM, intramuscular; IV, intravenous; PO, by mouth.

renal dysfunction, and they have unreliable activity against coagulase-negative staphylococci, *E coli*, other Enterobacteriaceae, and enterococci. Macrolides, though possessing good penetration into the prostate gland, low toxicity, and activity against *Chlamydia*, are not useful in gram-negative infections.[38] The majority of patients with infections due to *E coli* and other Enterobacteriaceae (60%–80%) can be cured with a 4- to 6-week course of therapy. However, prostatitis due to *Pseudomonas aeruginosa* and enterococci often fails to respond to treatment. Recurrent episodes of prostatitis are best managed by either intermittent treatment or continuous low-dose suppressive therapy.[39]

Antibiotics may be administered into the prostate directly through the transperineal, transrectal, or suprapubic transvesical routes to treat chronic recurrent bacterial prostatitis (NIH category II).[42] Some broad-spectrum antibiotics (aminoglycosides) achieve

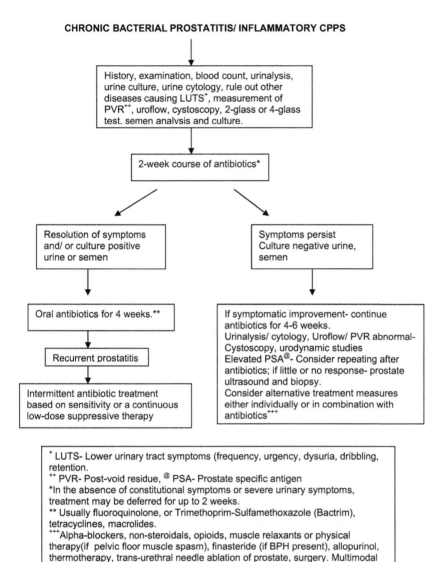

CHRONIC BACTERIAL PROSTATITIS/ INFLAMMATORY CPPS

History, examination, blood count, urinalysis, urine culture, urine cytology, rule out other diseases causing LUTS[+], measurement of PVR[++], uroflow, cystoscopy, 2-glass or 4-glass test. semen analysis and culture.

2-week course of antibiotics[*]

Resolution of symptoms and/ or culture positive urine or semen

Symptoms persist Culture negative urine, semen

Oral antibiotics for 4 weeks.[**]

Recurrent prostatitis

Intermittent antibiotic treatment based on sensitivity or a continuous low-dose suppressive therapy

If symptomatic improvement- continue antibiotics for 4-6 weeks.
Urinalysis/ cytology, Uroflow/ PVR abnormal- Cystoscopy, urodynamic studies
Elevated PSA[@]- Consider repeating after antibiotics; if little or no response- prostate ultrasound and biopsy.
Consider alternative treatment measures either individually or in combination with antibiotics[+++]

[+] LUTS- Lower urinary tract symptoms (frequency, urgency, dysuria, dribbling, retention.
[++] PVR- Post-void residue, [@] PSA- Prostate specific antigen
[*]In the absence of constitutional symptoms or severe urinary symptoms, treatment may be deferred for up to 2 weeks.
[**] Usually fluoroquinolone, or Trimethoprim-Sulfamethoxazole (Bactrim), tetracyclines, macrolides.
[+++]Alpha-blockers, non-steroidals, opioids, muscle relaxants or physical therapy(if pelvic floor muscle spasm), finasteride (if BPH present), allopurinol, thermotherapy, trans-urethral needle ablation of prostate, surgery. Multimodal approach to refractory pain, in consultation with specialists.

Fig. 2. Chronic bacterial prostatitis/inflammatory CPPS.

very low prostatic concentrations when administered intravenously or intramuscularly, while direct delivery enables high local concentrations to be achieved. Injected medications may also have an anti-inflammatory effect. Cure rates after 1 to 2 injections varies from 60% to 90%. Side effects include pain during injection, perineal discomfort (usually resolving in 24 hours), hematuria, dysuria, fever, and hematospermia lasting 1 to 2 weeks. This method should be reserved for patients who fail multiple courses of oral antibiotics.[42]

Patients with chronic prostatitis have high urethral closing pressures. Combination treatment with α-blockers (tamsulosin, terazosin, or alfuzosin) and antibiotics shows a higher cure rate than antibiotics alone in chronic prostatitis (NIH types IIIA and

B).[38] Men with more severe symptoms are significantly more likely to respond, with improved urinary symptoms and pain.[43] A placebo-controlled study of 90 patients with NIH type IIIB prostatitis treated with doxazosin (4 mg daily for 6 months, then followed for another 6 months) found good treatment response rates in nearly two-thirds.[44] Until larger definitive trials are completed, it seems reasonable to attempt treatment of CP/CPPS patients with an α-blocker for 3 to 6 months.[45]

Nonsteroidal anti-inflammatory drugs (NSAIDs) have been used in treating NIH category III prostatitis. Muscle relaxants in combination with NSAIDs are also thought to improve symptoms in patients with pelvic floor dysfunction. A systematic review of the literature showed some benefit from adding NSAIDs, and one randomized controlled trial using a combination of NSAIDs and muscle relaxants showed a 56% reduction in the NIH-CPSI scores in patients with type III prostatitis.[37,44,46]

Short-term opioids may be indicated for breakthrough or exacerbated pain and periodic flare-ups. Chronic opioid use for refractory pain will result in modest pain improvement but potentially poorer quality of life, and is ideally managed as part of multimodal therapy in consultation with a pain management specialist.[47]

Finasteride, a synthetic antiandrogen, has the potential to reduce the size and glandular component of the prostate and improve the urinary stream. In one randomized placebo-controlled trial, 64 patients with type III CPPS were randomized to finasteride or placebo for 6 months. Three-fourths of the patients on finasteride had mild improvement in symptoms; nearly half had moderate or marked improvement. Finasteride, however, is not typically recommended as monotherapy, except in men who also have benign prostatic hyperplasia.[48]

Phytotherapy with Cernilton (extract of rye pollen), quercetin (bioflavinoid found in red wine, green tea, and onions), or saw palmetto (a berry extract) is not approved for CPPS by the Food and Drug Administration. These plant and herbal substances are touted as having antioxidant, antiandrogenic, and anti-inflammatory properties. In one prospective, randomized trial, 64 patients with CP/CPPS treated with saw palmetto had no appreciable long-term improvement.[49] Quercetin at 500 mg twice daily for 1 month is well tolerated and results on average in a 35% improvement in the NIH-CPSI, with over two-thirds of patients experiencing a 25% improvement.[50]

Organisms sequestered in the prostate may be expressed by prostate massage and then eradicated by antibiotics. Massage may also open up occluded prostatic ducts, enable better antibiotic penetration, disrupt bacterial biofilms, and stimulate a neuro-muscular trigger point along the pelvic side wall. A systematic review of the literature suggests that prostate massage (2–3 times per week for 4–6 weeks) with concurrent antibiotic treatment provides relief in a quarter to a third of patients with CP/CPPS,[51] though it still lacks clear evidence of benefit.

Pentosan polysulfate, structurally similar to the glycosaminoglycans of the bladder that form a protective epithelial barrier, has anti-inflammatory effects. One trial involving 100 men with CP/CPPS randomized to oral pentosan polysulfate, 300 mg 3 times daily, or placebo for 16 weeks showed that the patients on pentosan polysulfate exhibited improvement in symptoms relative to placebo, but this did not achieve statistical significance.[52]

A pilot study involving acupuncture twice weekly for 6 weeks in patients with CP/CPPS resulted in a significant (>50%) improvement in the NIH-CPSI score in most patients.[53] Intraprostatic reflux of urine may cause prostatic inflammation by increasing the concentrations of purine- and pyrimidine-base–containing metabolites, including uric acid, in prostatic secretions. Because allopurinol should lower prostatic levels of uric acid, it could be beneficial in CP/CPPS. One randomized trial using allopurinol at 300 to 600 mg daily showed improvement in patient-reported pain, related symptoms, and biochemical parameters. However, the study was limited by small sample size, unvalidated outcome measures, and nonstandardized analyses. Routine use of allopurinol in treatment of CP/CPPS is currently not recommended.[54]

Pseudodyssynergia and pelvic floor muscle spasms cause overstimulation of the perineal and pelvic nerves and create a chronic neuropathic pain state. Symptomatic improvement of pelvic pain may result from relaxation and proper use of pelvic floor muscles through biofeedback, physical therapy, and pelvic floor reeducation. Many patients show improvement of pain, urgency, and frequency after 2 to 3 sessions, and no adverse reactions occur.[55]

Hyperthermia (42°–44°C) and thermotherapy (45°–50°C) delivered transrectally or transurethrally may induce fibrosis, kill occult bacteria, and modify pain perception in patients with CP/CPPS. In one small pilot study, patients with intractable CP/CPPS showed a 50% improvement in pain and quality of life scores as well as a 34% improvement in lower urinary tract symptom scores on the NIH-CPSI.[56] In the absence of large, randomized and controlled prospective studies, heat therapy for CP/CPPS should be considered only as a last resort for patients with symptoms refractory to standard treatments.[57] Transurethral needle ablation (TUNA) is another heat-based therapy using radiofrequency, creating a target temperature of 90° to 100°C in the central portion of the prostate. Although initial reports were favorable, a recent small, prospective, sham-controlled study did not demonstrate significant improvement in symptoms at 12 months.[58] A systematic review of the literature concluded that TUNA was not a suitable treatment choice in patients with intractable CP/CPPS.[59] Low-intensity laser radiation may diminish symptoms and improve prostatic function through anti-inflammatory and analgesic effects. Although some trials have shown benefit, conclusive proof of efficacy is still lacking.[57]

Surgical procedures have a limited though definite role in the management of prostatitis. Urinary retention due to bladder neck spasm in acute prostatitis resolves on catheterization. Suprapubic catheter placement minimizes periurethral complications, including abscess formation. However, it can cause bleeding, infection, injury to soft tissues and pelvic viscera, as well as risks of catheter blockage, recurrent cystitis, and upper tract infections.[60] Prostatic abscess may be drained through the urethra, perineum, or rectum; a percutaneous ultrasound-guided drainage is preferred. Patients with primary bladder neck obstruction and CPPS-related symptoms who fail medical therapy may benefit from transurethral incision of prostate (TUIP), with significant improvement in flow pattern and resolution of pain. Transurethral resection of the prostate (TURP) may be considered if all other less-invasive modalities fail, especially in patients who have prostatic calculi, persisting bacteria in prostatic secretions, or contraindications to antibacterial treatment.[57] Radical prostatectomy may benefit patients with nonbacterial prostatitis (category IIIA), prostatodynia (category IIIB), or both. However, aggressive surgeries for chronic prostatitis generally cause more problems, have not been critically assessed, and are neither encouraged nor recommended.[57]

The majority of patients with prostatitis have either nonbacterial prostatitis or prostatodynia. The NIH-CPSI (see **Table 4**) measures the intensity of symptoms in chronic prostatitis and their impact on quality of life. Acute bacterial prostatitis should be diagnosed on the basis of clinical presentation and cultures obtained; antibiotic treatment should be commenced and continued for 4 weeks. In the absence of fever and severe lower urinary tract symptoms, immediate antibiotics are not indicated in chronic prostatitis until other underlying causes have been excluded. In types II and IIIA prostatitis, antibiotics are recommended initially for 2 weeks, and then continued for 2 to 4 more weeks if organisms are grown or patients improve clinically. Finasteride is useful in patients with concomitant BPH. α-Blockers may help relieve bladder spasm and improve cure rates when combined with antibiotics. Benefits of phytotherapy, acupuncture, biofeedback, hyperthermia, TUNA, and other more invasive therapies are either unproven or have strictly limited roles in managing CP/CPPS.

REFERENCES

1. Krieger JN, Nyberg L Jr, Nickel JC. NIH consensus definition and classification of prostatitis. JAMA 1999;282(3):236–7.
2. Prostatitis and chronic pelvic pain syndrome In: Grabe M, Bishop MC, Bjerklund-Johansen TE, et al, editor, Guidelines on the management of urinary and male genital tract infections. Arnhem, The Netherlands: European Association of Urology (EAU); 2008 Mar. p. 79–88. Available at: http://www.guideline.gov/summary/summary.aspx?ss=15&doc_id=12586&string=. Accessed September 20, 2009.
3. Krieger JN, Egan KJ, Ross SO, et al. Chronic pelvic pains represent the most prominent urogenital symptoms of chronic prostatitis. Urology 1996;48(5): 715–21 [discussion: 721–2].
4. Schaeffer AJ. Epidemiology and demographics of prostatitis. Andrologia 2003; 35(5):252–7.
5. Nickel JC, Downey J, Hunter D, et al. Prevalence of prostatitis-like symptoms in a population-based study using the National Institutes of Health chronic prostatitis symptom index. J Urol 2001;165(3):842–5.
6. Clemens JQ, Meenan RT, O'Keeffe-Rosetti MC, et al. Prevalence of prostatitis-like symptoms in a managed care population. J Urol 2006;176(2):593–6 [discussion: 596].
7. Millan-Rodriguez F, Palou J, Bujons-Tur A, et al. Acute bacterial prostatitis: two different sub-categories according to a previous manipulation of the lower urinary tract. World J Urol 2006;24(1):45–50.
8. Collins MM, Stafford RS, O'Leary MP, et al. How common is prostatitis? A national survey of physician visits. J Urol 1998;159(4):1224–8.
9. Schaeffer AJ, Landis JR, Knauss JS, et al. Demographic and clinical characteristics of men with chronic prostatitis: the national institutes of health chronic prostatitis cohort study. J Urol 2002;168(2):593–8.
10. McNaughton-Collins M, Joyce GF, Wise M, et al. Prostatitis. NIH publication no. 07-5512. US Department of Health and Human Services, Public Health Service, National Institutes of Health, National Institute of Diabetes and Digestive and Kidney Diseases. In: Litwin MS, Saigal CS, editors. Urologic diseases in America. Washington, DC: US Government Publishing Office; 2007. p. 11–39.
11. McNaughton Collins M, Pontari MA, O'Leary MP, et al. Quality of life is impaired in men with chronic prostatitis: the Chronic Prostatitis Collaborative Research Network. J Gen Intern Med 2001;16(10):656–62.
12. Krieger JN, Riley DE, Cheah PY, et al. Epidemiology of prostatitis: new evidence for a world-wide problem. World J Urol 2003;21(2):70–4.
13. Rhee JJ, Piesman M, Costabile RA. Acute bacterial prostatitis and prostatic abscess. Emedicine 2008. Available at: http://emedicine.medscape.com/article/439968. Accessed September 5, 2009.
14. Shigehara K, Miyagi T, Nakashima T, et al. Acute bacterial prostatitis after transrectal prostate needle biopsy: clinical analysis. J Infect Chemother 2008;14(1):40–3.

15. Lindert KA, Kabalin JN, Terris MK. Bacteremia and bacteriuria after transrectal ultrasound guided prostate biopsy. J Urol 2000;164(1):76–80.
16. Lindstedt S, Lindstrom U, Ljunggren E, et al. Single-dose antibiotic prophylaxis in core prostate biopsy: impact of timing and identification of risk factors. Eur Urol 2006;50(4):832–7.
17. Lobel B, Rodriguez A. Chronic prostatitis: what we know, what we do not know, and what we should do! World J Urol 2003;21(2):57–63.
18. Benway BM, Moon TD. Bacterial prostatitis. Urol Clin North Am 2008;35(1):23–32.
19. Weidner W, Schiefer HG, Krauss H, et al. Chronic prostatitis a thorough search for etiologically involved microorganisms in 1461 patients. Infection 1991;19 (Suppl 3):S119–25.
20. Terai A, Yamomoto S, Mitsumori K, et al. *Escherichia coli* virulence factors and serotypes in acute bacterial prostatitis. Int J Urol 1997;4(3):289–94.
21. Etienne M, Chavanet P, Sibert L, et al. Acute bacterial prostatitis: heterogeneity in diagnostic criteria and management. Retrospective multicentric analysis of 371 patients diagnosed with acute prostatitis. BMC Infect Dis 2008;30(8):12.
22. Nickel JC. Recommendations for the evaluation of patients with prostatitis. World J Urol 2003;21(2):75–81.
23. Litwin MS, McNaughton-Collins M, Fowler FJ Jr, et al. The National Institutes of Health chronic prostatitis symptom index: development and validation of a new outcome measure. Chronic Prostatitis Collaborative Research Network. J Urol 1999;162(2):369–75.
24. Deville WL, Yzermans JC, van Duijn NP, et al. The urine dipstick test useful to rule out infections. A meta-analysis of the accuracy. BMC Urol 2004;4:1–4. Available at: http://www.ncbi.nlm.nih.gov/entrez/query.fcgi?cmd=Retrieve&db=PubMed&dopt=Citation&list_uids=15175113. Accessed September 14, 2009.
25. McMurray BR, Wrenn KD, Wright SW. Usefulness of blood cultures in pyelonephritis. Am J Emerg Med 1997;15(2):137–40.
26. Hara N, Koike H, Ogino S, et al. Application of serum PSA to identify acute bacterial prostatitis in patients with fever of unknown origin or symptoms of acute pyelonephritis. Prostate 2004;60(4):282–8.
27. Horcajada JP, Vilana R, Moreno-Martínez A, et al. Transrectal prostatic ultrasonography in acute bacterial prostatitis: findings and clinical implications. Scand J Infect Dis 2003;35(2):114–20.
28. Mateos JJ, Lomena F, Velasco M, et al. Diagnosis and follow-up of acute bacterial prostatitis and orchiepididymitis detected by In-111-labeled leukocyte imaging. Clin Nucl Med 2003;28(5):403–4.
29. Nickel JC. The Pre and Post Massage Test (PPMT): a simple screen for prostatitis. Tech Urol 1997;3(1):38–43.
30. Nickel JC, Shokses D, Wang Y, et al. How does the pre-massage and post-massage 2-glass test compare to the Meares-Stamey 4-glass test in men with chronic prostatitis/chronic pelvic pain syndrome? J Urol 2006;176(1):119–24.
31. Budía A, Luis Palmero J, Broseta E, et al. Value of semen culture in the diagnosis of chronic bacterial prostatitis: a simplified method. Scand J Urol Nephrol 2006;40(4):326–31.
32. Rothmann JR, Jaffe WI. Prostatitis: updates on diagnostic evaluation. Curr Urol Rep 2007;8(4):301–6.
33. Barozzi L, Pavlica P, Menchi I, et al. Prostatic abscess: diagnosis and treatment. AJR Am J Roentgenol 1998;170(3):753–7.

34. Leonhartsberger N, Pinggera G, Bektic J, et al. Percutaneous perineal drainage of prostatic abscesses using three-dimensional ultrasound guidance. Eur Urol Suppl 2008;7(3):159.
35. Aravantinos E, Kalogeras N, Zygoulakis N, et al. Ultrasound-guided transrectal placement of a drainage tube as therapeutic management of patients with prostatic abscess. J Endourol 2008;22(8):1751–4.
36. Bjerklund Johansen TE, Grüneberg RN, Guibert J, et al. The role of antibiotics in the treatment of chronic prostatitis: a consensus statement. Eur Urol 1998;34(6): 457–66.
37. Doble A. An evidence-based approach to the treatment of prostatitis: is it possible? Curr Urol Rep 2000;1(2):142–7.
38. Grabe M, Bishop MC, Bjerklund-Johansen TE, et al. Guidelines on urological infections. European association of urology 2009. Available at: http://www. uroweb.org/fileadmin/tx_eauguidelines/2009/Full/Urological_Infections.pdf. Accessed September 6, 2009.
39. Wagenlehner FM, Naber KG. Prostatitis: the role of antibiotic treatment. World J Urol 2003;21(2):105–8.
40. Nicolle LE. Urinary tract infection: traditional pharmacologic therapies. Am J Med 2002;113(Suppl 1A):35S–44.
41. Mombelli G, Pezzoli R, Pinoja-Lutz G, et al. Oral vs intravenous ciprofloxacin in the initial empirical management of severe pyelonephritis or complicated urinary tract infections: a prospective randomized clinical trial. Arch Intern Med 1999; 159(1):53–8.
42. Zvara P, Folsom JB, Plante MK. Minimally invasive therapies for prostatitis. Curr Urol Rep 2004;5(4):320–6.
43. Mishra VC, Browne J, Emberton M. Role of α-blockers in type III prostatitis: a systematic review of the literature. J Urol 2007;177(1):25–30.
44. Tugcu V, Tasci AI, Fazlioglu A, et al. A placebo-controlled comparison of the efficiency of triple- and monotherapy in category IIIB chronic pelvic pain syndrome (CPPS). Eur Urol 2007;51(4):1113–7 [discussion: 1118].
45. Duclos AJ, Lee C, Shoskes DA. Current treatment options in the management of chronic prostatitis. Ther Clin Risk Manag 2007;3(4):507–12.
46. Murphy AB, Macejko A, Taylor A, et al. Chronic prostatitis: management strategies. Drugs 2009;69(1):71–84.
47. Nickel JC. Opioids for chronic prostatitis and interstitial cystitis: lessons learned from the 11th World Congress on Pain. Urology 2006;68(4):697–701.
48. Nickel JC, Downey J, Pontari MA, et al. A randomized placebo-controlled multi-centre study to evaluate the safety and efficacy of finasteride for male chronic pelvic pain syndrome (category IIIA chronic nonbacterial prostatitis). BJU Int 2004;93(7):991–5.
49. Kaplan SA, Volpe MA, Te AE. A prospective, 1-year trial using saw palmetto versus finasteride in the treatment of category III prostatitis/chronic pelvic pain syndrome. J Urol 2004;171(1):284–8.
50. Shoskes DA, Zeitlin SI, Shahed A, et al. Quercetin in men with category III chronic prostatitis: a preliminary prospective, double-blind, placebo-controlled trial. Urology 1999;54(6):960–3.
51. Mishra VC, Browne J, Emberton M. Role of repeated prostatic massage in chronic prostatitis: a systematic review of the literature. Urology 2008;72(4):731–5.
52. Nickel JC, Forrest JB, Tomera K, et al. Pentosan polysulfate sodium therapy for men with chronic pelvic pain syndrome: a multicenter, randomized, placebo controlled study. J Urol 2005;173(4):1252–5.

53. Chen RC, Nickel JC. Acupuncture for chronic prostatitis/chronic pelvic pain syndrome. Curr Urol Rep 2004;5(4):305–8.
54. McNaughton CO, Wilt T. Allopurinol for chronic prostatitis. Cochrane Database Syst Rev 2002;4:CD001041.
55. Cornel EB, van Haarst EP, Schaarsberg RW, et al. The effect of biofeedback physical therapy in men with chronic pelvic pain syndrome type III. Eur Urol 2005;47(5):607–11.
56. Kastner C, Hochreiter W, Huidobro C, et al. Cooled transurethral microwave thermotherapy for intractable chronic prostatitis—results of a pilot study after 1 year. Urology 2004;64(6):1149–54.
57. El-Hakim A, Shah DK, Smith AD. Advanced therapy for prostatitis: minimally invasive and invasive therapies. Curr Urol Rep 2003;4(4):320–6.
58. Leskinen MJ, Kilponen A, Lukkarinen O, et al. Transurethral needle ablation for the treatment of chronic pelvic pain syndrome (category III prostatitis): a randomized, sham-controlled study. Urology 2002;60(2):300–4.
59. Kastner C. Update on minimally invasive therapy for chronic prostatitis/chronic pelvic pain syndrome. Curr Urol Rep 2008;9(4):333–8.
60. Ahluwalia RS, Johal N, Kouriefs C, et al. The surgical risk of suprapubic catheter insertion and long-term sequelae. Ann R Coll Surg Engl 2006;88(2):210–3.

Urinary Tract Stones

George R. Schade, MD[a], Gary J. Faerber, MD[a,b,c],*

KEYWORDS

- Urolithiasis • Urinary tract stones • Ureteral calculi
- Medical expulsive therapy • Nephrolithiasis • Lithotripsy

Approximately 13% of men and 7% of women in the United States will develop urinary tract stones at some time during their lives. Over the past 2 decades the prevalence of stones has increased by 37%.[1] The annual U.S. health care expenditure in 2001 for the treatment of urinary tract stones was $2.1 billion, which represents a 150% increase since 1980, and a 45% to 50% increase since 1994.[2]

EPIDEMIOLOGY

Stone formation is affected by gender, age, and geography. Men are more likely to form stones than women; however, the ratio has decreased from a 3:1 male to female predominance to less than 1.3:1.[1,3–5] Stone prevalence increases with age in both men and women, with the highest prevalence in the 4th and 5th decades. Historically, stones are three to four times more common in whites than in non-whites.[6,7] In the United States, the highest prevalence of stone disease was found in whites, followed in decreasing prevalence by Hispanics, Asians, and African Americans among men, and by Hispanics, African Americans, and Asians among women.[7,8] Other studies have suggested that lifestyle and diet may play a more significant role in stone formation than ethnicity.[9] Geography also seems to be a significant risk factor, with a higher prevalence of stone disease in hot, arid, or dry climates. Age-adjusted stone prevalence in the United States was highest in the South, followed by the East, Midwest, and West. Stone disease also seems to show a seasonal variation, which seems to be related to temperature. The highest incidence of stone disease in the United States occurs between July and September.[10] Water hardness does not seem to be associated with the incidence of stone episodes.[11]

[a] Department of Urology, University of Michigan Medical School, A. Alfred Taubman Health Care Center, 1500 East Medical Center Drive, Ann Arbor, MI 48109, USA
[b] Kidney Stone/Lithotriptor Program, A. Alfred Taubman Health Care Center, 1500 East Medical Center Drive, Ann Arbor, MI 48109, USA
[c] Michigan Center for Minimally Invasive Urology, A. Alfred Taubman Health Care Center, 1500 East Medical Center Drive, Ann Arbor, MI 48109, USA
* Corresponding author. Department of Urology, University of Michigan Medical School, A. Alfred Taubman Health Care Center, 1500 East Medical Center Drive, Ann Arbor, MI 48109.
E-mail address: gfaerber@med.umich.edu

Prim Care Clin Office Pract 37 (2010) 565–581
doi:10.1016/j.pop.2010.05.003
0095-4543/10/$ – see front matter © 2010 Elsevier Inc. All rights reserved.

The pathophysiology of stone formation within the kidney has not been fully elucidated, although a prerequisite for urinary stone formation is urinary crystal formation. Chemical and physical factors that play a role in crystal formation include supersaturated urine (overabundance of solute in a solution) and the presence or lack of urinary stone inhibitors (citrate, magnesium, zinc, macromolecules, and pyrophosphate) and matrix (a mucoprotein associated with stone formation). In normal human urine, the concentration of calcium oxalate (the most common stone composition) is four times higher than its solubility in water. Low urinary volume, low citrate, and increased calcium, oxalate, uric acid, and phosphate increase the chance of calcium oxalate supersaturation. Crystallization occurs when the concentration product exceeds the solubility product. According to the matrix theory, uromucoid activates the initial crystallization process by promoting formation of calcium oxalate and calcium phosphate.[12] Other possible explanations for stone formation include papillary vascular disease or Randall's plaques, resulting in crystal formation on cholesterol nidi.[13,14]

Inhibitory factors also mitigate these lithogenic factors. Citrate is a potent inhibitor of calcium oxalate and calcium phosphate stone formation because it can complex with calcium and reduce the availability of ionic calcium to bind oxalate or phosphate. In addition, citrate directly inhibits spontaneous precipitation of calcium oxalate.[15,16] Two glycoproteins are potent inhibitors of calcium oxalate crystal aggregation: nephrocalcin, which is synthesized in the proximal tubule, and Tamm-Horsfall protein, which is abundant in the loop of Henle and distal convoluted tubule.[17] Osteopontin is another glycoprotein excreted by the renal epithelial cells in the ascending loop of Henle; it works in conjunction with the Tamm-Horsfall protein to inhibit calcium oxalate crystallization.[18]

Additional lithogenic factors include a sedentary life style, obesity, certain dietary habits, a family history of stone disease, metabolic disorders (gout, hyperparathyroidism, type 1 renal tubular acidosis), and gastrointestinal diseases (colitis, Crohn's disease, ulcerative colitis). Obesity is a significant risk factor in stone formation. After adjusting for age, dietary factors, fluid intake, and thiazide use, the relative risk (RR) of stone formation was 1.33 in men with body mass index (BMI) greater than 30 compared with those with BMI less than 23. In women, the effect of BMI was even more pronounced, with an RR of 1.90. Weight gain also resulted in a higher risk: those who gained more than 35 pounds since the age of 18 to 21 years had an RR of stone disease of 1.92 (men) and 1.82 (women).[19] Obesity results in increased urinary excretion of uric acid, sodium, phosphate, and ammonium, and decreased urinary pH, all of which are associated with stone crystal formation.[19,20] Experimental studies have also shown a higher incidence of renal stone formation in animals fed a high fat diet.

STONE COMPOSITION

Most stones in the United States are calcium oxalate, calcium phosphate, or a combination of these components. **Table 1** shows the frequency of the various types of urinary tract stones. **Table 2** shows clinical factors that can be associated with each type of stone.

Calcium oxalate stones comprise 60% of all stones, whereas mixed calcium stones comprise another 20%. Hypercalciuria is the most common abnormality identified in calcium stone formers. It is defined as greater than 200 mg/d of urinary calcium after adherence to a 400 mg/d calcium and 100 mg/d sodium

Table 1
Frequency of types of urinary tract stones

Pure calcium oxalate	36%–70%
Pure calcium phosphate	6%–20%
Mixed calcium oxalate and phosphate	11%–31%
Struvite	6%–20%
Uric acid	6%–17%
Cystine	0.5%–3.0%
Miscellaneous	1%–4%

Adapted from Straub M, Hautman RE: Developments in stone prevention, Curr Opin Urol 2005;15:119–26; with permission.

diet for a 7-day period. Hypercalciuria may be from absorptive, resorptive, or renal leak abnormalities. Absorptive hypercalciuria is caused by an increased intestinal absorption of calcium, which may or may not be vitamin D–dependent. The elevated serum calcium results in PTH suppression, leading to increased calcium excretion. Resorptive hypercalciuria is most commonly seen in hyperparathyroidism, in which elevated PTH secretion from a parathyroid adenoma leads to bone resorption, enhanced intestinal absorption, and elevated serum and urinary levels of calcium. Hyperparathyroidism is the cause of urinary tract

Table 2
Clinical factors associated with various types of stones

Stone Type	Possible Clinical Associations
Calcium oxalate	Hypercalciuria
	Hypercalcemia
	Hyperoxaluria
	Hypocitraturia
	Gouty diathesis
	Low urinary volume
Calcium phosphate	Distal RTA
	Hyperparathyroidism
	Low urinary volume
	UTI
Uric acid	Gouty diathesis
	Gouty arthritis
	Gouty nephropathy
	Hyperuricosuria
	Hyperuricosemia
	Obesity
	Myeloproliferative disorders
	Tumor lysis syndrome
	Alcohol abuse
	Inborn errors of metabolism
Cystine	Cystinuria
Struvite	UTI (urea-splitting organisms)
Drug-induced stone	Indinavir, ephedrine, triamterene

stones for no more than 5% of patients. In renal leak hypercalciuria, there is impairment in renal tubular reabsorption, which leads to elevated PTH excretion. Patients with this secondary hyperparathyroid state maintain a homeostatic normal serum calcium by enhancing intestinal calcium absorption.

Hyperoxaluria is defined as urinary oxalate >40 mg/d. Enteric hyperoxaluria is the most common cause, and it is usually associated with chronic diarrheal states (Crohn's, ulcerative colitis, etc), small bowel resection, intestinal small bowel disease, jejuno-ileal bypass, and weight-reduction surgery (Roux-en-Y). In all of these conditions, there is fat malabsorption, which results in saponification of fatty acids and decreases the availability of calcium cations in the gut. As a result, the increased free enteric oxalate is absorbed, leading to higher urinary oxalate excretion. Dietary hyperoxaluria is caused by over-indulgence in oxalate-rich foods, such as nuts, chocolate, brewed teas, spinach, broccoli, strawberries, carrots, beans, dark beer, and colas. Some investigators have postulated that calcium oxalate stone-formers have decreased levels or absence of *Oxalobacter formigenes*, a gut bacteria which degrades oxalate.[21,22]

Hypocitraturia is defined as urinary citrate levels <200 mg/d. Causes of low urinary citrate levels include distal renal tubular acidosis, chronic diarrheal states, excessive animal protein ingestion, thiazide use, and strenuous activity resulting in lactic acidosis.

Uric acid stones comprise up to 10% of all stones. Uric acid is the end product of purine metabolism. The three main determinants of uric acid stone formation are: low urinary pH (<6), low urine volume, and hyperuricosuria. Congenital causes of uric acid stones include defects in renal tubular urate transport and uric acid metabolism. Acquired causes, which are much more common, include chronic diarrheal states, high animal protein diets, myeloproliferative disorders, and uricosuric medications. Interestingly, most patients with uric acid stones have normal urinary uric levels, but have low urinary pH.

Struvite stones, also called infection stones, are comprised of magnesium ammonium phosphate, and are caused by urea-splitting bacteria. Urea splitting produces ammonia and carbon dioxide and makes the urine alkaline. This highly alkaline state results in the precipitation of apatite and hydroxyapatite. The most common urea-splitting organisms are: Proteus, Klebsiella, Pseudomonas, and Staphylococcus species.[23] Struvite stones are twice as common in women as men. Patients at increased risk for the development of struvite stones include diabetics, those with urinary diversions, the elderly or the spinal cord injured with chronic urinary catheters. Struvite stones are often quite large at the time of diagnosis and may form a cast of the collecting system shaped somewhat like the horns of a stag, hence the common name "staghorn calculi" (**Fig. 1**).

Cystine stones make up a very small percentage of stones. They form as a result of a congenital defect in intestinal and renal tubular transport of the amino acids, cystine, ornithine, lysine, and arginine that increases their concentration in the urine. Cystine has poor solubility and is the only one of these amino acids that precipitates in the urine. Cystinuria is an autosomal recessive disorder associated with early onset stone disease, often presenting in children or teens.[24]

Medication-related stones are due to urinary precipitation and crystallization of the drug or its metabolite. Indinavir is a protease inhibitor used as an antiviral treatment for HIV or AIDS, which is only moderately soluble at normal urinary pH. Indinavir stones are unusual in that they are not seen on non-contrast CT imaging. Triamterene is a potassium-sparing diuretic that can precipitate in urine. Medication stones makes up a very small proportion (<0.4%) of stones.[25]

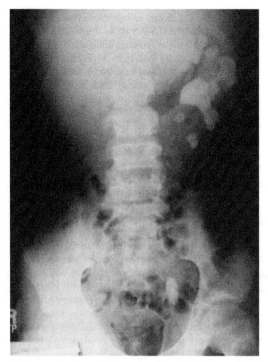

Fig. 1. Staghorn calculus and a large left ureteral calculus in a spinal cord injured 36 yo managed with a chronic foley catheter.

SIGNS AND SYMPTOMS

Patients with urinary tract stones present with a wide variation of symptoms, ranging from severe, agonizing pain to being completely asymptomatic. See **Box 1** for the differential diagnosis. Typical renal stone pain is chronic, episodic, flank discomfort. Ureteral colic, due to an acutely obstructing stone, is flank pain that is abrupt in onset, severe, colicky, and is often associated with nausea and emesis, which may mimic an acute gastrointestinal illness. Patients may complain of ipsilateral radiating groin pain. Approximately 10% will present with gross hematuria, while about 90% will have microscopic hematuria. In many cases, renal colic is associated with the inability of the patient to find a comfortable position, quite unlike patients with peritonitis who prefer to remain still.

Physical examination may show tachycardia and mild hypertension (due to pain), with ipsilateral costovertebral tenderness. Fever, if present, is an indication of an associated urinary tract infection and suggests a possible pyelonephritis.

A mild leukocytosis can be seen with an uncomplicated episode of renal colic. Significant leukocytosis may indicate a concomitant urinary tract infection. An elevated serum creatinine may indicate bilateral ureteral obstruction due to bilateral ureteral stones, an obstructing stone in a solitary kidney, or unilateral obstruction in a patient with pre-existing renal disease.

IMAGING FOR RENAL STONES

Plain abdominal x-ray is an excellent screening modality and is the most common radiologic method used to follow patients with known stone disease (see **Fig. 1**).

| Box 1 |
| Differential diagnosis of renal colic |

Abdominal aortic aneurysm

Appendicitis

Bowel obstruction

Cholecystitis

   Drug-seeking behavior

Gastritis

Mesenteric ischemia

Musculoskeletal pain

Ovarian abscess

Pelvic inflammatory disease

   Pyelonephritis

Ruptured ovarian cyst

   Ureteropelvic junction obstruction

Calcium oxalate and calcium phosphate stones, struvite stones, and cystine stones (to a lesser degree) can be seen on x-ray. Uric acid stones, however, are usually radiolucent. The intravenous pyelogram (IVP) was the study of choice before non-contrast spiral computed tomography (NCCT). NCCT has virtually supplanted the IVP, especially in the acute emergency room setting, for evaluation of a patient presenting with signs and symptoms consistent with urinary tract stones (**Figs. 2 and 3**). The advantages of the NCCT are: a rapid examination, no need for bowel prep or intravenous contrast, ability to diagnose non-urologic pathology, and superior accuracy for most types of renal stones.[26] However, there is an increased risk of radiation-induced cancer in patients who undergo recurrent CT imaging, so judicious use of CT should be practiced.[27] Renal ultrasound can be used for stone imaging and is preferred in children, pregnant women, and patients with uric acid stones.

MANAGEMENT OF ACUTE RENAL STONE DISEASE

Symptoms of obstructing stones can run the gamut from patients being in severe pain to being almost asymptomatic. Patients with severe renal colic should be encouraged to seek care at a local emergency room. Other indications for immediate emergency room evaluation are concomitant urinary tract infection, known solitary kidney or renal insufficiency, or significant co-morbid conditions. Patients who are otherwise healthy and are able to tolerate fluids for hydration can be treated with non-steroidal anti-inflammatory drugs, oral narcotic agents, and anti-emetics, if necessary. Patients should be encouraged to keep themselves vigorously hydrated and should strain their urine to retrieve the stone.

Most stones are less than 5 mm in diameter at the time of diagnosis. Approximately 60%–75% of stones 5 mm or less in diameter will pass without surgical intervention.[28] The larger a stone is, the lower the chance of spontaneous passage (**Table 3**). Ninety-five percent of distal ureteral stones <5 mm will pass spontaneously.[29] The average time for passage for stones <2 mm in diameter was 8.2 days (with a range of 2–11 days). Those that were 2–4 mm took on average 14.5 days (0–40) for distal stones,

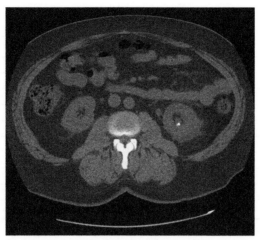

Fig. 2. Noncontrast CT Reveals a left renal stone. Note the soft tissue stranding around the kidney seen with acute obstruction. CT is the most accurate test to detect renal calculi. Calcium-containing stones, cystine, struvite, and uric acid stones are all radiopaque on CT.

and an average of 7 days (2–11) for proximal stones. Distal ureteral stones measuring 4–6 mm took an average of 5.5 days (0–17), while mid-ureteral and proximal stones of this size took an average of 6 and 53 days (15–105), respectively.[30]

Medical expulsive therapy (MET) has been developed to maximize the rate of spontaneous passage of ureteral stones, thereby minimizing the number of patients who require surgical intervention. At its most basic level, MET consists of pain control with NSAIDS and narcotics, and aggressive hydration to increase urine output and expel the stone. Non-steroidal anti-inflammatory medications (such as ketorolac) used in the acute setting appear to be equal or superior to narcotics for pain.[31] Substantial evidence over the last decade supports adding either an alpha blocker, generally tamsulosin, or a calcium channel blocker, to speed the expulsion of small

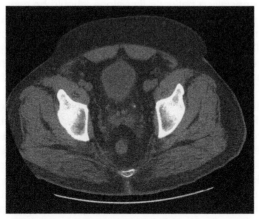

Fig. 3. Distal left ureteral calculus seen on noncontrast CT. Note the ureteral soft tissue around the stone.

Table 3
Spontaneous stone passage rate as a function of stone size

Stone Size (mm)	Number of Stones	Passage Rate (%)
1	15	87
2	43	72
3	23	83
4	18	72
5	15	60
6	18	72
7	17	47
8	9	56
9	3	33
10	11	27

Data from Coll DM, Varanelli MJ, Sith RC. Relationship of spontaneous passage of ureteral calculi to stone size and location as revealed by unenhanced helical CT. AJR Am J Roentgenol 2002;178:101–3; with permission.

ureteral stones. With a number needed to treat of less than 4, MET can increase the relative likelihood of spontaneous passage by 65% and decrease stone passage time by 10%–35%.[32] Secondary benefits of MET include decreased pain and narcotic usage, decreased time to spontaneous passage, and spontaneous passage of larger diameter stones.[33–35] Recently published cost analysis has shown that MET with tamsulosin saves more than $1100 per patient compared with observation alone, mainly by preventing unnecessary ureteroscopic interventions.[36] Additionally, there is some evidence to suggest that alpha blockers are superior to calcium channel blockers.[34] Patients with small ureteral stones (<8 mm), without evidence of infection or significant obstruction, in non-solitary kidneys, and who have satisfactory pain control, are routinely managed with a 10–14 day trial of tamsulosin at our institution.

METABOLIC EVALUATION AND TREATMENT

Knowing stone composition is essential for guiding treatment. For that reason, retrieved stones, especially a patient's first stone, should be sent for analysis. Risk factors mentioned earlier should be assessed. The initial laboratory evaluation should include urinalysis for urinary pH, specific gravity, and the presence of white blood cells, red blood cells, or crystals, as well as serum chemistries for creatinine, calcium, phosphorus, electrolytes, uric acid, and parathyroid hormone if serum calcium is high. Most patients who have passed a stone do not require any further metabolic evaluation.

About 50% of all stone formers will have an additional recurrence during their lifetimes, but if they follow the general lifestyle recommendations in **Box 2** the risk of repeated stone formation decreases to 10%–15%.[37,38] Approximately 10% of stone formers have more than 3 recurrences, and about 15% of all stone patients require specific metabolic measures for recurrence prevention.[39] For those with recurrent stones or other risk factors, additional metabolic evaluation should include a 24-urine collection for total urine volume, pH, phosphorus, calcium, oxalate, uric acid, magnesium, creatinine, citrate, and sodium, as well as a cystine spot urine test.

Medical management of urinary tract stones is a chronic endeavor that requires persistence and patience by both the health care practitioner and patient alike.

Box 2
Measures to prevent stone formation

Fluid intake, "drinking advice"

    Balanced

    Amount: 2.5–3.0 l/d

    Urine volume: 2.0–2.5 l/d

    Specific gravity of urine: <1.010

    Neutral beverages

    Circadian drinking

Balanced diet, "nutrition advice"

    Rich in vegetable fiber

    Rich in alkaline potassium

    Normal calcium content: 1,000–1,200 mg/d

    Limited sodium chloride content: 4–5 g/d

    Limited animal protein content: 0.8–1.0 g/kg/d

    Limited fat, oxalate, and sugar intake

Normalized general risk factors, "lifestyle advice"

    Adequate physical activity

    Balancing excessive fluid loss

    Normal BMI, between 18.5–24.9 kg/m^2

Adapted from Straub M and Hautman RE. Developments in stone prevention. Curr Opin Urol 2005;15:119–26; with permission.

Formation of stones is a complex biochemical process that is often multifactorial in nature. As a result, there is rarely a single solution in the medical management of urinary tract stones. Many of the therapies and dietary modifications are unpleasant and require significant sacrifice by the patients. Recommended medical therapies for specific types of stones are listed in **Table 4**.

We recommend screening all stone-forming patients to identify those at high risk who need urologic evaluation. Patients who present with stones and have a known genitourinary abnormality (solitary kidney, duplicated collecting system, hydronephrosis, etc), or a concomitant urinary tract infection should have urgent urologic consultation. Urologic consultation should also be considered in patients who have not had progression of a ureteral stone or continue to be symptomatic after 3–4 weeks of medical expulsive therapy.

Non-high risk patients should be counseled to increase their oral fluid intake to achieve a goal urine output of greater than 2.0–2.5 L per day, if co-morbidities permit. Additionally, dietary modifications including sodium restriction (<2 g per day) and limited protein intake (<80 g per day) have been shown to be of benefit. Dietary calcium restriction is not recommended as a general means of reducing stone recurrence. Several studies have indicated that dietary calcium supplementation may actually protect from further stone formation.[40–42] Ascorbic acid (Vitamin C) and cranberry juice may increase the risk of stone formation in calcium oxalate stone formers.[43,44]

Weight-loss strategies should be discussed with patients who are obese or morbidly obese. Those who embark on high protein diets should be counseled

Table 4
Medical therapies for stone-forming patients

Stone Type	Abnormality	Treatment
Calcium oxalate	Hypercalciuria	Potassium citrate, 30–60 mEq/d divided 3–4 x Alternative: sodium bicarbonate 1.5 g/d divided in 3 doses
	Hypocitraturia	Potassium citrate, 30–60 mEq/d divided 3–4 doses
	Hyperoxaluria	Calcium 500 mg/d with meals
	Hypomagnesuria	Magnesium 200–400 mg/d Caution: no replacement in renal insufficiency
Calcium phosphate	Hypercalciuria	Hydrochlorothiazide 25–50 mg/d
Uric acid	Urinary pH < 6	Potassium citrate 30–60 mEq/d divided 3–4 doses Alternative: sodium bicarbonate 1.5 g/d divided in 3doses
	Hyperuricosuria	Allopurinol 100 mg/d
	Hyperuricemia	Allopurinol 300 mg/d Cystine Daily fluid intake 3.5–4 L/d for urinary output 2.5–3.0 L/d Potassium citrate 30–120 mEq/d titrated for urine pH of 7.5–8.5 Penicillamine 1–4 gm/d divided in 4 doses Captopril 25–50 mg/d

regarding the potential risk of stone formation as a result of these diets. Diets high in sodium chloride are directly associated with significant increases in renal calcium excretion. When coupled with low levels of citrate and relative oliguria, such a diet further increases the risk of stone formation. Patients who have undergone Roux-en-Y gastric bypass develop increased urinary oxalate, decreased citrate excretion, and relative supersaturation of calcium oxalate within 3 months after surgery.[45–49] They are at increased risk of stone formation, with a relative risk of 1.7 compared with a control group of age- and sex-matched obese patients.

EXTRACORPOREAL SHOCK WAVE LITHOTRIPSY

Since its introduction in 1980, extracorporeal shock wave lithotripsy (SWL) has revolutionized the management of stone disease. It remains the preferred treatment for renal stones and proximal ureteral stones Despite a significant amount of work done in the physics of lithotripsy, the exact mechanism that causes stone fragmentation is not fully understood. All lithotriptors produce a characteristic waveform at the focal point, which produces both compressive and tensile forces on the stone. In addition, micro-bubble cavitation plays a role in stone fragmentation.[49,50]

All lithotripsy machines have similar components, consisting of *an energy source, a focusing system, an imaging system* and *a coupling mechanism.* Several types of systems have been used. The original method of shock wave generation, called the electrohydraulic technique, creates a high energy pressure wave using a spark gap, and the energy is focused with an ellipsoid reflector. In the piezoelectric method, the shockwave is generated and focused when a grid of ceramic or piezoelectric crystals is stimulated with a coordinated high-energy electrical pulse. The electromagnetic method uses an electromagnetic coil to vibrate a metallic membrane. Imaging systems can include fluoroscopy, ultrasound, or both. Coupling systems are necessary to effectively transmit the energy created by the shock wave across the skin surface, through the body, and to the stone. Originally, patients were immersed in water to provide air-free contact with the skin, but more contemporary machines use small water-filled cushions.

The most common indication for SWL is renal stone disease. Renal stones <20 mm in diameter, proximal ureteral stones <10 mm in diameter, and distal stones <10 mm in diameter can be treated with SWL. Some types of stones are more successfully fragmented with SWL, including calcium oxalate dihydrate, uric acid, and calcium apatite stones, while some stones are more resistant to SWL, including cystine and calcium oxalate monohydrate stones.

Contraindications to SWL can be categorized into medical and urologic. Absolute medical contraindications include uncorrected bleeding disorders, uncorrected hypertension, and pregnancy. Relative contraindications include aortic or renal artery aneurysm, and cardiac pacemakers. Urologic contraindications include untreated urinary tract infection, urinary obstruction or stricture distal to the stone being treated, anatomic or functional problems that prevent proper stone elimination (calyceal diverticulum, horseshoe kidney, ectopic kidney, duplicated kidney), and large stone burden. Morbid obesity and skeletal anomalies may also preclude treatment with SWL.

All potential lithotripsy patients need a thorough history and physical examination. If medically appropriate, patients should have a chest x-ray and electrocardiogram. Preoperative blood studies should include complete blood count, prothrombin time, partial thromboplastin time, and in some cases a bleeding time. Urine should be sterile before treatment. Patients with infection stones should be on appropriate antibiotics before treatment. Cardiology consultation should be requested for patients with cardiac pacemakers, and a cardiologist should stand by at the time of their procedure to address any concerns or correct any problems with the pacemaker during treatment. Patients should discontinue any drugs that can interfere with clotting (warfarin, aspirin, clopidogrel, etc), at least one week before treatment.

Postoperative care following SWL consists of vigorous hydration, return to usual physical activity as tolerated (usually in 3–7 days), and straining of the urine for stone collection if the stone type is unknown. Pain can be treated with oral narcotics or nonsteroidal anti-inflammatories. Patients can generally resume their anti-platelet or anticoagulant medications immediately after SWL treatment. Calcium channel blockers or selective alpha-1-blockers such as tamsulosin can be prescribed to facilitate stone passage.[51–54] Single-view abdominal x-ray in 4–6 weeks is routinely used to assess the degree of stone fragmentation and stone passage.

SWL is the most common first line treatment for the majority of renal stones. Several studies have demonstrated stone-free rates as follows: renal pelvis 76% (48%–85%), upper calyx 69% (46%–82%), middle calyx 68% (52%–76%), and lower calyx 59% (42%–73%). Stone free rates in all these series were dependent on stone size, with stones <10 mm allowing excellent stone-free rates.[55]

SWL or ureteroscopic (URS) treatments are both acceptable options for management of ureteral stones. Proponents of SWL cite its efficacy, non-invasiveness, and ability to be performed under conscious sedation. Proponents of URS cite its high stone-free success rate and the expediency with which the procedure can be performed. The American Urological Association (AUA) Ureteral Stones Guideline Panel meta-analysis showed SWL to have a stone clearance rate of 74% for stones <10 mm and 46% for stones 11–20 mm. More than one session is often required for stone clearance, and success rates decrease with successive treatments. Given these findings, the AUA panel recommended SWL as first line treatment for most patients with stones <10 mm in diameter. Distal stones <10 mm can be either treated with URS or SWL as first line therapy. Pre-stenting does not appear to improve stone-free rates, but it does reduce hospital readmission and emergency room visits.[56–60] Mid-ureteral stones can also be treated with SWL, as long as the stone can be localized either with flouroscopy or ultrasound. Lower ureteral stones can also be treated with SWL. The advantage of SWL over URS is the noninvasiveness of the treatment, and the disadvantages are the higher retreatment rate and the higher level of difficulty in localization of the stone. URS has superior stone free rates, is more cost effective, and the endoscopic equipment is readily available in most ambulatory surgery centers and hospital operating rooms.

Immediate complications of SWL include tissue injury, bleeding, adjacent organ injury, urinary tract obstruction, post-treatment obstruction, and urinary tract infection. Clinically significant subcapsular and perirenal hematomas occur infrequently, with reported rates between 0.24 and 4.1%.[61,62] Patients with hypertension, diabetes mellitus, obesity, and coronary artery disease are at increased risk.[61,63] The most common and important clinical sign of a hematoma is pain. Patients may also present with tachycardia, hypotension, and significant hematuria. Impaired renal function is uncommon and is typically seen only in patients with a solitary kidney or those with bilateral hematomas following bilateral treatment. A suspected hematoma can be confirmed by CT or ultrasound. Reported transfusion rates range from 0%–33%, but the vast majority of patients with hematoma can be managed conservatively. Lung injury occurs in <1%, but it is the most common non-urologic organ injury and is more common in children.[24] Obstruction of the urinary tract by fragments after SWL occur in 5%–10% of cases.[57,58]

Fortunately, long term complications of SWL are rare. Long term complications associated with SWL include renal insufficiency, hypertension, and possible metabolic abnormalities. Recently, Krambeck and colleagues[64] reported on a possible association between prior SWL and the development of diabetes.

URETEROSCOPY

Advances in fiberoptics, refinements in laser and lithotripsy technology, and miniaturization of the ancillary equipment used in ureteroscopic treatment of upper urinary tract mean that treatment of renal stone disease is one of the more common procedures that practicing urologists perform today. Semi-rigid and flexible ureteroscopes no larger than 2–3 mm in diameter are available and allow access to the entire upper urinary system. Holmium laser energy is the most commonly used ureteroscopic lithotripsy technology employed today. Fibers 200 to 100 microns in diameter are available and can tolerate the energy levels needed to fragment all types of urinary stones. Urinary baskets allow for stone or stone-fragment retrieval.

Routine use of ureteral stents after ureteroscopy is not necessary. However, certain factors suggest that stents be used. These include bilateral ureteroscopy, solitary kidney, ureteral perforation, impacted stone, ureteroscopy lasting >60 minutes, uncorrected bleeding diathesis, and ureteroscopy of a struvite (infection) stone.[65–71] Stents do result in hematuria, urinary urgency, frequency, and pelvic and flank discomfort, all of which resolve almost immediately with stent removal.

Distal ureteral stones are probably best treated using a semi rigid ureteroscope. A retrograde pyelogram can be performed to confirm the location of the stone(s) and can also delineate the degree of obstruction or impaction of the stone. If the stone is small enough to remove, then it is engaged in the basket and removed in

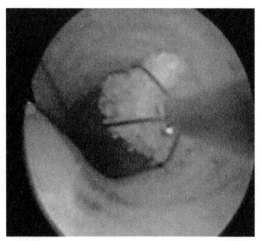

Fig. 4. Ureteroscopic view of a mid ureteral stone engaged in a basket. A safety wire is on the left.

one piece (**Fig. 4**). Stones which are large or in which the ureteral orifice was not dilated will require fragmentation. Holmium laser is the preferred ureteroscopic lithotripsy method. The fragments can be removed by using a basket to place them in the bladder, or the scope can be removed, allowing the fragments to spontaneously pass into the bladder. Mid-ureteral stones can be treated either with a semi rigid or flexible ureteroscope. Flexible ureteroscopy is the preferred technique in treating mid, proximal and renal stones. Complications of ureteroscopy can include ureteral injury and late ureteral stricture formation.[70,71]

PERCUTANEOUS STONE TREATMENT

For percutaneous nephrostolithotomy (PCNL) a tract is created via an incision in the flank, through which a scope can be placed to visualize the collecting system and stones within it. Using lithotripsy devices and stone-removal equipment, significant stone volume can then be safely and effectively removed. Indications for PCNL include stones >2 cm in diameter, staghorn calculi, and shockwave resistant stones, such as cystine or calcium oxalate monohydrate stones. Contraindications include bleeding diathesis, abdominal anatomy precluding percutaneous access, or unusual body habitus, such as morbid obesity or a very long flank kidney length.

PCNL has been proven to be safe and effective, with success rates from some series ranging from 90% 100%[72,73] It is the preferred method recommended by the AUA nephrolithiasis guideline panel for staghorn or partial staghorn calculi. The stone free success rate for PCNL, versus PCNL+SWL, versus SWL alone, was 78%, 66%, and 54%, respectively. Open stone surgery was less effective than PCNL, with a stone free rate of 71%.

Complications in PCNL can be categorized into: access related, endoscopic or stone removal related, immediate postoperative, and late complications. Intraoperative and post-operative bleeding is usually minimal, with reported transfusion rates of 2%–5%. Patients undergoing puncture above the 12th rib have an approximate 10% risk of pleural injury. The incidence of bowel injury is approximately 0.2% and is more likely to occur in thin patients in which the tract is made too lateral, or in the morbidly obese. Death associated with percutaneous nephrostolithotomy is very rare and is often related to other comorbid conditions, such as fatal arrhythmias or respiratory failure, rather than the procedure itself.[74,75]

REFERENCES

1. Stamatelou KK, Francis ME, Jones CA, et al. Time trends in reported prevalence of kidney stones in the United States. Kidney Int 2003;63:1817–23.
2. Pearle MS, Calhoun EA, Curhan GC, et al. Urologic diseases in America project: urolithiasis. J Urol 2005;173:848–57.
3. Pak CY. Should patients with single renal stone occurrence undergo diagnostic evaluation? J Urol 1982;127:855–7.
4. Johnson CM, Wilson DM, O'Fallon WM, et al. Renal stone epidemiology: a 25 year study in Rochester, Minnesota. Kidney Int 1979;16:624–31.
5. Scales CD Jr, Curtis LH, Norris RD, et al. Changing gender prevalence of stone disease. J Urol 2007;177:979–82.
6. Rous SN. A review of 171 consecutive patients with urinary lithiasis. J Urol 1981; 126:376–9.
7. Sarmina I, Spirnak JP, Resnick MI. Urinary lithiasis in the black population: an epidemiologic study and review of the literature. J Urol 1987;138:14–7.
8. Soucie JM, Thun MJ, Coates RJ, et al. Demographic and geographic variability of kidney stones in the United States. Kidney Int 1977;46:893–9.
9. Maloney ME, Springhart WP, Ekerou WO, et al. Ethnic background has minimal impact on the etiology of nephrolithiasis. J Urol 2005;173:2001–4.
10. Prince CL, Scardino PL. A statistical analysis of ureteral calculi. J Urol 1960;83: 561–5.
11. Schwartz B, Schenkman N, Bruce J, et al. Calcium nephrolithiasis: effect of water hardness on urinary electrolytes. Urology 2002;60:23–7.
12. van Aswegen CH, du Plessis DJ. Pathogenesis of kidney stones. Med Hypotheses 1991;36:368–70.
13. Stoller ML, Meng MV, Abrahams HM, et al. The primary stone event: a new hypothesis involving a vascular etiology. J Urol 2004;171:1920–4.
14. Matlaga BR, Coe FL, Evan AP, et al. The role of Randall's plaques in the pathogenesis of calcium stones. J Urol 2007;177:31–8.
15. Pak CY, Peterson R. Successful treatment of hyperuricosuric calcium oxalate nephrolithiasis with potassium citrate. Arch Intern Med 1986;146:863–7.
16. Nicar MJ, Hill K, Pak CY. Inhibition by citrate of spontaneous precipitation of calcium oxalate in vitro. J Bone Miner Res 1987;2:215–20.
17. Nakagawa Y, Ahmed M, Hall SL, et al. Isolation from human calcium oxalate renal stones of nephrocalcin, a glycoprotein inhibitor of calcium oxalate crystal growth. Evidence that nephrocalcin from patients with calcium oxalate nephrolithiasis is deficient in gamma-carboxyglutamic acid. J Clin Invest 1987;79:1782–7.
18. Asplin JR, Arsenault D, Parks JH, et al. Contribution of human uropontin to inhibition of calcium oxalate crystallization. Kidney Int 1998;53:194–9.
19. Taylor EN, Stampfer MJ, Curhan GC. Obesity, weight gain, and the risk of kidney stones. JAMA 2005;293:455–62.
20. Seiner R, Glatz S, Nicolay C, et al. The role of overweight and obesity in calcium oxalate stone formation. Obes Res 2004;12:106–13.
21. Kaufman DW, Kelly JP, Curhan GC, et al. Oxalobacter formigenes may reduce the risk of calcium oxalate kidney stones. J Am Soc Nephrol 2008;19:1197–203.

22. Troxel SA, Sidhu H, Kaul P, et al. Intestinal Oxalobacter formigenes colonization in calcium oxalate stone formers and its relation to urinary oxalate. J Endourol 2003; 17:173–6.
23. Griffith DP, Osborne CA. Infection (urease) stones. Miner Electrolyte Metab 1987; 13:278–85.
24. Faerber GJ. Pediatric urolithiasis. Curr Opin Urol 2001;11:385–9.
25. Ettinger B, Oldroyd NO, Sorger F. Triamterene nephrolithiasis. JAMA 1980;244: 2443–5.
26. Colistro R, Torreggiani WC, Lyburn ID. Unenhanced helical CT in the investigation of acute flank pain. Clin Radiol 2002;57:435–41.
27. Sodickson A, Baeyens PF, Andriole KP, et al. Recurrent CT, cumulative radiation exposure, and associated radiation-induced cancer risks from CT of adults. Radiology 2009;25:175–84.
28. Coll DM, Varanelli MJ, Sith RC. Relationship of spontaneous passage of ureteral calculi to stone size and location as revealed by unenhanced helical CT. AJR Am J Roentgenol 2002;178:101–3.
29. Segura JW, Preminger GM, Assimos DG, et al. Ureteral stones clinical guidelines panel summary report on the management of ureteral calculi. J Urol 1997;158: 1915–21.
30. Miller OF, Kane CJ. Time to stone passage for observed ureteral calculi: a guide for patient education. J Urol 1999;162:688–91.
31. Holdgate A, Pollock T. Systematic review of the relative efficacy of non-steroidal anti-inflammatory drugs and opioids in the treatment of acute renal colic. BMJ 2004;328:1401–4.
32. Hollingsworth J, Rogers M, Kaufman S, et al. Medical therapy to facilitate urinary stone passage: a meta-analysis. Lancet 2006;368:1171–9.
33. Agrawal M, Naja V, Singh S, et al. Is there an adjunctive role of tamsulosin to extracorporeal shockwave lithotripsy for upper ureteral stones: results of an open label randomized nonplacebo controlled trial. Urology 2009;74:989–92.
34. Dellabella M, Milanese G, Mussonigro G. Randomized trial of the efficacy of tamsulosin, nifedipine and phloroglucinol in medical expulsive therapy for distal ureteral calculi. J Urol 2006;174:167–72.
35. Porpiglia F, Ghignone G, Fiori C, et al. Nifedipine versus tamsulosin for the management of lower ureteral stones. J Urol 2004;172:568–71.
36. Bensalah K, Pearle M, Lotan Y. Cost-effectiveness of medical expulsive therapy using alpha-blockers for the treatment of distal ureteral stones. Eur Urol 2008; 53:411–9.
37. Strohmaier WL. Course of calcium stone disease without treatment. What can we expect. Eur Urol 2000;37:339–44.
38. Stoller ML. Urinary stone disease. In: Tanagho EA, McAnich JW, editors. Smith's general urology. 14th edition. Norwalk (CT): Appleton and Lange; 1995. p. 27–34.
39. Esen T, Marshall VR, Rao N, et al. Medical management of urolithiasis. In: Segura JW, Conort P, Khoury S, et al, editors. Stone disease. Paris: Health Publications; 2003. p. 133–49.
40. Curhan GC, Willett WC, Rimm EB, et al. A prospective study of dietary calcium and other nutrients and the risk of symptomatic kidney stones. N Engl J Med 1993;328:833–8.
41. Curhan GC, Willett WC, Knight EL, et al. Dietary factors and the risk of incident kidney stones in younger women: Nurses Health Study II. Arch Intern Med 2004;163:885–91.

42. Matlaga BR, Shore AD, Magnuson T, et al. Effect of gastric bypass surgery on kidney stone disease. J Urol 2009;181:2573–7.

43. Traxer O, Huet B, Poindexter J, et al. Effect of ascorbic acid consumption on urinary stone risk factors. J Urol 2003;170:397–401.

44. Gettman MT, Ogan K, Brinkley LJ, et al. Effect of cranberry juice consumption on urinary stone risk factors. J Urol 2005;174:590–4.

45. Park AM, Storm DW, Fulmer BR, et al. A prospective study of risk factors for neph-rolithiasis after Roux-en-Y gastric bypass surgery. J Urol 2009;182:2334–9.

46. Sinha MK, Collazo-Clavell ML, Rule A, et al. Hyperoxaluric nephrolithiasis is a complication of Roux-en-Y gastric bypass surgery. Kidney Int 2007;72:100–7.

47. Semins MJ, Matlaga BR, Shore AD, et al. The effect of gastric banding on kidney stone disease. Urology 2009;74:746–9.

48. Penniston KL, Kaplon DM, Gould JC, et al. Gastric band placement for obesity is not associated with increased urinary risk of urolithiasis compared to bypass. J Urol 2009;182:2340–6.

49. Pace KT, Ghiculete D, Harju M, et al. Shock wave lithotripsy at 60 or 120 shocks per minute: a randomized, double blind study. J Urol 2005;174:595–9.

50. Zhou Y, Cocks FH, Preminger GN, et al. Innovations in shock wave lithotripsy technology: updates in experimental studies. J Urol 2004;172:1892–8.

51. Kupeli B, Irkilata L, Gürocak S, et al. Does tamsulosin enhance lower ureteral stone clearance with or without shock wave lithotripsy? Urology 2004;64:1111–5.

52. Gravina GL, Costa AM, Ronchi P, et al. Tamsulosin treatment increases clinical success rate of single extra corporeal shock wave lithotripsy of renal stones. Urology 2005;66:24–8.

53. Porpiglia F, Destefanis P, Fiori, et al. Role of adjunctive medical therapy with nifed-ipine and deflazacort after extracorporeal shock wave lithotripsy of ureteral stones. Urology 2002;59:835–8.

54. Hollingsworth JM, Rogers MA, Kaufman SR, et al. Medical therapy to facilitate urinary stone passage: a meta-analysis. Lancet 2006;368:1138–9.

55. Weizer A, Preminger GM. Shock wave lithotripsy: current technology and evolving concepts. AUA Updates 2005;24(36):314–23.

56. Bierkens AF, Hendrikx AJ, Lemmens WA, et al. Extracorporeal shock wave litho-tripsy for large calculi: the role of ureteral stents. A randomized trial. J Urol 1991; 145:699–702.

57. Prior JL, Jenkins AD. Use of double pigtail stents in extracorporeal shock wave lithotripsy. J Urol 1990;143:475–8.

58. Chandhoke PS, Barqawi AZ, Wernecke C, et al. A randomized outcomes trial of ureteral stents for extracorporeal shock wave lithotripsy of solitary kidney or prox-imal ureteral stones. J Urol 2002;167:1981–3.

59. Knapp PM, Kulb TB, Lingeman JE, et al. Extracorporeal shock wave lithotripsy induced perirenal hematomas. J Urol 1988;139:700–3.

60. Dhar NB, Thornton J, Karafa MT, et al. A multivariate analysis of risk factors asso-ciated with subcapsular hematoma formation following electromagnetic shock wave lithotripsy. J Urol 2004;172:2271–4.

61. Kostakopoulos A, Stavropoulos NJ, Macrychoritis C, et al. Subcapsular hema-toma due to ESWL: risk factors. A study of 4,247 patients. Urol Int 1995;55:21–4.

62. Newman LH, Saltzman B. Identifying risk factors in development of clinically significant post shock wave lithotripsy subcapsular hematomas. Urology 1991; 38:35–8.

63. Coptcoat MJ, Webb DR, Kellett MJ, et al. The complications of extracorporeal shock wave lithotripsy: management and prevention. Br J Urol 1986;58:578.

64. Krambeck AE, Gettman MT, Rohlinger AL, et al. Diabetes mellitus and hypertension associated with shock wave lithotripsy of renal and proximal ureteral stones at 19 years of followup. J Urol 2006;175:1742–7.
65. Watterson JD, Girvan AR, Cook AJ, et al. Safety and efficacy of holmium: YAG laser lithotripsy in patients with bleeding diathesis. J Urol 2002;168:442–5.
66. Hollenbeck BK, Schuster TG, Faerber GJ, et al. Routine placement of ureteral stents is unnecessary after ureteroscopy for urinary calculi. Urology 2001; 57(4):639–43.
67. Srivastava A, Gupta R, Kumar A, et al. Routine stenting after ureteroscopy for distal ureteral calculi is unnecessary: results of a randomized clinical trial. J Endourol 2003;17(10):871–4.
68. Byrne RR, Auge BK, Kourambas, et al. Routine ureteral stenting is not necessary after ureteroscopy and ureteropyeloscopy: a randomized trial. J Endourol 2002; 16(1):9–13.
69. Borboroglu PG, Amling CL, Schenkman NS, et al. Ureteral stenting after ureteroscopy for distal ureteral calculi: a multi institutional prospective randomized controlled study assessing pain, outcomes and complications. J Urol 2001; 166(5):1651–7.
70. Johnson DB, Pearle MS. Complications of ureteroscopy. Urol Clin North Am 2004; 31:157–71.
71. Stoller ML, Wolf JS. Endoscopic ureteral injuries. In: McAninch JW, editor. Traumatic and reconstructive urology. Philadelphia: WB Saunders; 1996. p. 199–211.
72. Shah HN, Kausik VB, Hedge SS, et al. Tubeless percutaneous nephrolithotomy: a prospective feasibility study and review of previous reports. BJU Int 2005;96: 879–83.
73. Faerber GJ, Gow M. Percutaneous nephrolithotripsy in morbidly obese patients. Tech Urol 1997;3:2–7.
74. Kumar A, Banerjee GK, Tewari A, et al. Isolated duodenal injury during relook percutaneous nephrolithotomy. Br J Urol 1994;74(3):382–3.
75. Begun FP, Jacobs SC, Lawson RK. Small bowel perforation during percutaneous nephrolithotomy. J Endourol 1989;3:81.

Benign Prostatic Hyperplasia: Current Clinical Practice

Bob Djavan, MD, PhD*, Elisabeth Eckersberger, MPA,
Julia Finkelstein, BSc, Geovanni Espinosa, ND, LAc, Helen Sadri, MD,
Roland Brandner, MD, Ojas Shah, MD, Herbert Lepor, MD

KEYWORDS

- Benign Prostatic Hyperplasia • Lower Urinary Tract Symptoms
- Minimally Invasive Therapy

Published Studies		
Study	Level	Details
ARIA 3001 (US)	A	Randomized, double-blind, placebo controlled
ARIA 3002 (US)	A	Randomized, double-blind, placebo controlled
ARIA 3003 (19 Countries)	A	Randomized, double-blind, placebo controlled
CombAT, 2009	A	Randomized, double-blind, placebo controlled, parallel-group
Djavan, 2004	B	Meta-analysis
HYCAT, 1996	A	Randomized, double-blind, placebo controlled
MTOPS, 2008	A	Randomized, double-blind, placebo controlled
PLESS		
TRIUMPH	A	Randomized, double-blind, placebo controlled

Benign prostatic hyperplasia (BPH) is the most common benign adenoma in men, affecting nearly all of them. BPH represents a clinically significant cause of bladder outflow obstruction in up to 40% of men. The growing frequency of diagnosis is due to increasing life expectancy and a trend toward seeking medical advice at earlier stages of the disease.

Author Statement: There is no conflict of interest for any of the coauthors nor a funding source involved in the research mentioned.
Department of Urology, New York University School of Medicine, New York University Hospital, 150 East 32nd Street, New York, NY 10016, USA
* Corresponding author.
E-mail address: bdjavan@hotmail.com

Prim Care Clin Office Pract 37 (2010) 583–597
doi:10.1016/j.pop.2010.04.004
0095-4543/10/$ – see front matter © 2010 Elsevier Inc. All rights reserved.

OVERVIEW OF DIAGNOSIS, TREATMENT, AND MANAGEMENT

Advances in understanding of the epidemiology and pathophysiology of BPH have led to changes in treatment. Although treatment was previously based on ablative surgery, guidelines now emphasize pharmacotherapy and minimally invasive surgery. The advent of new medical therapies for BPH and the introduction of a range of minimally invasive therapies (MITs) now provide a wider range of therapeutic options for men with lower urinary tract symptoms (LUTS) secondary to BPH. The development of effective therapies such as alpha-adrenergic blockers and 5-alpha-reductase (5AR) inhibitors and the possibility of their combined use represent the most significant advance in the treatment of BPH.

Since 1991, the WHO international consensus meetings on BPH have facilitated continued discussion on the development of clinical research criteria for BPH. Outcomes include benefits and harms, which can be direct (such as changes in symptoms, magnitude of symptoms, bother, and quality of life as perceived by patients) or indirect (such as flow rate, residual urine, prostate size, and pressure flow parameters). The American Urological Association (AUA) is currently using a Symptom Index (SI) score (**Table 1**)[1] to establish the severity of clinical symptoms. Watchful waiting is recommended for patients whose clinical symptoms do not affect their quality of life.[2]

Evidence from several studies has highlighted the role of prostate enlargement in BPH progression, with strong relationships between prostate volume, need for

Table 1
International Prostate Symptom Score (IPSS)
During the last month or so, how often have you...
Not at all (0), less than 1 time in 5 (1) less than half the time (2), about half the time (3), more than half the time (4), almost always (5)
1. Had a sensation of not emptying your bladder completely after urinating?
0   1   2   3   4   5
2. Had to urinate again less than 2 hours after you have urinated?
0   1   2   3   4   5
3. Stopped and started several times when you urinated?
0   1   2   3   4   5
4. Found it difficult to postpone urination?
0   1   2   3   4   5
5. Had a weak urinary stream?
0   1   2   3   4   5
6. Had to push or strain to urinate?
0   1   2   3   4   5
During the last month...
7. How many times did you most typically get up to urinate from the time you went to bed at night until the time you got up in the morning?
0   1   2   3   4   5

From Barry MJ, Fowler FJ Jr, O'Leary MP, et al. The American Urological Association symptom index for benign prostatic hyperplasia. The Measurement Committee of the American Urological Association. J Urol 1992 Nov;148(5):1549–57; with permission.

BPH-related surgery, and risk of developing acute urinary retention.[3] The impor-tance of androgens in the development of prostate enlargement is now well under-stood based on several lines of evidence. BPH does not develop in men who have been castrated before puberty and therefore have greatly depleted levels of circu-lating androgens. Furthermore, in men with BPH, medical or surgical castration has been shown to cause a reduction in prostate volume.

ROLE OF DIHYDROTESTOSTERONE AND TESTOSTERONE

Dihydrotestosterone (DHT) is twice as potent as testosterone, and it plays the most important role in BPH progression, mediating androgenic effects in BPH. In the pros-tate, as opposed to blood, the level of DHT is higher than that of testosterone. Further-more, intraprostatic DHT levels remain high in aging men despite a decline in circulating testosterone, suggesting a central role for DHT in BPH.

Testosterone is converted to DHT, a reaction catalyzed by the 5AR isoenzymes type 1 and 2. Type 2 5AR is found predominantly in the prostate and other genital tissues. Type 1 5AR is more ubiquitous, found throughout the body wherever 5AR is expressed, including the skin, liver, and prostate. Tissues with a high concentration of these enzymes, such as the prostate, are therefore the major site of conversion of testosterone to DHT. It has long been argued that the prostatic conversion of testosterone to DHT amplifies the effects of circulating testosterone by converting it to the more potent androgen, DHT. Given the central role of DHT as the most potent androgen, predictably, men with genetic type 2 5AR deficiency have small and rudi-mentary prostates and do not develop BPH as adults, although they undergo viriliza-tion at puberty.[4]

This underlying prostate growth under androgenic control may be one of the key drivers of long-term BPH disease progression. Inhibition of testosterone conversion to DHT by targeting the 5AR isoenzymes is therefore a rational approach for the management of BPH. This can be done using 5AR inhibitors, which are a cornerstone of current medical therapy, along with α-blockers.

MEDICAL THERAPY
α-Blockers

Alpha(1)-adrenoceptor antagonists, or α-blockers, have become important compo-nents in the treatment of BPH. A better understanding of how adrenergic hormone receptors are involved in prostate disease has led to an increased use of α-blockers in treatment, shifting the focus from surgery to better uses of pharmacotherapy. Currently available α-blockers have similar effects on BPH, improving symptoms by approximately 35% and maximum urinary flow rate by 1.8 to 2.5 mL/s.[5]

Djavan, and Marberger[6,7] concluded that all α-blockers have comparable efficacy in improving symptoms and that those that require dose titration and are initiated at subtherapeutic doses (eg, terazosin) have a slower onset of action than those that can be initiated at their full therapeutic dose (eg, tamsulosin). The main difference between the α-blockers relates to their tolerability profiles, with alfuzosin and tamsu-losin better tolerated than doxazosin and terazosin. Patients with LUTS/BPH are more likely to discontinue α-blocker therapy because of vasodilatory adverse events, such as dizziness, than because of retrograde ejaculation.

Earlier placebo-controlled studies showed similar results. Lepor and colleagues[8] found that groups treated with 10 mg of terazosin exhibited significantly greater increases in peak and mean urinary flow rates than the group on the placebo. The improvements did not reach a plateau within the dose range evaluated, suggesting that higher doses could possibly be even more effective. In the Hytrin Community Assessment Trial study (HYCAT), Roehrborn and colleagues[9] evaluated terazosin in a community-based population under usual care conditions. Given in a daily dose of 2 to 10 mg, terazosin was more effective than placebo in reducing the symptoms of BPH, reducing the perception of bother, and in raising the disease-specific quality of life in men with moderate–to–severe symptoms of prostatism. These effects were maintained during a 12-month follow-up.

Although α-blocker therapy rapidly relieves BPH symptoms, there is no evidence that it reduces the long-term risks of acute urinary retention and surgery, probably because α-blockers do not reduce prostate volume.

5AR Inhibitors

The main circulating androgen, testosterone, is converted to DHT by the enzyme 5AR. Although DHT is necessary for normal growth and function, it is also involved in the development of BPH and, most likely, the initiation and maintenance of prostate cancer. Two 5AR inhibitors, finasteride and dutasteride, have been studied extensively in clinical trials of patients with BPH. Finasteride is a type 2 5AR inhibitor, whereas dutasteride is a dual 5AR inhibitor that inhibits both isoenzymes. Both compounds have been shown to inhibit serum DHT, although dutasteride is more effective.[10] In large-scale clinical trials in men with symptomatic BPH, 5AR inhibitors reduce prostate volume, improve symptoms, reduce the risk of acute urinary retention, and decrease the likelihood of BPH-related surgery.[11,12] These medications reduce serum prostate-specific antigen (PSA) by approximately 50% at 6 months and reduce total prostate volume by 25% in 2 years.[13] The 5AR inhibitors also have the potential to reduce the risk of prostate cancer as a secondary benefit in men receiving treatment for symptomatic BPH.[14]

The first placebo-controlled study on dutasteride was published in 2002, pooling patients from 3 randomized trials: ARIA 3001 and ARIA 3002 in the United States, and ARIA 3003 in 19 countries in which 2167 men received 0.5mg/d and 2158 received placebos.[12] At 24 months, serum PSA had increased by 15.8% in the placebo group, compared with a decrease of 52.4% in the dutasteride group. Assessing the BPH Impact Index (BII) in the same cohort, O'Leary and colleagues[15] showed that dutasteride resulted in clinically and statistically significant improvements from 6 months. BII scores improved by 2.41 in men with a high baseline BII (≥5 [greatest symptomatic burden]), whereas in patients treated with the placebo, they only improved by 1.64.

Combination Therapy

Combination therapy for BPH is the combination of drugs that have proved useful as monotherapy and are able to give the patient even great relief when combined. In the case of BPH, α-blockers and 5AR inhibitors have been shown to be effective individually[9,16,17] and are now being investigated in combination, especially in those patients reluctant to undergo surgery and getting no relief from monotherapy. A 2008 analysis of the Medical Therapy of Prostatic Symptoms (MTOPS) assessed the long-term treatment with doxazosin, an α-blocker, and finasteride, a 5AR inhibitor.[18] Three thousand forty-seven patients were randomized to placebo, doxazosin (4 to 8 mg), finasteride (5mg), or a combination of doxazosin and finasteride. Treatment with finasteride led to a reduction of approximately 25% in prostate volume in those with relatively small, moderate–sized, and enlarged prostates at baseline. The reductions in risk of acute urinary retention and surgery with finasteride were statistically significant ($P = .009$ and $P<.001$, respectively). The rates of acute urinary retention and surgery in the α-blocker arm were 0.4 and 1.3 per 100 person-years, respectively, which were not significantly different from placebo. The results lead to the conclusion that combination therapy is most functional when the patient's PSA level is more than 1.5ng/mL, his prostate volume greater than 30cc, and his LUTS significant.[16]

Because MTOPS was designed with drugs that are less used today, such as terazosin and doxazosin, the Combination of Avodart and Tamsulosin (CombAT) study published first results on the effect of combined therapy with dutasteride and tamsulosin as opposed to each as monotherapy, and results were assessed using the BII [17] (**Table 2**) and International Prostate Symptom Score (IPSS; see **Table 1**).[19] Results show that at 24 months, BII scores were best reduced (symptoms improved) from baseline in the combination and second best in the dutasteride and tamsulosin groups, and the improvement in BII was statistically ($P<.001$) greater with the combined therapy than with either monotherapy. The results on the IPSS show that, at 24 months, change in baseline IPSS was greatest with the combination, and again, the reduction in score was significantly greater with the combination than with each monotherapy ($P<.001$). The BII continued to improve with the combination and with dutasteride alone over the 2-year study period but seemed to decline with tamsulosin after 15 months. Additionally, the improvement in BII from the baseline was greater than previously reported for dutasteride in the Phase III trials, probably due to the lack of a placebo arm and a higher mean baseline BII in CombAT. It can be concluded from these trails that combination therapy has significant benefits for patients in terms of reduction in symptoms and prostate volume.

Phytotherapy

Medical therapy with α-blockers and 5AR inhibitors has been extended with the growing interest in phytotherapy; around one in 5 men are currently using complementary and alternative methods.[20,21] The most commonly used phytotherapies for BPH are extracts of Serenoa repens (saw palmetto), thought to have antiandrogenic, antiproliferative, and antiinflammatory effects, and extracts of the African plum tree's bark.[22,23] Because BPH is not a life-threatening condition, using drugs composed of natural ingredients with low side-effects is attractive to many patients. The

Table 2 BPH Impact Index
Q1. Over the past month, how much physical discomfort did any urinary problems cause you?
None (0), only a little (1), some (2), a lot (3)
Q2. Over the past month, how much did you worry about your health because of any urinary problems?
None (0), only a little (1), some (2), a lot (3)
Q3. Overall, how bothersome has any trouble with urination been during the past month?
Not at all bothersome (0), bothers me a little (1), bothers me some (2) bothers me a lot (3)
Q4. Over the past month, how much of the time has any urinary problem kept you from doing the kinds of things you would normally do?
None of the time (0), a little of the time (1), some of the time (2), most of the time (3), all of the time (4)

From AUA Guideline on the management of benign prostatic hyperplasia (BPH) 2003. Updated 2006, with permission. Available at: http://www.auanet.org/content/guidelines-and-quality-care/clinical-guidelines.cfm?sub=bph. Accessed April 2010.

effectiveness of phytotherapies compared with placebos is still debated, and studies are proving difficult to execute. A randomized, double-blind, placebo-controlled study did not show any benefit of Serenoa repens over the placebo arm in respect to symptom relief at 1 year.[24] As a result of this trial, the Complementary and Alternative Medicine for Urological Symptoms (CAMUS) trial with 3300 participants testing Serenoa repens, African plum tree extract, an alpha-adrenergic blocker, and a placebo shifted its endpoint from a measure of long-term efficacy to determining any short-term (6–8 months) symptom relief.[25] The results are anticipated in 2011.

Role of Anticholinergic Therapy

In patients with overactive bladder symptoms, anticholinergic drugs can be considered. As an alternative to bladder retraining, anticholinergics block the parasympathetic pathway, thereby abolishing or reducing the severity of detrusor muscle contractions. Unfortunately no current anticholinergics target the bladder muscles specifically, and they often cause side effects, such as dry mouth or dry eyes, because of their effect on muscarinic receptors in other body parts. In a review of 32 placebo controlled trials of anticholinergics, Herbison and colleagues[26] found small but statistically significant differences in symptoms. Anticholinergic drugs improved symptoms of overactive bladder, such as number of leakages, episodes per day, number of voids per day, and urodynamic measures. It is still unclear which anticholinergic drugs work best, what is the most effective route of administration and which population groups would benefit most.

Additionally, studies have shown that Botulinum toxin can be effective in cases of detrusor overactivity and overactive bladder syndrome not effectively treated by anticholinergenics.[27] This treatment is not yet approved by the US Food and Drug Administration but warrants further study.

PATIENT ASSESSMENT AND TREATMENT ALLOCATION

The last decade has witnessed significant changes in the therapeutic approach to BPH. Before the early 1990s, choice of therapy was limited; watchful waiting was advised if the symptoms and their impact on quality of life did not warrant surgical intervention or if surgery was impractical because of comorbidity or patient preference. Transurethral resection of the prostate (TURP) had become the surgical treatment of choice over open resection. Phytotherapy was available, although over-the-counter use of such preparations was not well characterized until later. The advent of medical therapy with alpha(1)-antagonists and 5AR inhibitors resulted in a significant change in practice. There was a steady decline in the use of TURP accompanied by a dramatic increase in the use of medical therapy and, to a lesser extent, MIT.[28,29]

USE OF SYMPTOM QUESTIONNAIRE

The most commonly used symptom index for BPH is the SI score questionnaire developed by the AUA. The index comprises 7 questions on frequency, nocturia, weak urinary stream, hesitancy, intermittence, incomplete emptying, and urgency. Patients are asked to score all 7 categories on a range from 0 (not at all) to 5 (almost always). Scores are added, and classification of symptoms is either mild (0–7), moderate (8–19), or severe (20–35). This evaluation of symptoms is superior to unstructured interviews. The index has been shown to be internally consistent and sensitive to change with treatment, showing practicality and reliability for use in practice.[1]

COMPARING MEDICAL TREATMENT APPROACHES: TRIUMPH STUDY

A large-scale international study, the Trans European Research into the use of Management Policies for BPH in Primary Health Care (TRIUMPH) study, has sought to characterize assessment and treatment practices for BPH across Europe. This prospective, cross-sectional, observational study was conducted in 6 European countries, enrolling newly and previously diagnosed patients with LUTS suggestive of BPH.[30] One-year follow-up data were available for 5057 patients.

The study demonstrated that initial assessment varied significantly between countries; for example, the use of PSA testing in the total study population was 73%, but for individual countries, it ranged from 41% in Germany to 88% in Spain.[31] The use of serum creatinine measurements, digital rectal examinations (DRE), and uroflow measurements also varied considerably between countries. When initial assessment of 4979 newly presenting patients in the TRIUMPH study was examined, the use of different tests was found to vary between general practitioners and office-based urologists, with urologists performing more tests than general practitioners on average.[32] Serum creatinine measurements, DRE, and uroflow measurements are all recommended for routine use in the current European Association of Urology (EAU) guidelines for management of BPH,[33] whereas PSA testing is recommended for men with a greater than 10-year life expectancy where knowledge of prostate cancer status would change patient management.

WATCHFUL WAITING

Watchful waiting is usually decided on through a combination of the patient's preference and the physician's assessment of the disease and its progression, without strict criteria existing and with individual feeling paramount to the decision. Overall, it seems that patients with mild symptom and bother scores, those with low PSA scores and prostate volume, and those with stable postvoid residual volumes (PVRs) are deemed the best candidates for watchful waiting.[34]

One study on watchful waiting, the Olmstead County Study of Urinary Symptoms and Health Status enrolled 2115 men aged 40 to 79 years over a course of 6 years.[35] The study found that age was a significant factor in seeking treatment; the incidence of treatment in men aged 40 to 49 years was 3.3 per 1000 person-years, which rose to 30 per 1000 person-years in men older than 70 years. This suggests that as a progressive disease, watchful waiting is more likely to be an option in younger patients with BPH. A study following patients in 6 European countries found that the number of patients treated with watchful waiting was 30% of the study population, with figures ranging from 20% in Italy to 69% in the United Kingdom.[32]

However, some men eventually require surgical intervention. In a Veterans Affairs' study, 556 men with moderate BPH symptoms were randomized to receive TURP or watchful waiting. The findings demonstrated high rates of crossover (conversion) from watchful waiting to surgery in men with high or low degrees of bother during 5 years of follow-up.[36] Higher bother at baseline was associated with a higher crossover rate than lower bother. These findings have been confirmed in a longitudinal study of 397 men with mild LUTS (IPSS < 8) due to BPH who were followed over a 4-year period of watchful waiting.[37] At the end of follow-up, 31% of patients had clinical progression, defined as a worsening of symptoms with migration to the moderate (IPSS 8–18) or severe (IPSS 19–35) symptom group and an increase of at least 3 points on the IPSS. At 4 years, 84% of patients had a worse IPSS than at baseline. When baseline characteristics for patients with and without clinical progression were compared, PSA ($P<.001$), obstructive symptom score ($P = .04$), and transitional zone volume ($P<.001$)

were found to be significantly higher in men with progression compared with those without progression.

The evidence from these and other studies suggests that watchful waiting may not always be the optimal approach for men with mild symptomatic BPH.[32,33,38] It may therefore be more appropriate to identify those men at risk of progression so that they can be managed more effectively, reducing the risk of progression, symptom deterioration, and acute urinary retention and surgery. The combination of several risk factors into nomograms may have clinical utility in helping physicians identify at-risk men. One such example was constructed to predict the risk of BPH progression using data from the dutasteride phase III program, and it showed a predictive accuracy of approximately 71%.[39] However, given that prostate volume is strongly related, in an age-dependent manner, to serum PSA in men with BPH but with no evidence of prostate cancer,[40] serum PSA alone may be sufficient for risk stratification.[41]

Treatment costs per patient were also examined in the TRIUMPH study.[42] Medication was the most important cost driver, accounting for 72% of total treatment costs. Treatment of patients with worse voiding and filling/storage symptoms was associated with greater costs ($P<.001$). Linear regression showed that certain medication choices, acute urinary retention, urinary tract infections (UTIs), renal dysfunction, and surgery were associated with higher treatment costs.

The TRIUMPH study serves to highlight the differences in current clinical practice that exist across Europe, with considerable disparity between the choices of watchful waiting and medical therapy and in the types of medical therapy selected (classes of drugs and monotherapy vs combination therapy).[28] An examination of patient characteristics from the study found that patient heterogeneity did not account for the variations in patient management between countries.[29] The authors concluded that choice of therapy seems to be influenced by local clinical practice preferences, differences in national health care systems, and possibly, drug availability and pricing rather than by evidence-based clinical guidelines.[29,31] Another potential driver of therapeutic choice, patient preference, was not examined in this study. It is important that patient expectations of therapy and adverse events are included in treatment decisions to ensure that therapy is tailored to individual patient needs and that health-related quality of life is addressed.[42]

RISK OF PROGRESSION AS A DRIVER FOR TREATMENT ALLOCATION

BPH is a progressive disease in some men.[43] BPH progression has been studied using various measures, including increased symptom severity or bother, decreased urinary flow, prostate enlargement, development of acute urinary retention, obstructive nephropathy, occurrence of UTI or incontinence, and need for surgical intervention. Longitudinal community-based studies provide key insights into the natural history of the disease. In the Olmsted County Study, a cohort of 631 randomly selected men aged 40 to 79 years was followed for 5 years. Their average baseline prostate volume significantly increased with increasing age, with a mean annual increase of 1.6% reported across all age groups.[44] Data for urinary symptoms were reported for the entire baseline study population of 2115 men, with a mean increase in AUA-SI score of 0.18 points per year observed during 42 months of follow-up.[45] The mean increase in score ranged from 0.05 points for men in their forties to 0.44 points for men in their sixties. A median decrease in peak urinary flow rate of 2.1% per year was also reported.[46] Again, this was found to be age-related, with men aged 70 years and more showing a faster decline (6.2% per year) than men in their forties (1.1% per year).

Randomized controlled trials also provide evidence of the progressive nature of BPH. For example, in the MTOPS study,[42] a composite measure of any of the following was used to define progression: 4-point increase in AUA-SI score, acute urinary retention, incontinence, UTI/urosepsis, or renal insufficiency. This study enrolled 3047 men aged at least 50 years, with an AUA-SI score of 8 to 35, a peak urinary flow rate between 4 and 15 mL/s, and a voided volume of at least 125 mL. The MTOPS study demonstrated that over a 4-year period, of the 737 men who received placebo, 17% had a BPH progression event, 14% had a 4-point increase in AUA-SI score, 2% had acute urinary retention, and 5% had surgery. Prostate volume also increased by a median of 24% after a mean follow-up of 4.5 years.[47]

A subsequent analysis of data from the placebo arm in the MTOPS study was used to determine the risk factors for BPH progression.[48] In this study population, prostate volume of 31 mL or more, PSA level of 1.6 ng/mL or more, maximum flow rate less than 10.6 mL/s, PVR of 39 mL or more, or age 62 years or older were found to significantly increase the risk of overall BPH progression. These findings are in agreement with those from previous community-based studies and randomized clinical trials in which PSA level and total prostate volume are well-defined risk factors for BPH progression.[49] Knowing the clinical characteristics that may predict the progression of BPH allows physicians to identify symptomatic men at risk of progression at an early stage and treat them appropriately.

INTERVENTIONAL THERAPY
Surgical Intervention Options

Surgery remains an important part of treatment for BPH. Different forms of surgery, broadly classified into TURP, open surgery, and minimally invasive procedures, are currently used. TURP has become the most common form of contemporary surgery and is the reference standard for the treatment of LUTS secondary to BPH. Obstructing adenomatous tissue is removed using a cutting diathermy current applied via a loop. The distal end of the incision is the verumontanum, which represents the proximal extremity of the distal sphincter mechanism. Bleeding vessels can also be easily visualized and coagulated. An option for patients with prostate glands of 25 g or less is to perform a transurethral incision of the prostate (TUIP). Men in their forties and fifties who present with a lifelong history of voiding difficulty that seems to be principally related to narrowing at the bladder neck (bladder neck dyssynergia) are seen to benefit most for TUIP. This technique may also be effective in men with a combination of mild prostatic enlargement and bladder neck obstruction. Open prostatectomy (retropubic prostatectomy[RPP]) aims to remove the central obstruction by shelling it out along the cleavage plane between the adenoma and compressed normal prostatic tissue. In contrast, radical prostatectomy comprises excision of the whole prostate gland and seminal vesicles, perineally or via a suprapubic approach. This procedure is used to treat localized prostatic adenocarcinoma. A modified form of TURP, bipolar TURP (B-TURP), can be done in normal saline, a conductive medium, instead of the conventional nonconductive irrigation fluid. This should help eliminate the dilutional hyponatremia and transurethral resection syndrome caused by hypotonic/hypoosmolar fluid irrigation.[50] A lack of homogenous trials has so far hampered the comparisons between TURP and B-TURP. One meta-analysis of 16 trials with a total of 1406 patients found no clinically relevant differences in short-term efficacy.[51] Patients unsuitable for transurethral or open surgery due to comorbid disease and those who wish to avoid the recognized morbidity—particularly relating to sexual function—may choose minimally invasive surgery.

Minimally Invasive Surgery

Compared with other procedures, minimally invasive surgery is associated with shorter postoperative hospitalizations and decreased morbidity. Although there is a plethora of shorter-term data on minimally invasive techniques, there are limited long-term data, so these procedures have not yet replaced TURP as the gold standard for the surgical management of BPH.

Minimally invasive surgery includes several promising treatments, such as Holmium laser resection, plasma kinetic vaporization, and GreenLight laser vaporization. Holmium laser resection enables complete enucleation of the prostate gland (as does RPP) and is considered to be a serious contender for the gold standard for large prostates (>100 g). This technique has been shown to be safe and effective, and it is associated with decreased blood loss and complications compared with TURP. However, it has high start-up costs, longer operative times, and a steep learning curve. Long-term randomized prospective studies comparing laser treatments with other treatments for BPH are ongoing. Another option is using Green-Light laser to vaporize prostatic tissue. A study by Coz and Domenech[52] showed very good results in the use of GreenLight laser to treat BPH; AUA score was reduced from a mean of 22 before treatment to a mean of 11.4 after 30 days, and urine flow rate increased. Complications included delayed removal of the catheter (11.1%), dysuria (16.6%), and late hematuria (11.1%). The few trials comparing GreenLight laser to TURP[53] show divergent results, and more trials with longer follow-up are needed.

Cooled transurethral microwave thermotherapy (TUMT) has emerged as an alternative to medical treatment for patients unsuitable for surgery. Microwaves are used to heat obstructive prostatic tissue under topical urethral anesthesia to a temperature of $40\,°C \pm 1°C$ for 45 minutes to 1 hour. A single 1-hour outpatient treatment can result in significant improvements. In a 2003 study, Osman and colleagues[54] showed that microwave therapy was well tolerated and that there was an overall subjective success rate in 83% of patients after at least 1 year. In more than 55% of patients, the improvements were marked and showed a successful urodynamic change to unobstructed. It was also found that TUMT achieved better results in those with higher grades of bladder outlet obstruction, lower age, and larger prostates. These findings are in line with earlier studies showing that the improvement is not due to the placebo effect,[55] is not temporary, and can last for up to 5 years.[56] The fast onset of action with α-blockers and the long-term efficacy of TUMT point to combining the 2 treatment options. This possibility was explored in a 1999 study of 41 patients who were treated with TUMT with or without neoadjuvant and adjuvant tamsulosin administration.[57] The combination of the 2 treatment modalities resulted in significantly lower mean IPSS at 2 weeks and 6 weeks than those in the TUMT-only group. TUMT can therefore be considered a promising treatment option alone and in combination with other established treatments.

EFFECTS OF TREATMENTS ON SEXUAL FUNCTION

Treatment for BPH can cause deterioration in sexual function, which can have a significant impact on patients' quality of life. The risks should be discussed with each patient before beginning treatment. Libido, erectile function, and ejaculatory function can all be affected in different ways by different treatment approaches. Alpha-adrenergic blockers and 5AR inhibitors can affect sexual and ejaculatory function.[58] The MTOPS study'[47] found slightly decreased libido and erectile and ejaculatory function with finasteride and combination therapy.

Box 1
Indications for intervention in clinical BPH

A. Absolute indications for intervention in clinical BPH (mostly surgery)

  1. Chronic retention: patients with impaired renal function, hydronephrosis (high-pressure chronic retention), or overflow incontinence

  2. Acute retention: patients receive a trial of medical therapy before surgery is considered

  3. Stone formation

  4. Recurrent hematuria: patients who are unresponsive to 5AR therapy and recurrent infection caused by residual urine

B. Relative indications for intervention in clinical BPH (mostly pharmacotherapy)

  1. Patients with moderate-to-severe symptoms and abnormal flow less than 15 mL/s

  2. Recurrent urinary infections associated with bladder outflow obstruction and high PVR urine

Adapted from AUA and EAU guidelines.[45,64]

α-Blocker therapy rarely contributes to a decrease in libido or sexual function.[59–61] Surgical treatments carry additional risks to sexual function, and as with medical treatment, different aspects of sexual function can be affected by different treatments. Transurethral resection involving cauterization can potentially damage the ejaculatory ducts. Although erectile dysfunction now occurs in less than 5% of cases,[62] ejaculatory function is negatively affected in more than half of all treatment cases.[63] Patients receiving minimally invasive procedures report disruption of sexual function less frequently, but effects vary for every patient. Patients being treated surgically are likely to have more severe urinary symptoms than those being treated medically. This means that for every patient, the balance between improving poor urinary function and retaining sexual function must be found.

AUA/EAU GUIDELINES SUMMARY

Current guidelines on the management of BPH published by the AUA and the EAU include systematic reviews of data to support the different assessments and interventions available.[32,45] However, although the 2 sets of guidelines provide guidance on absolute indications for treatment (for example renal impairment), they contain little guidance on the identification of men at risk of progression and the choice of watchful waiting versus active therapy. For example, the EAU guidelines state that "Watchful waiting is recommended for patients with mild symptoms that have minimal or no impact on their quality of life."[45] In contrast, the AUA guidelines state that "Watchful waiting is the preferred management strategy for patients with mild symptoms. It is also an appropriate option for men with moderate to severe symptoms who have not yet developed complications of BPH" (**Box 1**).[64]

SUMMARY

The last decade has witnessed a significant shift in emphasis in the management of BPH, with medical therapies and, to a lesser extent, MITs becoming the predominant active therapy choice.

Current guidelines may lag behind available evidence in their guidance on assessment and management of men with BPH. A critical review of guidelines for BPH found considerable differences in the overall quality of the available guidelines, particularly concerning methodology of guideline development.[65] Examination of risk factors for BPH progression has identified that baseline prostatic enlargement is a precursor and that PSA level is a reliable surrogate for prostate volume and therefore represents a robust measure of future progression risk. Taken together, this evidence demonstrates that men at risk of progression can be identified through PSA assessment.

Watchful waiting may prove inadequate for many men with mild symptomatic BPH at risk of progression. The lack of therapeutic intervention in these men exposes them to a greater risk of symptom deterioration, acute urinary retention, and surgical intervention. Data from large-scale clinical studies have demonstrated that treatment with 5AR inhibitors significantly ameliorates symptoms of BPH and, in contrast to α-blockers, reduces the long-term risks of acute urinary retention and BPH-related surgery in men at risk of progression. However, despite the large body of clinical evidence that demonstrates the benefits of 5AR inhibitors in reducing the risk of BPH progression, it seems that they are often underprescribed in at-risk men in everyday clinical practice, especially as a first-choice therapy to ameliorate symptoms and reduce the risk of BPH progression. In order for men at risk of BPH progression to be managed effectively, clinical practice should change to reflect the level 1 evidence for 5AR inhibitors in reducing their risk of progression.

REFERENCES

1. Barry MJ, Fowler FJ Jr, O'Leary, et al. The American Urological Association symptom index for benign prostatic hyperplasia. The Measurement Committee of the American Urological Associate. J Urol 1992;148(5):1549–57.
2. Neal RH, Keiser D. What's best for your patient with BPH? J Fam Pract 2009;58: 241–7.
3. Fong YK, Milani S, Djavan B. Natural history and clinical predictors of clinical progression in benign prostatic hyperplasia. Curr Opin Urol 2005;15:35–8.
4. Imperato-McGinley J, Zhu YS. Androgens and male physiology the syndrome of 5alpha-reductase-2 deficiency. Mol Cell Endocrinol 2002;198:51–9.
5. Schwinn D, Roehrborn C. Alpha (1)-adrenoceptor subtypes and lower urinary tract symptoms. Int J Urol 2009;15:193–9.
6. Djavan B, Marberger M. A meta-analysis on the efficacy and tolerability of Alpha (1)-adrenoceptor antagonists in patients with lower urinary tract symptoms suggestive of benign prostatic obstruction. Eur Urol 1999;36:1–13.
7. Djavan B, Chapple C, Milani S, et al. State of the art on the efficacy and tolerability of alpha(1)-adrenoceptor antagonists in Patients with Lower Urinary Tract Symptoms Suggestive of Benign Prostatic Hyperplasia. Urology 2004;64: 1081–8.
8. Lepor H, Auerbach S, Puras-Baez A, et al. A randomized, placebo-controlled multicenter study of the efficacy and safety of terazosin in the treatment of benign prostatic hyperplasia. J Urol 1992;148:1467–74.
9. Roehrborn CG, Oesterling JE, Auerbach S, et al. The Hytrin Community Assessment Trial study: a one-year study of terazosin versus placebo in the treatment of men with symptomatic benign prostatic hyperplasia. HYCAT Investigator Group. Urology 1996;47:159–68.

10. Frye SV. Discovery and clinical development of dutasteride, a potent dual 5alpha-reductase inhibitor. Curr Top Med Chem 2006;6:405–21.

11. McConnell JD, Bruskewitz R, Walsh P, et al. The effect of finasteride on the risk of acute urinary retention and the need for surgical treatment among men with benign prostatic hyperplasia. N Engl J Med 1998;338:557–63.

12. Roehrborn CG, Boyle P, Nickel JC, et al. Efficacy and safety of a dual inhibitor of 5-alpha-reductase types 1 and 2 (dutasteride) in men with benign prostatic hyperplasia. Urology 2002;60:434–41.

13. Marihart S, Mike H, Djavan B. Dutasteride: a review of current data on a novel dual inhibitor of 5alpha reductase. Rev Urol 2005;7:203–10.

14. Roehrborn CG, Lotan Y. The motion: prevention of prostate cancer with a 5alpha-reductase inhibitor is feasible. Eur Urol 2006;49:396–400.

15. O'Leary MP, Roehrborn CG, Andriole G, et al. Improvements in benign prostatic hyperplasia-specific quality of life with dutasteride, the novel dual 5-alpha-reductase inhibitor. BJU Int 2003;92:262–6.

16. Barkin J. Management of benign prostatic hyperplasia by the primary care physician in the 21st century: the new paradigm. Can J Urol 2008 Aug;15(Suppl 1): 21–30 [discussion: 30].

17. AUA Guideline on the management of benign prostatic hyperplasia (BPH) 2003. Updated 2006. Available at: http://www.auanet.org/content/guidelines-and-quality-care/clinical-guidelines.cfm?sub=bph. Accessed Febuary 2010.

18. Kaplan S, Roehrborn C, McConnell J. Long-term treatment with finasteride results in a clinically significant reduction in total prostate volume compared to placebo over the full range of baseline prostate sizes in men enrolled in the MTOPS trial. J Urol 2008;180:1030–3.

19. Barkin J, Roehrborn C, Siami P, et al. Effect of dutasteride, tamsulosin and the combination on patient-reported quality of life and treatment satisfaction in men with moderate-to-severe benign prostatic hyperplasia: 2-year data from the CombAT trial. BJU Int 2009;103:919–26.

20. Bautista OM, Kusek JW, Nyberg LM, et al. Study design of the Medical Therapy of Prostatic Symptoms (MTOPS) trial. Control Clin Trials 2003;24:224–43.

21. Gardiner P, Graham R, Legedza AT, et al. Factors associated with herbal therapy use by adults in the United States. Altern Ther Health Med 2007;13:22–9.

22. Fourcade RO, Theret N, Taieb C. Profile and management of patients treated for the first time for lower urinary tract symptoms/benign prostatic hyperplasia in four European countries. BJU Int 2008;101:1111–8.

23. Dedhia RC, McVary KT. Phytotherapy for lower urinary tract symptoms secondary to benign prostatic hyperplasia. J Urol 2008;179:2119–25.

24. Bent S, Kane C, Shinohara K, et al. Saw palmetto for benign prostatic hyperplasia. N Engl J Med 2006;354:557–66.

25. Lee J, Andriole G, Avins A, et al. Redesigning a large-scale clinical trial in response to negative external trial results: the CAMUS study of phytotherapy for benign prostatic hyperplasia. Clin Trials 2009;6(6):628–36.

26. Herbison P, Hay-Smith J, Ellis G, et al. Effective of anticholinergic drugs compared with placebo in the treatment of overactive bladder: systematic review. BMJ 2003; 326(7394):841–4.

27. Nitti V. Botulinum toxin for the treatment of idiopathic and neurogenic overactive bladder: state of the art. Rev Urol 2006;198–208.

28. Sarma AV, Jacobson DJ, McGree ME, et al. A population based study of incidence and treatment of benign prostatic hyperplasia among residents of Olmsted County, Minnesota: 1987 to 1997. J Urol 2005;173:2048–53.

29. Wei JT, Calhoun E, Jacobsen SJ. Urologic diseases in America project: benign prostatic hyperplasia. J Urol 2005;173:1256–61.

30. Chapple CR. Lower urinary tract symptoms suggestive of benign prostatic obstruction–Triumph: design and implementation. Eur Urol 2001;39(Suppl 3):31–6.

31. van Exel NJ, Koopmanschap MA, McDonnell J, et al. Medical consumption and costs during a one-year follow-up of patients with LUTS suggestive of BPH in six European countries: report of the TRIUMPH study. Eur Urol 2006;49:92–102.

32. Hutchison A, Farmer R, Chapple C, et al. Characteristics of patients presenting with LUTS/BPH in six European countries. Eur Urol 2006;50:555–61 [discussion: 62].

33. de la Rosette JJ, Alivizatos G, Madersbacher S, et al. European Association of Urology: guidelines on benign prostatic hyperplasia. Update March 2004. Available at: www.uroweb.org/fileadmin/tx_eauguidelines/2004/Full/BPH_2004.pdf. Accessed June 2010.

34. Wiygul J, Babyan RK. Watchful waiting in benign prostatic hyperplasia. Curr Opin Urol 2009;19(1):3–6.

35. Jacobsen SJ, Jacobsen DJ, Girman CJ, et al. Treatment for benign prostatic hyperplasia among community dwelling men: the Olmsted County study of urinary symptoms and health status. J Urol 1999;162:1301–6.

36. Flanigan RC, Reda DJ, Wasson JH, et al. 5-year outcome of surgical resection and watchful waiting for men with moderately symptomatic benign prostatic hyperplasia: a Department of Veterans Affairs cooperative study. J Urol 1998; 160:12–6 [discussion: 16–7].

37. Djavan B, Fong YK, Harik M, et al. Longitudinal study of men with mild symptoms of bladder outlet obstruction treated with watchful waiting for four years. Urology 2004;64:1144–8.

38. Djavan B, Fong YK, Chaudry A, et al. Progression delay in men with mild symptoms of bladder outlet obstruction: a comparative study of phytotherapy and watchful waiting. World J Urol 2005;23:253–6.

39. Slawin KM, Kattan MW. The use of nomograms for selecting BPH candidates for dutasteride therapy. Rev Urol 2004;6(Suppl 9):S40–45.

40. Roehrborn CG, Boyle P, Gould AL, et al. Serum prostate-specific antigen as a predictor of prostate volume in men with benign prostatic hyperplasia. Urology 1999;53:581–9.

41. Roehrborn CG, McConnell J, Bonilla J, et al. Serum prostate specific antigen is a strong predictor of future prostate growth in men with benign prostatic hyperplasia. PROSCAR long-term efficacy and safety study. J Urol 2000;163:13–20.

42. Montorsi F, Moncada I. Safety and tolerability of treatment for BPH. Eur Urol Suppl 2006;5:1004–12.

43. Emberton M, Andriole GL, de la Rosette J, et al. Benign prostatic hyperplasia: a progressive disease of aging men. Urology 2003;61:267–73.

44. Rhodes T, Girman CJ, Jacobsen SJ, et al. Longitudinal prostate growth rates during 5 years in randomly selected community men 40 to 79 years old. J Urol 1999;161:1174–9.

45. Jacobsen SJ, Girman CJ, Guess HA, et al. Natural history of prostatism: longitudinal changes in voiding symptoms in community dwelling men. J Urol 1996;155:595–600.

46. Roberts RO, Jacobsen SJ, Jacobson DJ, et al. Longitudinal changes in peak urinary flow rates in a community based cohort. J Urol 2000;163:107–13.

47. McConnell JD, Roehrborn CG, Bautista OM, et al. The long-term effect of doxazosin, finasteride, and combination therapy on the clinical progression of benign prostatic hyperplasia. N Engl J Med 2003;349:2387–98.

48. Crawford ED, Wilson SS, McConnell JD, et al. Baseline factors as predictors of clinical progression of benign prostatic hyperplasia in men treated with placebo. J Urol 2006;175:1422–6 [discussion: 1426–7].
49. Roehrborn CG. Definition of at-risk patients: baseline variables. BJU Int 2006; 97(Suppl 2):7–11 [discussion: 21–2].
50. Reich O. Bipolar transurethral resection of the prostate: what did we learn, and where do we go from here? Eur Urol 2009;56:796–7.
51. Mamoulakis C, Ubbink DT, de la Rosette JJ. Bipolar versus monopolar transurethral resection of the prostate: a systematic review and meta-analysis of randomized controlled trials. Eur Urol 2009;I(56):798–809.
52. Coz F, Domenech A. [KTP (green light) laser for the treatment of benign prostatic hyperplasia. Preliminary evaluation]. Prog Urol 2007;17:950–3 [in French].
53. Herrmann TR, Georgiou A, Bach T, et al. Laser treatments of the prostate vs TURP/ open prostatectomy: systematic review of urodynamic data. Minerva Urol Nefrol 2009;61(3):309–24.
54. Osman Y, Waidie T, El-Diasty T, et al. High-energy transurethral microwave thermotherapy: symptomatic vs urodynamic success. BJU Int 2003;91:365–70.
55. de Wildt MJ, Hubregtse M, Ogden C, et al. A 12-month study of the placebo effect in transurethral microwave therapy. Br J Urol 1996;77:221–7.
56. Baba S, Nakamura K, Tachibana M, et al. Transurethral microwave thermotherapy for management of benign prostatic hyperplasia: durability of response. Urology 1998;47:664–71.
57. Djava B, Shariat S, Fakhari M, et al. Neoadjuvant and adjuvant á-blockade improves early results of high-energy transurethral microwave thermotherapy for lower urinary tract symptoms of benign prostatic hyperplasia: a randomized, prospective clinical trial. Urology 1999;53:251–9.
58. Skolarus TA, Wei JT. Measurement of benign prostatic hyperplasia treatment effects on male sexual function. Int J Impot Res 2009;21:267–74.
59. Roehrborn CG, Rosen RC. Medical therapy options for aging men with benign prostatic hyperplasia: focus on alfuzosin 10 mg once daily. Clin Interv Aging 2008;3:511–24.
60. Chung BH, Lee JY, Kim CI, et al. Sexuality and the management of BPH with alfuzosin (SAMBA) trial. Int J Impot Res 2009;21:68–73.
61. Kaplan SA, DE Rose AF, Kirby RS, et al. Beneficial effects of extended-release doxazosin and doxazosin standard on sexual health. BJU Int 2006;97:559–66.
62. Fowler FJ Jr, Wennberg JE, Timothy RP, et al. Symptom status and quality of life following prostatectomy. JAMA 1988;259:3018–22.
63. Schulman C. Impact of treatment of BPH on sexuality. Prostate Cancer Prostatic Dis 2001;4(S1):S12–6.
64. AUA Practice Guidelines Committee. AUA guideline on management of benign prostatic hyperplasia (2003). Chapter 1: Diagnosis and treatment recommendations. J Urol 2003;170:530–47.
65. Novara G, Galfano A, Gardi M, et al. Critical review of guidelines for BPH diagnosis and treatment strategy. Eur Urol Suppl 2006;5:418–29.

Urinary Incontinence

Eva Fong, MD, Victor W. Nitti, MD*

KEYWORDS
- Urinary incontinence • Pathophysiology • Diagnosis
- Treatment

OVERVIEW OF INCONTINENCE

Urinary incontinence is defined by the International Continence Society as the "complaint of involuntary loss of urine." Urinary incontinence is a major health problem at population and individual levels.

The prevalence of urinary incontinence has been investigated in several large epidemiologic studies. In 2002, Hunskaar and colleagues,[1] reporting on their survey of women from 29,000 households in 4 European countries, found that between 15% and 34% had experienced urinary leakage in the previous 30 days. A 2005 survey of 45,000 households in the United States with a mixed respondent population, 82% female, found a 34% prevalence of urinary incontinence in the last 30 days.[2] The prevalence of urinary incontinence increases significantly as women and men age. It is uncommon in young women but becomes common in the perimenopausal period. For men, incontinence is approximately half as common as in women at all ages, with an overall prevalence of 3% to 11%.[3–6]

A helpful concept in urinary incontinence is that of "bother." Bother determines how much incontinence has an impact on patients physically, socially, and emotionally. Although the severity of incontinence can be quantified by measuring the amount of leakage, the degree of bother is crucial in determining how much intervention a patient desires and how successful that intervention may be.

Several types of urinary incontinence can be distinguished[7]:

1. Stress urinary incontinence is the complaint of involuntary leakage on effort or physical exertion or on sneezing or coughing.
2. Urgency urinary incontinence is the complaint of involuntary leakage accompanied by or immediately preceded by urgency, where urgency is a sudden compelling desire to pass urine, which is difficult to defer.
3. Mixed incontinence is where the symptoms and signs of stress and urgency incontinence coexist.

Department of Urology, NYU Langone Medical Center, 150 East 32nd Street, New York, NY 10016, USA
* Corresponding author.
E-mail address: Victor.Nitti@nyumc.org

Prim Care Clin Office Pract 37 (2010) 599–612
doi:10.1016/j.pop.2010.04.008
0095-4543/10/$ – see front matter © 2010 Elsevier Inc. All rights reserved.

The urodynamic classification of incontinence is based on measurements of pressures in the bladder, sphincter, and abdomen. Urodynamic stress urinary incontinence is when there is loss of urine with a rise in abdominal pressure, without a detrusor (bladder) contraction. Urodynamic detrusor overactivity is when there is loss of urine with an involuntary detrusor contraction, which is often accompanied by urgency.

Some patterns of incontinence are not easily classified into the above categories:

Extraurethral incontinence is the observation of urine leakage through channels other than the urethra (such as a fistula or an ectopic ureter).

Unconscious (unaware) incontinence is incontinence unaccompanied by urge or stress. It can be caused by severe urodynamic stress urinary incontinence, detrusor overactivity incontinence without urgency, impaired bladder compliance, or extraurethral incontinence.

Continuous urinary incontinence is the complaint of a continuous urinary leakage.

Nocturnal enuresis is the complaint of loss of urine occurring during sleep.

Postmicturition dribble is the complaint of an involuntary loss of urine immediately after passing urine.

Overflow incontinence is not a symptom or condition but rather a term used to describe leakage of urine associated with urinary retention.

NORMAL CONTINENCE AND MICTURITION

Normal continence requires coordination between bladder, sphincter, and peripheral and central nervous systems. In the healthy bladder, the particular mix of smooth muscle, collagen, and elastin produces a highly compliant structure. This gives the bladder the special viscoelastic properties that allow accommodation, so that normal bladder filling occurs with a minimal increase in detrusor pressure.[8] These properties can be affected by insults, however, such as radiation or bladder outlet obstruction.

Normal storage of urine is dependent on spinal reflex mechanisms that activate sympathetic and somatic pathways to the bladder outlet and on tonic inhibitory systems in the brain that suppress parasympathetic excitatory outflow to the bladder.[9] Distention of the bladder walls during filling leads to sympathetic stimulation of the bladder outlet smooth musculature and pudendal outflow to the external urethral sphincter. Sympathetic stimulation also inhibits the bladder body musculature and transmission in the bladder parasympathetic ganglia.[10,11] These responses occur by spinal reflex pathways and represent guarding reflexes that promote continence. Damage to central inhibitory pathways or sensitization of peripheral afferent terminals in the bladder can unmask primitive voiding reflexes and trigger bladder overactivity.[10]

Normal voiding is accomplished by activation of the micturition reflex. This is triggered when intense bladder afferent activity activates the pontine micturition center, which inhibits the spinal guarding reflex. The first event is relaxation of the striated urethral sphincter, followed by a rise in detrusor pressure and opening of the bladder neck and urethra as voiding begins. The micturition reflex is normally under voluntary control and is organized in the pontine micturition center. It requires integration and modulation by the parasympathetic and somatic components of the sacral spinal cord (the sacral micturition center) as well as the thoracolumbar sympathetic components.[12–15]

Normal Sphincter Function

In men and women, the sphincter can be conceptualized as having two parts: the first is the smooth muscle bladder neck and proximal urethral component,[16] and the second is the striated muscle external sphincter component. The principles underlying the function of a sphincter are (1) watertight apposition of the urethral lumen,

(2) compression of the wall around the lumen, (3) structural support to keep the proximal urethra from moving during increases in pressure, (4) a means of compensating for abdominal pressure changes, and (5) neural control. Normal sphincter function results from the integrated interaction among all these factors.

The Sphincter in Women

The watertight seal in women is thought to be due to mucus on the mucosa, the effects of the submucosal vascular cushions, and estrogenic effects. There has been a significant shift in the understanding of the function of the female sphincter in the past 20 years due to the emergence of midurethral synthetic slings and from research during and after their development. The most commonly held theory of urethral support is now the hammock theory developed by DeLancey.[17] He proposes that urethral support is provided by an intact backboard comprised of the anterior vaginal wall and its fascial and muscular attachments. In health, the urethra is compressed against these structures during rises in abdominal pressure and thus remains shut. Anterior support of the bladder neck is provided by the pubourethral ligaments (**Fig. 1**). Thus, in women, intrinsic sphincter function and urethral support are important for maintaining continence.

The Sphincter in Men

In men, there is a proximal and distal urethral sphincter mechanism.[18] The proximal sphincter approximately corresponds to the smooth muscle of the bladder neck. The distal urethral sphincter complex is composed of the prostatomembranous urethra, the cylindrical external sphincter muscle, and the extrinsic paraurethral musculature and connective tissue structures of the pelvis. The external sphincter, or rhabdosphincter, is a concentric muscular structure consisting of longitudinal smooth muscle and slow-twitch (type I) skeletal muscle fibers that can maintain resting tone and preserve continence. In contrast, some periurethral fibers of the levator ani are fast twitch fibers that can contract rapidly in response to sudden rises in intra-abdominal pressure, such as coughing.[19,20] In men, at least one sphincteric mechanism must be fully functional to maintain continence. The proximal sphincter is lost during operations for benign and malignant diseases of the prostate.

PATHOPHYSIOLOGY OF URINARY INCONTINENCE

Urinary incontinence can be thought of in two parts: bladder dysfunction and sphincter dysfunction. The 2-by-2 square devised by Alan Wein summarizes this (**Table 1**).[21]

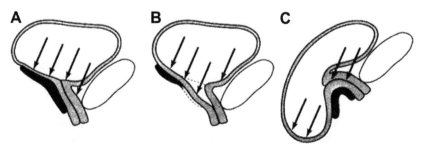

Fig. 1. Hammock theory of sphincter function and urethral support in women. (*From* DeLancey JO. Structural support of the urethra as it relates to stress urinary incontinence: the hammock hypothesis. Am J Obstet Gynecol 1994;170:1713–20; with permission.)

Table 1	
Weis square for urinary incontinence	
Bladder Dysfunction	**Sphincter Dysfunction**
Detrusor overactivity	Urethral support defect (women)
Impaired compliance	Intrinsic sphincter deficiency

Data from Wein AJ. Classification of neurogenic voiding dysfunction. J Urol 1981;125:605–9.

Bladder Dysfunction

Bladder dysfunction is the urodynamic diagnosis, which is suspected when patients have the symptom of urgency or have urgency incontinence. When the bladder fails to act as a low-pressure storage system, then urinary incontinence can occur. This can be due to low compliance or detrusor overactivity, and these can be distinguished urodynamically. When associated with urgency, this is classified as urgency urinary incontinence. The cause may be neurogenic or idiopathic (non-neurogenic). In men, detrusor overactivity is commonly associated with benign prostatic hyperplasia (BPH) and its associated bladder outlet obstruction. This often is the reason why men with BPH experience urgency and urgency urinary incontinence.

Low bladder compliance can be due to neurologic disease or to non-neurologic conditions. Neurologic causes include spinal cord injury, spina bifida and other congenital conditions, spinal stenosis, multiple sclerosis, cerebrovascular accident, and denervation injuries that can occur with radical pelvic surgery. Non-neurologic causes of low bladder compliance alter the structural makeup of the bladder and include radiation cystitis, long-term bladder outlet obstruction, long-term indwelling catheter, or tuberculosis of the bladder. If low bladder compliance is suspected, patients should be referred to a urologist for a full investigation, including urodynamic testing, because these patients may store urine at high pressure and are at risk for consequent renal damage.

Sphincter Dysfunction

In women, sphincter dysfunction occurs commonly after childbirth or with aging. It may also be associated with previous bladder and urethral surgeries or may occur after radiation therapy. In men, sphincter dysfunction is uncommon, except after prostatectomy. Sphincter dysfunction can also be caused by neurologic diseases that affect neural innervations below the sacral spinal cord. Special consideration needs to be given to incontinence in patients with neurologic disease, because the problem may go beyond simple bladder dysfunction.

Sphincter dysfunction may be caused by lesions above the brainstem, including cerebrovascular accident, brain tumor, Parkinson disease, and multiple system atrophy. These patients show detrusor overactivity and may have decreased sensation for lower urinary tract events, but the external sphincter is coordinated. In Parkinson disease, patients may have sphincter bradykinesia, with difficulty initiating voiding.

In suprasacral spinal cord injury, there is detrusor overactivity without sensation, but detrusor striated sphincter dyssynergia can also occur. This can lead to incomplete emptying, high storage pressures, and, if untreated, renal damage. Patients with spinal lesions above T6 may also experience autonomic dysreflexia, with resulting bladder or bowel distension. A sacral spinal cord injury causes absent detrusor activity with a fixed striated sphincter. Peripheral lesions, as in patients with sacral lesions or after radical pelvic surgery, are associated with an atonic bladder. Multiple sclerosis has variable presentations, most commonly detrusor overactivity, with some having sphincter dyssynergia with impaired emptying.

DIAGNOSING INCONTINENCE

In taking the history of incontinence, the authors aim to classify the type of incontinence symptoms and the severity and bother to the patient and to take a comprehensive medical and surgical history of comorbidities that have an impact on the urinary tract. A review of neurologic symptoms is particularly important, because urinary incontinence may be the first presentation of neurologic disease. It is also wise to exclude transient and reversible causes of incontinence before doing further investigation. These can be remembered using the mnemonic, DIAPPERS (**Box 1**).[22]

The authors often ask patients to describe a typical day and night. It is important to ask about the fluids patients are drinking, including amounts, types of fluid, and times of ingestion.

The questions listed in **Box 2** cover a wide range of symptoms in depth.

It is important to elicit not only the presence of the symptom but also the degree of bother and effect on lifestyle. A good history often allows for accurate characterization of incontinence. Voiding and intake diaries are helpful when patients cannot clearly recall a typical day or when nocturia or nocturnal incontinence is a major complaint. A voiding diary that covers 2 typical days should be adequate.

Physical Examination

The physical examination is directed toward urologic, neurologic, and transient causes of incontinence. Observation of gait, ability to stand and lie on the examination couch, and speech and cognition suffice to classify most patients as grossly neurologically normal or abnormal. A more focused neurologic examination can be performed in a select group. This includes lower limb examination, anal tone and sphincter tone, and the bulbocavernosus reflex, which examines the sacral nerves S2, 3 and 4.

The abdomen and inguinal areas should be palpated for masses, a distended bladder, and hernias.

In men, the external genitalia should be inspected and palpated for abnormalities. The prostate and rectal tone should be assessed with a digital rectal examination.

Box 1
DIAPPERS mnemonic

_D_elirium

_I_nfection (urinary tract infection)

_A_trophic vaginitis/urethritis

_P_sychological (eg, severe depression or neurosis)

_P_harmacologic

_E_xcess urine production

_R_estricted mobility

_S_tool impaction

Data from Resnick NM. Urinary incontinence in the elderly. Medical Grand Rounds 1984;3: 281–90.

Box 2
Urinary incontinence symptoms

How often do you void during the day and how often during the night?

How long can you comfortably wait between urinations?

Why does voiding occur as often as it does (urgency, convenience, or attempt to prevent incontinence)?

How severe is incontinence (only a few drops or enough to saturate outer clothing)?

Do you wear protective pads?

Do pads become saturated?

How often and why do you change pads?

Are you aware of incontinence occurring, or do you just find yourself wet?

Do you have a sense of urgency before incontinence occurs?

When you have a sense of urgency, how long can you postpone urinating?

Does incontinence occur during coughing, sneezing, while rising from sitting, or during heavy physical exercise?

Is urine lost only for an instant during activity, or does activity lead to uncontrollable voiding?

Is the incontinence positional?

Does incontinence ever occur in the lying or sitting position?

Do you have difficulty starting the urine stream, requiring pushing or straining?

Is your urine stream weak or interrupted?

Do you have dribbling after urinating?

Have you ever had urinary retention?

From Nitti VW, Blaivas JG. Urinary incontinence: epidemiology, pathophysiology, evaluation, and management overview. In: Wein AJ, Kavoussi LR, Novick AC, editors. Campbell-Walsh urology, vol. 3. 9th edition. Philadelphia: Saunders Elsevier; 2007. p. 2046–78; with permission.

In women, the vulva and perineum should be inspected for atrophy, excorations, and abnormal anatomy, such as prolapse at or beyond the introitus. In the estrogenized state, the vagina is pink and thick with rugae whereas in the atrophic state, it is paler and thinner, with loss of rugae. Initially the pelvic examination should be performed with the bladder full. With a patient in the lithotomy position, she is asked to cough, as a stress test for incontinence. This can also show if the urethra is mobile. Then vaginal examination is performed, first with a digital examination to palpate for prolapse. Speculum examination can help differentiate anterior and posterior prolapse by using the posterior blade to first hold the posterior then anterior walls away while asking the patient to strain. Rectal examination may also be useful to look for a rectocele.

Prolapse can be graded according to the Baden-Walker system[23] or the more complex pelvic organ prolapse quantification (POP-Q) system,[24] but in the primary care setting, it may be more appropriate to note the presence of prolapse and describe its extent within or below the introitus.

Simple Diagnostic Tests

Urinalysis is a mandatory test for all patients with incontinence. Dipstick testing can indicate need for culture and sensitivity. Urinary tract infection should be ruled out as a reversible cause of incontinence. Testing can also reveal glucose or blood in the urine, which necessitates investigation for diabetes or urologic work-up for hematuria.[25]

Postvoid residual is the amount of urine left in the bladder immediately after a patient voids. This can be measured using catheterization or by ultrasound. Measurement of postvoid residual is helpful when retention with overflow is suspected from history or due to physical findings of a distended bladder.

There are several standardized, validated questionnaires that are helpful in assessing incontinence, such as the Incontinence Symptom Index. Voiding diaries can be used to clarify symptoms, and they can provide a useful starting point for discussion.

Advanced Diagnostic Tests

Further testing that may be performed on referral to a urologist includes uroflow, pad tests, multichannel urodynamic testing, and cystoscopy. Uroflow curves are generated when a patient urinates into a calibrated measurement device that plots urine flow over time. This simple, noninvasive measure of flow rate may suggest an etiology for symptoms, such as bladder outlet obstruction. Recording the weights of incontinence pads for 24 hours can quantify the severity of incontinence and is often used before surgical intervention.[26]

Urodynamic testing is used to confirm symptomatic diagnoses or when symptoms are unclear, as in patients with unaware incontinence. Urodynamic testing measures bladder and abdominal pressures and allows calculation of detrusor pressures during filling and voiding. The pressure-flow relationship is measured during filling and voiding. This may be combined with fluoroscopy to demonstrate anatomic abnormalities, such as bladder neck obstruction. Stress incontinence can be tested for with cough or Valsalva maneuver. Cystoscopy is advised for patients with hematuria, those with a suspected anatomic abnormality, and those who fail to respond to appropriate therapy.

Indications for Referral

Patients with stress urinary incontinence, particularly if mild, can be managed initially in the primary care setting. Patients who have overactive bladder and urgency urinary incontinence can also be managed in a primary care setting. Patients with more complex incontinence or those who fail to respond to simple treatment should be referred to a specialist if they wish further treatment. Patients who should be referred early are those with a history of coexistent neurologic disease, pelvic irradiation, radical pelvic surgery, previous prolapse, or incontinence procedures and those with continuous incontinence. In addition, patients with hematuria should be referred for work-up of the hematuria.

Incontinence Associated with BPH and its Treatment

BPH is associated with lower urinary tract symptoms, which are differentiated into voiding and storage symptoms. Voiding symptoms include slow flow, hesitancy, and incomplete emptying. Storage symptoms include nocturia, frequency, urgency, and urgency urinary incontinence. Medical treatments are the first line of therapy for BPH. Historically, α-blockers and 5α-reductase inhibitors (such as finasteride) have been used to relieve the obstructive symptoms. More recently, several randomized trials have shown that is safe and efficacious to also use anticholinergic medications in this population, with minimal risk of precipitating urinary retention. These medications are discussed in more detail later. Surgical treatments for BPH include various modes of resecting or vaporizing the adenomatous tissue of the transitional zone of the prostate. Stress urinary incontinence occurs in approximately 1% of patients who have had endoscopic treatment for BPH. These patients usually not improve with conservative means, such as pelvic floor (Kegel) exercises, and they may require surgical interventions (discussed later).

TREATMENT OF URINARY INCONTINENCE

In the primary care setting, treatments for urinary incontinence may include behavioral and lifestyle modifications, pelvic floor exercises, medications, intermittent catheterization, and other treatments.

Behavioral and Lifestyle Modifications

Making systematic changes in behavior and lifestyle is most useful for patients with frequency, urgency, and urgency urinary incontinence, but it also helps some patients with stress urinary incontinence. Recommendations can include changes in diet and fluid intake, bladder training, and timed voiding.[27-30]

Patients' daily fluid intake can be assessed with an initial voiding diary. Patients should reduce nighttime fluid intake to reduce nocturia. Bladder irritants, such as caffeine, tea, coffee, and cola, should be reduced or eliminated.[31,32] Alcohol can act as a diuretic, so patients should expect greater urinary volumes if they consume it. Advice about maintaining regular bowel habits should also be given. Simple suggestions, such as increased fiber via food or fiber supplements, should be given if patients are constipated. Patients who drink large volumes of fluid may be able to improve their symptoms by reducing their intake.

Bladder training can improve existing voiding habits. Patients with frequency should be encouraged to gradually increase their voiding interval by half-hour increments. If they experience urgency and frequency they should be advised to

Not rush—stop and stay still
Concentrate on suppressing the urge
Perform several quick pelvic floor contractions
Wait until the urge subsides
Walk to the bathroom at a normal pace.

Pelvic Floor Exercises

Pelvic floor, or Kegel, exercises are useful as a first-line measure for stress, urge, and mixed incontinence (**Box 3**). Considerable heterogeneity and study design problems have affected attempts at benefit analysis; however, a systematic review of four randomized controlled trials (n = 229), published in 2008, concluded that continence rates and improvement in stress urinary incontinence were higher after pelvic floor muscle training.[33] Patients can be given a simple set of instructions on how to identify and contract their pelvic floor muscles. During the pelvic examination, patients can be asked to squeeze to verify that they can correctly identify and contract these muscles. Referral to a physical therapist specializing in pelvic floor physical therapy may help patients learn the correct technique.

Pharmacologic Therapy for Urinary Incontinence

There are no currently approved drug therapies for stress urinary incontinence available in the United States. Oral drug therapies for overactive bladder and urge urinary incontinence include antimuscarinics, musculotropic relaxants, and tricyclic antidepressants. Only antimuscarinics have a grade A recommendation from the International Consultation on Incontinence based on level 1 evidence,[34] and they are the

---

Box 3
Patient instructions for pelvic floor (Kegel) exercises

Pelvic floor exercises strengthen the supporting structures of the bladder and urethra to help with the problem of stress urinary incontinence. They also can help relax the bladder and reduce unwanted bladder contractions.

The easiest way to learn which muscles to exercise is to stop and start the urinary stream several times. Once you know the feeling of contracting these muscles, practice tightening and holding for approximately 10 seconds and then relax for 10 seconds. Repeat this approximately 10 times, and that is 1 session. Try to do at least 4 sessions per day. Do not practice while urinating. That is done only in the beginning to help identify the correct muscles. Also, when you get the urge to urinate, do the exercises. This starts a reflex that relaxes the bladder.

Do not tighten the abdominal muscles when doing pelvic floor exercises. That just increases the urge to urinate and may even force urine out. Consciously relax the abdominal muscles. If you have difficulty learning this technique, it can be taught in the office using biofeedback techniques.

---

mainstay of treatment for overactive bladder and urgency urinary incontinence. These agents are competitive inhibitors of acetylcholine at muscarinic receptors. Some drugs have mixed action, with a poorly defined direct action on bladder muscle (musculotropic relaxation) in addition to their predominant antimuscarinic action. **Box 4**[34] lists commonly used antimuscarinics, according to level of evidence.

Generally dosing is increased according to efficacy and is limited by dose-related side effects, such as constipation and dry mouth. These side effects can cause patients to discontinue the medication. A recent study found that the cumulative discontinuation rate for antimuscarinic drugs at 6 months was 58.8%, varying from 71% for oxybutynin to 54% for extended release tolterodine tartrate.[35] The authors recommend starting patients on low doses and titrating upwards while closely monitoring for side effects. Although specific theoretic advantages may be associated with some medications, none has superior efficacy, and all are associated with typical side effects. Patients may find one medication, however, is more tolerable than another

---

Box 4
Commonly used antimuscarinics

Darifenacin A

Oxybutynin (mixed action) A

Propiverine (mixed action) A

Tolterodine A

Trospium A

Solifenacin A

Propantheline B

Hyoscyamine C

From Abrams P, Cardozo L, Khoury S, et al. Incontinence. 3rd International Consultation on Incontinence. Recommendations of the International Scientific Committee. Evaluation and treatment of urinary incontinence, pelvic organ prolapse, and faecal incontinence. In: Abrams P, Cardozo L, Khoury S, et al, editors. Incontinence, vol. 2. Plymouth (UK): Health Publication Ltd; 2005. p. 809–54.

Table 2
Clinical properties of antimuscarinic medications

Name	Formulation	Dosages (Maximum)	Side Effects	Clearance	Dose Adjustment
			Dry mouth		
Oxybutynin	Oral IR	5 mg (15 mg)	−	Hepatic	No data
	Oral ER	10 mg (30 mg)	+		
	Patch	10% (1 sachet)	+++		
	Gel		+++		
Tolterodine	Oral IR	2mg	++ (2 mg)	R/H	2 mg/d in R/H
	Oral ER	2 mg (4 mg)	+ (4 mg)		impairment
Solifenacin	Oral ER	5 mg (10 mg)	++	R/H	R/H impairment: 5 mg
Darifenacin	Oral	7.5 (15 mg)	++	Hepatic	Moderate hepatic impairment: 7.5 mg
Trospium	Oral IR	20 mg (40 mg)	+++	Renal	Renal impairment: 20 mg/d at bedtime, possible extension of dosing to every 2 days.
	Oral ER	60 mg	+++		
Fesoterodine	Oral	4 mg (8 mg)	++ (4 mg) + (8 mg)	R/H	4 mg (8 mg with caution)

Abbreviations: ER, extended release; IR, immediate release; R/H, renal/hepatic; −, poor; +, acceptable; ++, good; +++, excellent.
　Side effects, tolerability, and withdrawal columns modified from Kirby M, et al. Int J Clin Pract 2006.
　Data from Kirby M, Artibani W, Cardozo L, et al. Overactive bladder: The importance of new guidance. Int J Clin Pract 2006;60(10):1263–71 and Witte LP, Mulder WM, de la Rosette JJ, et al. Muscarinic receptor antagonists for overactive bladder treatment: does one fit all? Curr Opin Urol 2009;19(1):13–9.

within this class, so that it is worthwhile to try switching them to a different medication for side effects. The clinical properties of available antimuscarinic medications are summarized in **Table 2**.

Intermittent Catheterization

Clean intermittent self-catheterization is advised for patients who do not empty consistently and thus suffer from overflow incontinence, frequency, or urgency incontinence. This technique, which is clean as opposed to sterile, is performed as needed up to 4 to 5 times per day and during the night for a few select patients.[36] The most common problem with intermittent self-catheterization is urinary tract infection. Estimates of bacteriuria vary widely, but most show that it is common. Estimates of the rate of clinical urinary tract infection also vary. One large series found that in 77 spinal cord injury patients using intermittent self-catheterization for 5 years, 81% had been treated for at least one urinary tract infection, 22% had two or three infections per year, and 12% had four or more infections per year. The risk of rarer problems, such as urethral strictures and false passages, increases with longer use of intermittent self-catheterization.[37]

Other Treatments

Second-line therapies for refractory urgency urinary incontinence and detrusor overactivity include botulinum toxin, sacral neuromodulation, and bladder augmentation.

Botulinum toxin, injected into the detrusor muscle, can reduce symptoms of urgency and urgency urinary incontinence in the neurogenic population.[38] Fewer data exist for its use in the non-neurogenic setting. It is not approved by the Food and Drug Administration for use in the bladder, although it is commonly used off-label. It is important to warn patients of the risk of transient urinary retention and the potential need for intermittent self-catheterization.

Sacral neuromodulation for detrusor overactivity involves placing leads in the S3 foramina, with a neurostimulator in the upper buttock. The principle is to induce somatic afferent inhibition of sensory processing in the spinal cord. Pudendal afferent input to the sacral cord is thought to inhibit, or turn off, supraspinally mediated hyperactive voiding. A clinical study published in 2007 reported that 56–71% of patients are successful at 5 yrs.[39]

Bladder augmentation and urinary diversion are surgical procedures for very refractory cases, most often used for patients with neurogenic bladders.

TREATMENTS FOR STRESS URINARY INCONTINENCE

The initial treatment for stress urinary incontinence is behavioral and lifestyle modifications (discussed previously). Further treatment may include urethral bulking agents or surgery.

Urethral Bulking Agents

Urethral bulking agents are most commonly used in older patients who are not surgical candidates. They probably work by augmenting the submucosal layer of the urethra, thus increasing the compressive force inward toward the urethral lumen. There are several substances used, including collagen, calcium hydroxyapatite, carbon-coated zirconium beads, polytetrafluoroethylene, silicones, such as polydimethylsiloxane, and autologous tissues, such as fat and cartilage. Most published trials have small numbers and short follow-up (<1 year). Martins and colleagues[40] published a series of 40 patients showing that cure or improvement was achieved on urodynamic studies in 46% of patients with bladder hypermobility and in 40.7% with intrinsic sphincter deficiency. Corcos and Fournier[41] published medium-term data (50 months) showing similar results, 40% improvement and 30% cure. Results for coapatite are similar to these.

Surgical Treatment in Women

The goals of surgical treatment for stress urinary incontinence in women are to restore urethral support and recreate a proper backboard to resist increases in abdominal pressure, to restore the coaptative forces of the urethra, or both. Midurethral slings have become the most common surgical intervention in recent years. These are minimally invasive ambulatory procedures where a synthetic sling is placed under the midurethra and brought out through the thigh (transobturator) or abdomen (retropubic). Long-term cure rates for this procedure are 80% to 90% by subjective and objective criteria. Generally, these are low morbidity procedures. Up to 30% of patients, however, may develop new irritative bladder symptoms, a few patients may have obstructed voiding requiring sling lysis or takedown, and approximately 1% have vaginal erosion of the sling.[42] Rare but serious adverse effects can include urethral or bladder erosion of the sling, necessitating removal of part or all of the sling and reconstructive surgery. Other surgical options include autologous fascial slings and Burch colposuspension, which avoid the use of synthetics and may be preferable in some patients.

Surgical Treatment in Men

Surgical options in men include the artificial urinary sphincter and male perineal slings. The artifical urinary sphincter has three parts: a cuff that wraps around the bulbar urethra, a pump in the scrotum, and a reservoir. The fluid-filled system has an inflated cuff at rest. To urinate, a patient presses the pump to shift fluid out of the cuff. Cure rates are approximately 80% to 90%. The major drawback is that components of the device may need to be replaced at a relatively high cumulative rate, approximately 30% to 45% at 10 years. One series with a mean follow-up of 8.1 years had median device duration of 6.9 years.[43]

Male perineal slings are a more recent innovation. A mesh sling is placed around the bulbar urethra via a perineal incision, with transobturator, pubic bone, or transobturator and prepubic fixation, depending on the type. There are few published data on these procedures. One report describes 13 patients, the other 102. In the larger of the two studies, 64 patients were cured, 18 were improved, and 20 were not improved.[44] Further follow-up and published data are needed to truly establish the efficacy and safety of these procedures.

REFERENCES

1. Hunskaar S, Gunnar L Lars V, et al. Prevalence of stress incontinence in women in four European countries. Presented at ICS Annual Meeting, August 2002. Heidelberg, Germany: Neurourol Urodyn 2002;21(4):275–42.
2. Kinchen K, et al. Prevalence and frequency of stress urinary incontinence among community-dwelling women. Presented at European Association in Urology (EAU) Annual meeting, February 2002, Birmingham UK. European Urology (Suppl 1):85, 2002.
3. Feneley RC, Sheperd AM, Powell PH, et al. Urinary incontinence: prevalence and needs. Br J Urol 1979;51:493–6.
4. Yarnell JW, St Leger AS. The prevalence, severity and factors associated with urinary incontinence in a random sample of the elderly. Age Ageing 1979;8:81–5.
5. Malmsten UG, Milsom I, Molander U, et al. Urinary incontinence and lower urinary tract symptoms: an epidemiological study of men aged 45 to 99 years. J Urol 1997;158:1733–7.
6. Schulman C, Claesm H, Matthijs J. Urinary incontinence in Belgium: a population-based epidemiological survey. Eur Urol 1997;32:315–20.
7. Abrams P, Cardozo L, Fall M, et al. The standardisation of terminology of lower urinary tract function: report from the standardisation sub-committee of the International Continence Society. Neurourol Urodyn 2002;21(2):167–78.
8. Klevmark B. Motility of the urinary bladder in cats during filling at physiologic rates: I. Intravesical pressure patterns studied by a new method of cystometry. Acta Physiol Scand 1974;90:565–77.
9. Morrison J, Birder L, Craggs M, et al, editors. Incontinence (Edition 2005) 3rd International Consultation on Incontinence. Plymmouth (UK): Health Publications; 2005. p. 363–422.
10. de Groat WC. A neurologic basis for the overactive bladder. Urology 1997; 50(Suppl):36–52.
11. de Groat WC, Fraser MO, Yoshiyama M, et al. Neural control of the urethra. Scand J Urol Nephrol Suppl 2001;207:35–43.
12. Bradley WE, Conway CJ. Bladder representation in the pontine-mesencephalic reticular formation. Exp Neurol 1966;16:237–49.

13. Blaivas JG. The neurophysiology of micturition: a clinical study of 550 patients. J Urol 1982;127:958–63.
14. Morrison JF. Bladder control: role of higher levels of the central nervous system. In: Torrens M, Morrison JF, editors. The physiology of the lower urinary tract. London: Springer-Verlag; 1987. p. 237–74.
15. de Groat WC, Steers WD. Autonomic regulation of the urinary bladder and sex organs. In: Loewy AD, Spyer KM, editors. Central regulation and autonomic functions. London: Oxford University Press; 1990. p. 310–33.
16. Tanagho EA. Anatomy of the lower urinary tract and mechanical interpretation of storage and voiding. Curr Opin Urol 1992;2:245–7.
17. DeLancey JO. Structural support of the urethra as it relates to stress urinary incontinence: the hammock hypothesis. Am J Obstet Gynecol 1994;170: 1713–20.
18. Hadley HR, Zimmern PE, Raz S. The treatment of male urinary incontinence. In: Walsh PC, Gittes RF, Perlmutter AD, editors. Campbell's Urology. 5th edition. Philadelphia: WB Saunders; 1986. p. 2658.
19. Gosling JA, Dixon JS, Critchley HO, et al. A comparative study of the human external sphincter and periurethral levator ani muscles. Br J Urol 1981;53: 35–41.
20. Turner-Warnick R. The sphincter mechanisms: their relation to prostatic enlargement and its treatment. In: Hinman F Jr, editor. Benign prostatic hypertrophy. Newyork: Springer Verlag; 1983. p. 809.
21. Wein AJ. Classification of neurogenic voiding dysfunction. J Urol 1981;125: 605–9.
22. Resnick NM. Urinary incontinence in the elderly. Medical Grand Rounds 1984;3: 281–90.
23. Baden W, Walker T. Surgical repair of vaginal defects. Philadelphia: JB Lippincott; 1992.
24. Bump RC, Mattaisson A, Bo K, et al. The standardization of terminology of female pelvic organ prolapse and pelvic floor dysfunction. Am J Obstet Gynecol 1996; 175:10–7.
25. Staskin D, Hilton P, Emmanuel A, et al. Initial assessment of incontinence. In: Abrams P, Cardozo L, Khoury S, et al, editors. Incontinence (Edition 2005) 3rd International Consultation on Incontinence. Plymmouth (UK): Health Publications; 2005. p. 485–517.
26. Groutz A, Blaivas JG, Chaikin DC, et al. Noninvasive outcome measures of urinary incontinence and lower urinary tract symptoms: a multicenter study of micturition diary and pad tests. J Urol 2000;164:698–701.
27. Burgio KL, Goode PS. Behavioral interventions for incontinence in ambulatory geriatric patients. Am J Med Sci 1997;314:257–61.
28. Fantl JA. Behavioral intervention for community-dwelling individuals with urinary incontinence. Urology 1998;51(Suppl):30–4.
29. O'Donnell PD. Behavioral modification for institutionalized individuals with urinary incontinence. Urology 1998;51(Suppl):40–2.
30. Wilson PD, Hay-Smith J, Nygaard I, et al. Adult conservative management. In: Abrams P, Cardozo L, Khoury S, et al, editors. Incontinence (Edition 2005) 3rd International Consultation on Incontinence. Plymmouth (UK): Health Publications; 2005. p. 855–964.
31. Creighton SM, Stanton SL. Caffeine: does it affect your bladder? Br J Urol 1990; 66:613–4.

32. Dallosso HM, McGrother CW, Matthews RJ, et al. The association of diet and other lifestyle factors with overactive bladder and stress incontinence: a longitudinal study in women. BJU Int 2003;92:69–77.

33. Shamliyan T, Kane RL, Wyman J, et al. Systematic review: randomized, controlled trials of nonsurgical treatments for urinary incontinence in women. Ann Intern Med 2008;148(6):459.

34. International Continence Society. 3rd International Consultation on Incontinence. Recommendations of the International Scientific Committee 2005. Available at: publishing/page.accueil.pub.html; http://www.congress-urology.org/. Accessed January 10, 2010.

35. Gopal M, Haynes K, Bellamy SL, et al. Discontinuation rates of anticholinergic medications used for the treatment of lower urinary tract symptoms. Obstet Gynecol 2008;112(6):1311–8.

36. Lapides J, Diokno AC, Silber SJ. Clean, intermittent self-catheterization in the treatment of urinary tract disease. J Urol 1972;107(3):458–61.

37. Biering-Sorensen F, Nielans HM, Dørflinger T, et al. Urological situation five years after spinal cord injury. Scand J Urol Nephrol 1999;33:157–61.

38. Schurch B, Stöhrer M, Kramer G, et al. Botulinum-A toxin for treating detrusor hyperreflexia in spinal cord injured patients: a new alternative to anticholinergic drugs? Preliminary results. J Urol 2000;164(3 Pt 1):692–7.

39. van Kerrebroeck PE, van Voskuilen AC, Heesakkers JP, et al. Results of sacral neuromodulation therapy for urinary voiding dysfunction: outcomes of a prospective, worldwide clinical study. J Urol 2007;178(5):2029–34.

40. Martins SB, Oliveira RA, Castro RA, et al. Clinical and urodynamics evaluation in women with stress urinary incontinence treated by Periurethral collagen injection. Int Braz J Urol 2007;33:695–703.

41. Corcos J, Fournier C. Periurethral collagen injection for the treatment of female stress urinary incontinence: 4 year follow up results. Urology 1999;54:815–8.

42. Novara G, Ficarra V, Boscolo-Berto R, et al. Tension-free midurethral slings in the treatment of female stress urinary incontinence: a systematic review and meta-analysis of randomized controlled trials of effectiveness. Eur Urol 2007;52(3):663–78.

43. Petero VG Jr, Diokno AC. Comparison of the long-term outcomes between incontinent men and women treated with artificial urinary sphincter. J Urol 2006;175:605–9.

44. Cornu JN, Sèbe P, Ciofu C, et al. The advance transobturator male sling for postprostatectomy incontinence: clinical results of a prospective evaluation after a minimum follow-up of 6 months. Eur Urol 2009. [Epub ahead of print].

Common Scrotal and Testicular Problems

Stephen M. Wampler, MD*, Mikel Llanes, MD

KEYWORDS

- Scrotal pain • Testicular torsion • Epididymitis
- Cryptorchidism • Hydrocele • Varicocele • Testicular cancer

Scrotal and testicular problems range from the benign and painless to the malignant and debilitating. The primary care physician should be able to triage these problems, and know when to give reassurance and when to initiate a targeted workup that may lead to specialist intervention. This article focuses on scrotal pain and palpable abnormalities. Scrotal pain includes well-defined acute causes such as torsion and infection, and the less well-defined chronic orchialgia. Palpable abnormalities covered here include cryptorchidism, hydrocele, spermatocele, varicocele, and testicular cancer.

TESTICULAR TORSION

Testicular torsion is a twisting of the testis, blocking blood flow from the spermatic cord and causing acute scrotal pain. Malformations that allow scrotal rotation increase the risk of torsion. The most common is when the tunica vaginalis wraps improperly around the spermatic cord and does not allow the testis to attach to the posterior scrotum.[1] Other predisposing factors include increase in testicular volume, testicular tumor, testicles with horizontal lie, a history of cryptorchidism, and a spermatic cord with a long intrascrotal portion.[1] Trauma is a less common cause. Testicular torsion annually affects 1 in 4000 males younger than 25 years.

The first step in diagnosing torsion is a thorough history, including onset, location, and intensity of the pain. Testicular torsion usually causes sudden onset of pain as compared with other causes of acute scrotum. The duration of pain is critical in determining the risk of prolonged ischemia and subsequent testicular loss. There is a 90% chance of salvaging the testicle when ischemia has been present for less than 6 hours, which decreases to 50% at 12 hours and 10% at 24 hours.[1]

Assessing the cremasteric reflex is a key component of the physical examination. An absent cremasteric reflex in patients with testicular torsion has a sensitivity of 100% in some studies; however, there have been case reports describing patients

Department of Family Medicine, University of Michigan, Room L2003, Box 5239, Ann Arbor, MI 48109-5239, USA
* Corresponding author.
E-mail address: stepwamp@med.umich.edu

with a positive cremasteric reflex and testicular torsion.[2] Other examination findings such as an elevated scrotum on the affected side, an enlarged, painful testis, and an abnormal testicular lie are also useful but less reliable.

Because no examination finding can completely rule out torsion, ultrasound with Doppler should always be done to confirm or rule out the diagnosis.[3] Scintigraphy is another imaging option, with sensitivity near 100%.[1,4,5] However, scintigraphy is used less because of the time required for testing and limited availability. If suspicion for torsion is high, it is reasonable to proceed directly to surgery.[6]

Manual detorsion is possible but should not delay surgical intervention. Because of the high frequency of congenital abnormalities resulting in testicular torsion, bilateral orchidopexy should be performed once blood flow has been reestablished to the affected side.[1] Orchiectomy is performed if the testis cannot be salvaged.

ACUTE EPIDIDYMITIS

Epididymitis is inflammation of the epididymis, the tightly coiled tube that connects the testicle with the vas deferens. Epididymitis is the most common cause of acute scrotal pain in all age groups, although most cases occur in men 14 to 35 years of age. In the acute phase, symptoms are present for less than 6 weeks.[7]

Most cases are infectious, caused by bacteria that reflux from the vas deferens to the epididymis. In sexually active men younger than 35 years, *Chlamydia trachomatis* and *Neisseria gonorrhoeae* are the most common causes. In men older than 35 and in men who practice anal intercourse, coliform bacteria such as *Escherichia coli* are common culprits.[7,8] Tuberculosis and sarcoidosis can cause granulomatous epididymitis. In boys younger than 14, noninfectious causes such as postviral inflammation or Henoch-Schönlein vasculitis should be considered. Some medications, such as amiodarone, can cause a chemical epididymitis.[7]

Risk factors include sexual activity, bladder outlet obstruction, urogenital malformation, strenuous physical activity, and bicycle or motorcycle riding.[7] Symptom onset tends to be slower and more gradual than the pain of testicular torsion. If the patient has urinary symptoms, epididymitis is more likely. Swelling is usually localized to the epididymis but can progress to the testicle.

A urethral swab, urine analysis, and urine culture are recommended in all patients, although cultures often are negative. Ultrasound with Doppler can help establish the diagnosis of epididymitis and rule out testicular torsion.[8]

Treatment with antibiotics is directed toward the most likely pathogens, based on age and risk factors. Analgesics, ice, and scrotal elevation can provide symptomatic relief. If the patient does not steadily improve, he should be reevaluated for possible complications such as abscess formation, sepsis, or continued infection.[7]

TORSION OF THE TESTICULAR AND EPIDIDYMAL APPENDAGES

The testicular and epididymal appendages are part of the scrotal anatomy and subject to torsion; this is the most common cause of acute scrotum in prepubertal children. Because appendageal torsion can mimic testicular torsion, it should be considered in all patients presenting with sudden onset of scrotal pain.

The pain is usually localized to a specific area in the testis. These patients lack any signs or symptoms of urinary tract infection or sexually transmitted disease. In these patients, the cremasteric reflex is intact and there is no pain on testicular palpation. A bluish nodule at the superior aspect of the testicle, found in as many as 40% of patients, makes the diagnosis of appendageal torsion highly likely.[4]

Doppler ultrasound is important in ruling out testicular torsion if the diagnosis is not clear, based on history and physical examination alone. Laboratory workup is usually unnecessary.

Because appendageal torsion is a benign condition, it is treated conservatively with analgesics. On rare occasions when pain persists, the appendage can be surgically removed.

CHRONIC SCROTAL PAIN

Chronic scrotal pain is pain lasting longer than 3 months, which interferes with daily activity and affects quality of life.[9] This condition occurs in 15% to 19% of postvasectomy patients, but in the general population the incidence is unknown. Causes are many and varied, and include prior or ongoing infection (including epididymitis, prostatitis, and orchitis), vasectomy or other previous inguinal surgery, referred pain from the back or abdomen, inguinal hernia, tumor, prior trauma or testicular torsion, varicocele, hydrocele, spermatocele, polyarteritis nodosa, epididymal or testicular cysts, and idiopathic origin (25%).

The history should include past surgeries or trauma, sexual history including infections, psychiatric history, history of other types of chronic pain, prior treatments, and medications used. The physical examination should include detailed genital, inguinal, and prostate examinations, and back and abdominal examinations.[10,11]

Urine analysis and testing for gonorrhea and Chlamydia are recommended in all patients, regardless of history. Ultrasound can reassure patient and physician by ruling out testicular cancer as the cause of pain. In selected patients, a computed tomography (CT) scan for renal stones or a magnetic resonance imaging (MRI) scan of the lower back can be useful.

Management of chronic scrotal pain is challenging for the patient and the physician. The initial treatment consists of a trial of nonsteroidal anti-inflammatory drugs and antibiotics, in addition to scrotal elevation. Although this strategy has not been shown to effectively treat most patients, it is cost-effective and can avoid more invasive therapy in the few patients who receive partial or complete relief.[9–11] If pain does not improve, a trial of neuromodulators can be pursued. Gabapentin and nortriptyline are the two that have been studied, but it is reasonable to try medications in the same drug category based on the patient's preference, medication tolerance, and insurance coverage.[12] Other conservative options include transcutaneous electrical nerve stimulation or alpha blockers. Pulsed radiofrequency has been suggested, but research is lacking in the use of this modality.

Minimally invasive techniques are the next step if conservative management fails. Spermatic cord blocks with lidocaine and methylprednisolone have been shown to provide relief for weeks up to several months in small case studies, and can be repeated at several-month intervals if modest temporary relief is achieved.[13,14] Transrectal ultrasound-guided periprostatic local injections is another option for temporary relief in patients who do not respond to spermatic cord blocks.[15] More invasive therapy using microsurgical denervation is a good option in patients willing to undergo the procedure. Research shows limited complications with a good response rate in a significant percentage of patients. This treatment is recommended only for those patients who experience temporary relief with anesthetic injection into the spermatic cord.[16,17]

Surgical options should be a last resort because they are not always effective and are nonreversible. The two most common options are epididymectomy and orchiectomy (inguinal or scrotal). When pain is localized to the epididymis, an epididymectomy may be a good testicular-sparing option. In general, studies of surgical intervention are few with limited number of patients, and data are conflicting regarding relief experienced.[9,18] Therefore, candidates for surgery should have multiple evaluations, including one by a mental health professional, and have exhausted all other treatment options. It is important that patients understand that surgical intervention does not always provide relief.

Although many modalities exist for treating chronic scrotal pain, none are 100% effective. The best care uses a multifactorial approach throughout the course of treatment, and addresses the psychological factors (such as depression, anxiety, sexual dysfunction) and social stressors that accompany and contribute to chronic pain. Addressing these issues can improve long-term outcomes, regardless of what treatment is used.

CRYPTORCHIDISM

Cryptorchidism is a developmental defect whereby the testis fails to descend completely into the scrotum. Undescended testes can be found anywhere from their origin near the inferior pole of the kidney to just outside the external inguinal ring. A normally descended testis can also retract to become cryptorchid later in childhood. Cryptorchid testes can be palpable or nonpalpable,[19] with palpable testes accounting for 70% to 80% of cases.

Cryptorchidism is actually a group of abnormalities, with numerous proposed etiologies, many of which are poorly understood. Proposed mechanisms include hormonal influences, uteroplacental dysfunction, environmental factors, and genetics. Issues such as low birth weight, gestational diabetes, preeclampsia, breech presentation, delivery by cesarean section, complicated delivery, and a family history of cryptorchidism increase the infant's risk of cryptorchidism.[20–27]

Cryptorchidism is a common congenital anomaly, with an incidence of approximately 3% in full-term infants. However, this rate increases significantly with low birth weight. One prospective study found the rate of cryptorchidism at 3 months to be 7.7% for infants with birth weights less than 2000 g, 2.5% for birth weights of 2000 to 2500 g, and 1.41% for birth weights of 2500 g or more.[28]

Cryptorchidism is diagnosed by physical examination. With the patient undressed and supine, identify the external inguinal ring and carefully palpate it and the path of the inguinal canal. Soap applied to the examiner's hand can decrease friction and increase the chances of identifying a testis in the canal. If a testis is not found, palpate for ectopic testes in front of the pubis, in the perineum, and in the upper thigh.[29] Other findings that can accompany an undescended testis include hypospadias, inguinal hernia, and hydrocele.

Imaging studies are traditionally not believed to be beneficial in the workup of cryptorchidism. Ultrasound and MRI can identify testes in or distal to the inguinal canal. However, for intra-abdominal testes, the sensitivity of ultrasound is only 12% to 45%.[30,31] MRI is somewhat better at identifying intra-abdominal testes,[32] but it requires general anesthesia in young children. Because cryptorchid testes that fail to descend will require surgical intervention, laparoscopy serves as a diagnostic and therapeutic modality for those with nonpalpable testes.

Infertility is a major complication of cryptorchidism. Because few studies follow boys from the time of orchidopexy through adulthood to find true fertility rates, sperm parameters are often used as a surrogate to predict future fertility. Unfortunately, studies often have median ages of orchidopexy much higher than the current recommendations. Cortes and colleagues[33] showed normal sperm counts in 80% of

unilateral and 20% of bilateral cryptorchid patients, but the median age of orchidopexy was 11 and 13 years, respectively. An earlier study revealed that if orchidopexy
is performed by 1 year of life, there is no significant abnormality in sperm parameters.[34] More recent data show histologic changes as early as 9 months of age, suggesting that even earlier intervention may prevent future infertility.[35,36] Unfortunately,
sperm parameters do not always correlate well with fertility studies, which show
that men with a history of unilateral cryptorchidism have fertility rates up to 90%
compared with 94% in controls, while men treated for bilateral cryptorchidism show
a paternity rate of 62%.[37] Considering that a unilaterally absent testis or unilateral
orchiectomy does not alter paternity rates,[38] cryptorchidism seems to affect both
testes. Use of hormonal therapies to improve the prospect of fertility later in life is
an ongoing area of research.[37]

Testicular cancer is also a well-established complication of cryptorchidism. Farrer
and colleagues[39] showed that a history of cryptorchidism increased the risk of
a germ cell tumor to 1:2550 from the 1:100,000 seen in the general population, giving
a relative risk of nearly 40. The reason is a matter of debate, and exposure of the cryptorchid testis to higher temperatures has been traditionally blamed. However, in men
with a history of unilateral cryptorchidism, neoplasms also develop more commonly
in the contralateral testis, with a relative risk of 3.6.[40] This finding suggests cryptorchidism affects the testes, and is a process more significant than simply the position of
the testis in childhood. Fortunately, there is good evidence that early surgical intervention mitigates the risk of developing a neoplasm. One study showed a relative risk of 2
with early intervention,[41] whereas another noted no increase in cancer rates if orchidopexy was performed by the age of 10 years.[42] The risk of testicular cancer goes up
with the age at time of orchidopexy,[43] supporting the current practice of early
intervention.

Treatment for cryptorchidism is primarily surgical. However, because 70% to 77%
of cryptorchid testes descend spontaneously by 3 months of age, the initial
approach can be optimistic.[44] From 3 to 6 months of age only a small percentage
of testes will descend on their own,[45,46] and these patients should be referred for
definitive treatment, namely orchidopexy. Although there are several surgical
approaches, they all involve identification and mobilization of the cryptorchid testis
and spermatic cord, fixation of the testis in the scrotum, and correction of comorbid
conditions such as indirect inguinal hernia or a patent processus vaginalis. Orchidopexy is typically done as an outpatient by laparoscopy, although open techniques
with a high scrotal or inguinal approach are also used. Overall, the success rate
approaches 98%.

Hormonal therapies for cryptorchidism are based on the premise that testicular
descent is regulated by androgens and may be accelerated by using luteinizing
hormone-releasing hormone 1 or human chorionic gonadotropin (hCG) to increase
testosterone production. Success rates have ranged from 6% to 75%,[29] with better
results in boys older than 5 years, those with bilateral cryptorchidism, and those
with retractile testes.[29,46,47] Although hormone therapy is generally unsuccessful
and therefore seldom used, there is mounting evidence that it improves fertility
indices.[48–50]

HYDROCELE

A hydrocele is a fluid collection between the layers of the tunica vaginalis. A communicating hydrocele occurs when a patent processus vaginalis allows fluid to pass from
the peritoneal space into the scrotum, whereas a noncommunicating or simple

hydrocele has no such connection. The incidence of neonatal hydroceles is as high as 4.7%,[51] while only about 1% of adult males have hydroceles.

Congenital hydroceles are present at birth or within the first year of life, and are typically caused by an incomplete or delayed closure of the processus vaginalis. Hydroceles acquired after the first year of life may occur in response to venous or lymphatic obstruction caused by trauma or infection. Most hydroceles, however, have no identifiable cause. In a study of children older than 1 year with new-onset hydrocele, a clear cause was found in only 20 out of 302 patients.[52] In North America, common infectious causes of hydroceles include epididymitis and viruses. Worldwide, however, filariasis is a major cause of hydroceles and should be considered in patients from or with recent travel to tropical nations. Other conditions causing hydroceles include trauma, torsion of the testicle or testicular appendage, and recent scrotal surgery. Testicular cancer has an etiology not to be missed, especially in a man presenting with a new-onset hydrocele in his third or fourth decade. About 10% of testicular tumors are accompanied by a hydrocele, which can obscure the testicle and prevent a thorough examination.

Hydroceles vary in size, but most are asymptomatic. Acquired hydroceles usually develop slowly and are often not alarming to the patient. In early childhood, most hydroceles are found by the parents or on routine physical examination. Larger hydroceles can cause an aching pain in the scrotum or lower back. A communicating hydrocele may be smaller each morning but grow larger throughout the day as the patient is upright. The hallmark feature on physical examination is a tense, smooth, scrotal mass that easily transilluminates. Transillumination can help distinguish a hydrocele from a hernia or a solid mass. Communicating hydroceles may be accompanied by an indirect inguinal hernia. The entire surface of both testes should be palpated to evaluate for a mass.

If the size of the hydrocele prohibits a thorough examination of other scrotal structures, or if the hydrocele does not fully transilluminate, ultrasound can rule out testicular tumor as the cause.[53] Imaging should also be ordered if the patient is symptomatic or if the history and physical examination suggest a causative process. Ultrasound can show an inguinal hernia, which often accompanies a communicating hydrocele.

In infants, noncommunicating hydroceles often resolve by 2 years of age, and new-onset hydroceles in boys older than 1 year resolve within 6 months in about 75% of cases.[52] Watchful waiting is appropriate in this population. In adults, as long as there is a normal testicle and the patient remains asymptomatic, hydroceles do not need treatment. However, symptomatic or communicating hydroceles need definitive treatment. Noncommunicating hydroceles can be treated with surgical resection via an inguinal approach, or with aspiration and sclerotherapy. In a small, nonrandomized trial, surgical resection was slightly more effective than aspiration and sclerotherapy, but had a higher rate of complications (mostly hematoma) and was significantly more expensive.[54] Communicating hydroceles are treated surgically, by resection and correction of the anatomic defect, causing the persistent connection with the peritoneal cavity. The surgical approach is similar to correction of an indirect inguinal hernia.

SPERMATOCELE

Spermatoceles (epididymal cysts) are benign cystic collections of fluid that arise from the epididymis, usually at the superior pole of the testis. Spermatoceles are typically smooth, painless masses, found incidentally by the patient or on routine physical examination, that transilluminate. Spermatoceles require no treatment unless they are significantly painful, and they require no further workup in most cases. Scrotal ultrasound can be used if the diagnosis is in question. If treatment is needed, a simple excision can be performed, but patients should be aware of the risks of infertility or chronic pain.[55]

VARICOCELE

A varicocele is a dilation of the testicular vein and pampiniform plexus within the scrotum. Varicoceles are one of the most commonly identified scrotal abnormalities, found in 15% of adult men and in 40% of men with infertility. Varicoceles are thought to be the most common cause of male infertility worldwide.[56] Due to discrepancies in venous drainage, 90% of varicoceles occur on the left side. The cause is poorly understood. Most develop in adolescence, so physiologic changes in testosterone levels may contribute by increasing blood flow to the testicle, causing venous dilation. Varicoceles are less frequent in obese men, possibly because abdominal fat protects the left renal vein from becoming compressed between the aorta and superior mesenteric artery.[57,58]

Varicoceles are typically asymptomatic, and are found on routine physical examination or by the patient. In a minority of patients, an aching pain is present that improves when the patient lies down. The classic finding is a left-sided scrotal mass with a "bag of worms" consistency that increases in size with standing or a Valsalva maneuver, and decompresses when supine. Grade I varicoceles are small and palpable only with Valsalva, Grade II are easily palpable while the patient is standing without use of a Valsalva maneuver, and Grade III are large enough to be detected visually with the patient standing.[59] If the diagnosis is in question, ultrasound is the test of choice, with a sensitivity of 97% and specificity of 94%.[59] Varicoceles can rarely be caused by retroperitoneal masses that obstruct the spermatic vein. Further imaging with CT or ultrasound of the abdomen and pelvis is indicated for varicoceles that are of sudden onset, do not reduce in size with the patient supine, or occur on the right side.

Varicoceles are the leading cause of infertility. There are several proposed mechanisms for this phenomenon. The prevailing theory is that poor venous drainage disrupts heat exchange from the spermatic cord, elevating scrotal temperatures and impairing spermatogenesis.[56] Varicoceles can alter testosterone and follicle-stimulating hormone levels,[60] cause oxidative stress,[61] decrease sperm count, and adversely affect sperm morphology and motility.

Varicocele repair is generally performed when the male partner of an infertile couple has a grade II or III varicocele and an abnormal semen analysis,[62] and the female partner has no known reversible cause of infertility. The 3 main surgical techniques are open inguinal, laparoscopic, and subinguinal microscopic varicocelectomy. Each is equally effective at reversing abnormal sperm parameters, but complication rates are lowest with subinguinal microscopic varicocelectomy.[63] Hydrocele development and varicocele recurrence are the most common complications. Less-invasive methods include retrograde embolization and anterograde sclerotherapy. These percutaneous methods have similar complication rates, but higher rates of failure than laparoscopy.[64]

There is active controversy concerning the repair of varicoceles. Although varicoceles cause abnormal semen analysis, and varicocelectomy can normalize these abnormalities,[65] there is no irrefutable evidence that this translates into higher rates of pregnancy,[66,67] possibly because of a lack of good randomized data, improper study protocols, and poor reporting of data.[68] A Cochrane review gave an odds ratio (OR) of 1.1 favoring treatment, but with a confidence interval (CI) of 0.73 to 1.68. Isolating the most relevant studies from this meta-analysis, the OR improves to

2.08, but the CI is 0.60 to 4.25.[67] As a result, the evidence does not currently support varicocele repair as a reliable treatment for male infertility.

TESTICULAR CANCER

Although testicular cancer is a rare cancer, accounting for only about 1% of all male cancers, it is the leading cause of cancer in men between the ages of 15 and 35 years, with an average age at diagnosis of 34. The annual incidence of 4 cases per 100,000 men is rising and has nearly doubled in the past 40 years. Germ cell testicular tumors (seminomas and nonseminomas) are the most common, whereas sex cord-stromal tumors account for only 4% of testicular tumors[69] and are not further addressed here.

Risk factors include cryptorchidism, family history, tobacco use, white race, previous testicular cancer, and infertility. Testicular cancer caused by cryptorchidism is decreasing with earlier orchidopexy. Family history is important; having a brother with testicular cancer increases the risk by 6- to 10-fold.[70] Smoking doubles a man's risk of testicular cancer, and this increased risk may not improve with smoking cessation.[71] In the United States, Caucasians develop testicular cancer at a rate 4 times that of African Americans, although African Americans have a higher stage of cancer at the time of diagnosis.[72]

Testicular cancer is often believed to present with a discrete painless mass on the testicle. Although this does occur, the most common presenting feature is testicular swelling in 73% of men, with testicular pain in 18% to 46%.[73] Scrotal heaviness and firmness of the affected testicle are also presenting complaints. Some have symptoms identical to epididymitis, so patients who fail to respond to treatment for epididymitis should be reassessed for testicular cancer. Examination should include a thorough evaluation of the scrotum, and a survey of lymph nodes, particularly inguinal nodes. Scrotal masses should be carefully palpated and checked for transillumination. Signs and symptoms of metastatic disease are present in about 5% of patients. Back pain secondary to retroperitoneal spread is the most common symptom of metastatic disease, but abdominal pain, chest pain, shortness of breath, or hemoptysis can be present in more advanced cases. If the tumor produces hCG, the patient may develop gynecomastia.

Diagnosis of a presumed testicular mass begins with a scrotal ultrasound. If the lesion is confirmed as intratesticular, it is presumed to be cancerous and should proceed to surgery for a unilateral radical orchiectomy. Before surgery, serum marker is obtained including α-fetoprotein (AFP), hCG, and lactate dehydrogenase (LDH). Nonseminoma tumors typically elevate the AFP and hCG except in early stages, whereas seminomas occasionally raise hCG and typically do not raise AFP levels. LDH levels increase with the activity level of metastatic disease.[74] Once the diagnosis is confirmed on pathologic examination, a CT of the chest, abdomen, and pelvis is obtained to evaluate for metastasis. CT or MRI of the brain can be considered in patients with widespread disease or with neurologic signs or symptoms.

Routine screening for testicular cancer in asymptomatic men has not been shown to reduce mortality from testicular cancer. As a result, the US Preventive Services Task Force and the American Cancer Society recommend against routine screening by patients or clinicians,[75,76] based on the low rate of testicular cancer and the excellent prognosis once a diagnosis is made. This recommendation applies to asymptomatic men only, and should not diminish the consideration of testicular cancer in men with scrotal complaints or findings on examination.

The mainstay of treatment for both seminomas and nonseminomas is radical inguinal orchiectomy, where testicle and spermatic cord are removed.[77] Transscrotal approaches are not recommended, because they can cause the cancer to spread. Treatment after orchiectomy depends on staging, as shown in **Table 1**. Lower-grade seminomas (Stages I and IIA) are often treated with radiation after orchiectomy. Nonseminomas may require retroperitoneal lymph node dissection and chemotherapy. Higher-grade lesions in histologic categories are typically treated with chemotherapy, with or without further surgery.

With appropriate treatment, survival rates from testicular cancer are excellent. According to the National Cancer Institute, the overall 5-year survival rate from testicular cancer was 95.3% between 1999 and 2005. If the cancer was confined to the testis at the time of diagnosis, the survival rate was 99.2% and dropped only slightly to 95.9% with regional extension. For patients with distant metastases, the survival rate was 71%.[78]

With the survival rates for testicular cancer so high, it is important to be mindful of the long-term complications of treatment, as shown in **Table 2**. These complications include infertility, recurrent or secondary malignancy, and cardiac disease.

Infertility can be a result of the cancer and the treatment. Subfertility is common at the time of diagnosis,[79] due to local destruction of tissue, secretion of hCG, and other paracrine factors, and changes in blood flow and temperature.[80] These factors affect

Table 1
Treatment options after surgery for the stages of testicular cancer

Stage	Seminoma	Nonseminoma
I	Usually irradiation, although observation and limited chemotherapy are also options	Retroperitoneal lymph node dissection or observation with monthly follow-up IB: Consider 2 cycles of chemotherapy IS: Full-dose chemotherapy if serum tumor marker levels do not rapidly decrease after surgery
II	IIA: irradiation of the regional lymph nodes IIB or IIC: 3 cycles of 3-drug chemotherapy	IIA: Retroperitoneal lymph node dissection followed by observation with monthly follow-up and frequent laboratory testing or 2 cycles of 2-drug chemotherapy IIB or IIC: 3 or 4 cycles of 3-drug chemotherapy followed by retroperitoneal lymph node dissection if computed tomography still shows lymph nodes High serum tumor marker levels: chemotherapy followed by lymph node dissection
III	Three-drug chemotherapy; if there is no response, consider clinical trials of other chemotherapy drug combinations Brain metastasis is present: Treat with radiation of the brain or surgical removal	Three-drug chemotherapy; surgical removal of persistent tumors High serum tumor-marker levels: These patients often do not respond to usual chemotherapy; therefore, more aggressive clinical trials may be considered

Note: Two-drug chemotherapy usually includes cisplatin (Platinol AQ) and etoposide (Vepesid); 3-drug chemotherapy usually includes cisplatin, etoposide, and bleomycin (Blenoxane).

Adapted from Shaw J. Diagnosis and treatment of testicular cancer. Am Fam Physician 2008;77(4):472; with permission.

Table 2 Potential long-term risks of treatments for testicular cancer	
Treatment	**Risks**
Surgical	Infertility Ventral hernia Bowel obstruction
Chemotherapy	Secondary malignancy Infertility Cardiotoxicity Nephrotoxicity Neurotoxicity Ototoxicity Pulmonary toxicity Vascular toxicity
Radiotherapy	Secondary malignancy Infertility Cardiotoxicity

Data from Kaufman MR, Chang S. Short- and long-term complications of therapy for testicular cancer. Urol Clin N Am 2007;34:259–68; with permission.

spermatogenesis in the testes. Treatment with irradiation and chemotherapy has an even greater adverse effect on fertility than the cancer itself. One study showed a 91% pretreatment fertility rate, which declined to 67% after treatment.[81] Men should be encouraged to bank sperm prior to treatment.

Secondary or recurrent cancer is another major risk after testicular cancer. The risk of developing a second testicular cancer increased by a factor of 12 in one study when compared with men who had no history of testicular cancer.[82] This risk is greatest within the first 5 years after the primary diagnosis. One of the major complications of chemotherapy is the increased risk of leukemia. One risk-benefit analysis calculated that 1 man would develop leukemia for every 20 men cured with the use of standard chemotherapeutic regimens in the 1990s.[83] However, the risk of leukemia is dose related, so with current practice calling for smaller doses and fewer cycles, there should be a decrease in leukemia risk.[84] Chemotherapy recipients are also at a higher risk of secondary nongerm-cell tumors, including lung, biliary, gastrointestinal, bladder, and stomach cancers, and sarcomas.[84]

The ways chemotherapy and radiation cause cardiotoxicity are poorly understood.[85,86] One study found the relative risk of cardiac disease to be 2.7 with irradiation and 2.6 with chemotherapy.[87] Men with a history of testicular cancer should be educated to watch for symptoms of cardiac disease and to reduce their risk through lifestyle modifications.

REFERENCES

1. Ringdahl E, Teague L. Testicular torsion. Am Fam Physician 2006;74(10): 1739–43.
2. Schmitz D, Safranek S. Clinical inquiries. How useful is a physical exam in diagnosing testicular torsion? J Fam Pract 2009;58(8):433–4.
3. Lavallee ME, Cash J. Testicular torsion: evaluation and management. Curr Sports Med Rep 2005;4(2):102–4.
4. Abul F, Al-Sayer H, Arun N. The acute scrotum: a review of 40 cases. Med Princ Pract 2005;14(3):177–81.

5. Marcozzi D, Suner S. The nontraumatic, acute scrotum. Emerg Med Clin North Am 2001;19(3):547–68.
6. Cavusoglu YH, Karaman A, Karaman I, et al. Acute scrotum—etiology and management. Indian J Pediatr 2005;72(3):201–3.
7. Trojian TH, Lishnak T, Heiman D. Epididymitis and orchitis: an overview. Am Fam Physician 2009;79(7):583–7.
8. Centers for Disease Control and Prevention. Sexually transmitted diseases. Treatment guidelines 2006. Epididymitis. Available at: http://www.cdc.gov/std/treatment/2006/epididymitis. Accessed January 23, 2009.
9. Davis B, Noble MJ, Weigel JD, et al. Analysis and management of chronic testicular pain. J Urol 1990;143:936–9.
10. Granitsiotis P, Kirk D. Chronic testicular pain: an overview. Eur Urol 2004;45:430–6.
11. Masarani M, Cox R. The aetiology, pathophysiology and management of chronic orchialgia. BJU Int 2003;91:435–7.
12. Wiffen PJ, McQuay HJ, Rees J, et al. Gabapentin for acute and chronic pain. Cochrane Database Syst Rev 2005;3:CD005452.
13. Fuchs E. Cord block anesthesia for scrotal surgery. J Urol 1982;128:718–9.
14. Issa M, Hsiao K, Bassel Y, et al. Spermatic cord anesthesia block for scrotal procedures in the outpatient clinic setting. J Urol 2004;172(6):2358–61.
15. Zorn B, Rauchenwald M, Steers WD. Periprostatic injection of local anesthesia for relief of chronic orchialgia. J Urol 1994;151:411, A735.
16. Choaa RG, Swami KS. Testicular denervation. A new surgical procedure for intractable testicular pain. Br J Urol 1992;70:417–9.
17. Strom KH, Levine LA. Microsurgical denervation of the spermatic cord for chronic orchialgia: long-term results from a single center. J Urol 2008;180:949–53.
18. Costabile RA, Hahn M, McLeod DG. Chronic orchialgia in the pain prone patient: the clinical perspective. J Urol 1991;146:1571–4.
19. Kaplan GW. Nomenclature of cryptorchidism. Eur J Pediatr 1993;152(Suppl 2):S17–9.
20. Mayr JM, Lawrenz K, Berghold A. Undescended testicles: an epidemiological review. Acta Paediatr 1999;88:1089–93.
21. Virtanen HE, Tapanainen AE, Kaleva MM, et al. Mild gestational diabetes as a risk factor for congenital cryptorchidism. J Clin Endocrinol Metab 2006;91(12):4862–5.
22. Hjertkvist M, Damber JE, Bergh A. Cryptorchidism: a registry based study in Sweden on some factors of possible aetiological importance. J Epidemiol Community Health 1989;43:324–9.
23. Mori M, Davies TW, Tsukamoto T, et al. Maternal and other factors of cryptorchidism—a case-control study in Japan. Kurume Med J 1992;39:53–60.
24. Berkowitz GS, Lapinski RH. Risk factors for cryptorchidism: a nested case-control study. Paediatr Perinat Epidemiol 1996;10:39–51.
25. Jones ME, Swerdlow AJ, Griffith M, et al. Prenatal risk factors for cryptorchidism: a record linkage study. Paediatr Perinat Epidemiol 1998;12:383–96.
26. Akre O, Lipworth L, Cnattingius S, et al. Risk factor patterns for cryptorchidism and hypospadias. Epidemiology 1999;10:364–9.
27. Elert A, Jahn K, Heidenreich A, et al. The familial undescended testis. Klin Padiatr 2003;215:40–5.
28. John Radcliffe Hospital Cryptorchidism Study Group. Cryptorchidism: a prospective study of 7500 consecutive male births, 1984–8. Arch Dis Child 1992;67:892–9.

29. Esposito C, Caldamone AA, Settimi A, et al. Management of boys with nonpalpable undescended testis. Nat Clin Pract Urol 2008;5(5):252–60.
30. Weiss RM, Carter AR, Rosenfield AT. High resolution real-time ultrasonography in the localization of the undescended testis. J Urol 1986;135:936–8.
31. Stéfaniu M, Lefebure B, Liard-Zmuda A, et al. Laparoscopic surgery for undescended testicles. Arch Pediatr 2004;11(4):315–8.
32. Muglia V, Tucci S Jr, Elias J Jr, et al. Magnetic resonance imaging of scrotal diseases: when it makes the difference. Urology 2002;59:419–23.
33. Cortes D, Thorup J, Lindenberg S, et al. Infertility despite surgery for cryptorchidism in childhood can be classified by patients with normal or elevated follicle-stimulating hormone and identified at orchidopexy. BJU Int 2003;91:670–4.
34. McAleer IM, Packer MG, Kaplan GW, et al. Fertility index analysis in cryptorchidism. J Urol 1995;153:1255–8.
35. Hadziselimovic F, Herzog B. The importance of both an early orchidopexy and germ cell maturation for fertility. Lancet 2001;358:1156–7.
36. Lee PA, O'Leary LA, Songer NJ, et al. Paternity after unilateral cryptorchidism: a controlled study. Pediatrics 1996;98(4):676–9.
37. Hadziselimovic F. Successful treatment of unilateral cryptorchid boys risking infertility with LH-RH analogue. Int Braz J Urol 2008;34(3):319–26.
38. Lee PA. Fertility after cryptorchidism: epidemiology and other outcome studies. Urology 2005;66:427–31.
39. Farrer JH, Walker AH, Rajfer J. Management of the postpubertal cryptorchid testis: a statistical review. J Urol 1985;134:1071–6.
40. Prener A, Engholm G, Jensen OM. Genital anomalies and risk for testicular cancer in Danish men. Epidemiology 1996;7:14–9.
41. Pettersson A, Richiardi L, Nordenskjold A, et al. Age at surgery for undescended testis and risk of testicular cancer. N Engl J Med 2007;356(18):1835–41.
42. United Kingdom Testicular Cancer Study Group. Aetiology of testicular cancer: association with congenital abnormalities, age at puberty, infertility and exercise. BMJ 1994;308:1393–9.
43. Moller H, Prener A, Skakkebaek NE. Testicular cancer, cryptorchidism, inguinal hernia, testicular atrophy, and genital malformations: case-control studies in Denmark. Cancer Causes Control 1996;7:264–74.
44. Berkowitz GS, Lapinski RH, Dolgin SE, et al. Prevalence and natural history of cryptorchidism. Pediatrics 1993;92:44–9.
45. Wenzler DL, Bloom DA, Park JM. What is the rate of spontaneous testicular descent in infants with cryptorchidism? J Urol 2004;171:849–51.
46. Canavese F, Cortese MG, Gennari F, et al. Non-palpable testes: orchiopexy in single stage. Eur J Pediatr Surg 1995;5(2):104–7.
47. Esposito C, De Lucia A, Palmieri A, et al. Comparison of five different hormonal treatment protocols for children with cryptorchidism. Scand J Urol Nephrol 2003;37(3):346–9.
48. Hadziselimovic F, Herzog B. Treatment with a luteinizing hormone-releasing hormone analogue successful orchiopexy markedly improves the chance of fertility later in life. J Urol 1997;158(3):1193–5.
49. Sahin C, Artan M, Aksoy Y. The effects of one- and two-stage orchiopexy on postoperative serum testosterone levels and testicular volume in adult patients with bilateral nonpalpable testes. J Laparoendosc Adv Surg Tech A 2002;12(5):327–31.
50. Jallouli M, Rebai T, Abid N. Neoadjuvant gonadotropin-releasing hormone therapy before surgery and effect on fertility index in unilateral undescended testes: a prospective randomized trial. Urology 2009;73(6):1251–4.

51. Osifo OD, Osaigbovo EO. Congenital hydrocele: prevalence and outcome among male children who underwent neonatal circumcision in Benin City, Nigeria. J Pediatr Urol 2008;4(3):178–82.
52. Christensen T, Cartwright PC, Devries C, et al. New onset of hydroceles in boys over 1 year of age. Int J Urol 2006;13(11):1425–7.
53. Coley B. The acute pediatric scrotum. Ultrasound Clin 2006;1(3):485–96.
54. Beiko DT, Kim D, Morales A. Aspiration and sclerotherapy versus hydrocelectomy for treatment of hydroceles. Urology 2003;61(4):708–12.
55. Hagerty J, Yerkes E. Pediatric scrotal masses. Clin Ped Emerg Med 2009;10: 50–5.
56. Khera M, Lipshultz L. Evolving approach to the varicocele. Urol Clin North Am 2008;35(2):183–9.
57. Nielsen ME, Zderic S, Freedland SJ, et al. Insight on pathogenesis of varicoceles: relationship of varicocele and body mass index. Urology 2006;68(2):392–6.
58. Practice Committee of the American Society for Reproductive Medicine. Report on varicocele and infertility. Fertil Steril 2006;86:S93–5.
59. Trum JW, Gubler FM, Laan R, et al. The value of palpation, varioscreen contact thermography and colour Doppler ultrasound in the diagnosis of varicocele. Humanit Rep 1996;11:1232–5.
60. Cayan S, Kadioglu A, Orhan I, et al. The effect of microsurgical varicocelectomy on serum follicle stimulating hormone, testosterone and free testosterone levels in infertile men with varicocele. BJU Int 1999;84(9):1046–9.
61. Agarwal A, Sharma RK, Desai NR, et al. Role of oxidative stress in pathogenesis of varicocele and infertility. Urology 2009;73:461–9.
62. Male Infertility Best Practice Policy Committee of the American Urological Association; Practice Committee of the American Society for Reproductive Medicine. Report on varicocele and infertility [abstract]. Fertil Steril 2004;82(Suppl 1): S142–5.
63. Al-Kandari AM, Shabaan H, Ibrahim HM, et al. Comparison of outcomes of different varicocelectomy techniques: open inguinal, laparoscopic, and subinguinal microscopic varicocelectomy: a randomized clinical trial. Urology 2007; 69:417–20.
64. Beutner S, May M, Hoschke B, et al. Treatment of varicocele with reference to age: a retrospective comparison of three minimally invasive procedures. Surg Endosc 2007;21:61–5.
65. Segenreich E, Israilov SR, Shmueli J, et al. Correlation between semen parameters and retrograde flow into the pampiniform plexus before and after varicocelectomy. Eur Urol 1997;32:310–4.
66. Evers JL, Collins JA. Assessment of efficacy of varicocele repair for male subfertility: a systematic review. Lancet 2003;361:1849–52.
67. Evers JL, Collins JA, Evers Johannes. Surgery or embolisation for varicocele in subfertile men (Cochrane Review). Chichester, UK: John Wiley and Sons, Ltd; 2007. The Cochrane Library Issue 1.
68. Richardson I. Outcomes of varicocelectomy treatment: an updated critical analysis. Urol Clin North Am 2008;35:191–209.
69. Kocakoc E, Bhatt S, Dogra V. Ultrasound evaluation of testicular neoplasms. Ultrasound Clin 2007;2:27–44.
70. Dearnaley D, Huddart R, Horwich A. Regular review: managing testicular cancer. BMJ 2001;322(7302):1583–8.
71. Srivastava A, Kreiger N. Cigarette smoking and testicular cancer. Cancer Epidemiol Biomarkers Prev 2004;13(1):49–54.

72. Gajendran VK, Nguyen M, Ellison LM. Testicular cancer patterns in African-American men. Urology 2005;66:602.

73. Sesterhenn IA, Weiss RB, Mostofi FK, et al. Prognosis and other clinical correlates of pathologic review in stage I and II testicular carcinoma: a report from the Testicular Cancer Intergroup study. J Clin Oncol 1992;10:69.

74. Shaw J. Diagnosis and treatment of testicular cancer. Am Fam Physician 2008; 77(4):469–74.

75. Screening for testicular cancer: update of the evidence for the U.S. Preventive Services Task Force. Rockville, MD: Agency For Healthcare Research and Quality; 2004. Available at: http://www.ahrq.gov/clinic/3rduspstf/testicular/testiculrs.htm. Accessed October 24, 2009.

76. American Cancer Society. Can testicular cancer be found early? Available at: http://www.cancer.org/docroot/CRI/content/CRI_2_4_3X_Can_Testicular_Cancer_Be_Found_Early_41.asp?rnav=cri. Accessed October 24, 2009.

77. American Cancer Society. Detailed guide: testicular cancer. Treatment options by stage. Available at: http://www.cancer.org/docroot/CRI/content/CRI_2_4_4X_Treatment_Options_by_stage_41.asp?sitearea=. Accessed October 23, 2009.

78. National Cancer Institute. Surveillance epidemiology and end results. Available at: http://seer.cancer.gov/statfacts/html/testis.html. Accessed October 24, 2009.

79. Raman JD, Nobert CF, Goldstein M. Increased incidence of testicular cancer in men presenting with infertility and abnormal semen analysis. J Urol 2005; 174(5):1819–22.

80. Sabanegh ES Jr, Ragheb AM. Male fertility after cancer. Urology 2009;73:225–31.

81. Huyghe E, Matsuda T, Daudin M, et al. Fertility after testicular cancer treatments: results of a large multicenter study. Cancer 2004;100:732–7.

82. Fosså SD, Chen J, Schonfeld SJ, et al. Risk of contralateral testicular cancer: a population-based study of 29,515 U.S. men. J Natl Cancer Inst 2005;97(14): 1056–66.

83. Kollmannsberger C, Kuzcyk M, Mayer F, et al. Late toxicity following curative treatment of testicular cancer. Semin Surg Oncol 1999;17:275–81.

84. Kaufman MR, Chang S. Short- and long-term complications of therapy for testicular cancer. Urol Clin North Am 2007;34(2):259–68.

85. Meinardi MT, Gietema JA, van der Graaf WT, et al. Cardiovascular morbidity in long term survivors of metastatic testicular cancer. J Clin Oncol 2000;18:1725–32.

86. Fossa SD. Long-term sequelae after cancer therapy—survivorship after treatment for testicular cancer. Acta Oncol 2004;43:134–41.

87. Huddart RA, Norman A, Shahidi M, et al. Cardiovascular disease as a long-term complication of treatment for testicular cancer. J Clin Oncol 2003;21(8):1513–23.

Common Penile Problems

Julian Wan, MD[a],*, Karl T. Rew, MD[b,c]

KEYWORDS

- Hypospadias • Chordee • Priapism • Phimosis
- Paraphimosis • Peyronie disease

Patients from infancy to adulthood can present with a variety of penile problems, ranging from congenital to acquired conditions. This article reviews some of the more common conditions that are encountered in a typical primary care office practice. Although surgical procedures are discussed, the emphasis is on diagnosis, evaluation, and a general discussion of treatment options.

PENILE ANATOMY AND EMBRYOLOGY; A BRIEF REVIEW
Terminology and Pertinent Embryology

The penis is not a single solid structure. Unlike other parts of the human body that extend outward from the trunk, there is no central bone or cartilage around which are layered muscles, fat, and skin. Instead, the penis is composed of 3 major deep structures wrapped by skin: 2 corpora cavernosa bodies and a single corpus spongiosum. All 3 bodies contain erectile tissue that can become distended with blood. Surrounding this entire package of erectile bodies is Buck fascia. In normal situations, there is free flow of blood between the corpora cavernosa, so they function as a single unit. The corpora cavernosa are responsible for the primary structural integrity of erection. When engorged with blood, they inflate and become rigid. This rigidity is maintained by the tunica albuginea, a tough sheath of tissue that envelopes the corpora cavernosa. The 2 corpora cavernosa share a common wall formed by the tunica albuginea from each side. The posterior quarter of each corpus as it nears the pubic symphysis becomes the crura, a tough tendonlike tissue that acts as the anchoring point of the penis to the ischiopubic rami. The corpus spongiosum surrounds the

---

The authors received no external funding for this work.

[a] Department of Urology, University of Michigan, 3875 Taubman Center, 1500 East Medical Center Drive, Ann Arbor, MI 48109-0330, USA

[b] Department of Family Medicine, University of Michigan, 24 Frank Lloyd Wright Drive, Lobby H, SPC 5795, Ann Arbor, MI 48106-5795, USA

[c] Department of Urology, University of Michigan, 24 Frank Lloyd Wright Drive, Lobby H, SPC 5795, Ann Arbor, MI 48106-5795, USA

* Corresponding author.

E-mail address: juliwan@med.umich.edu

urethra and distally enlarges to form the head of the penis, also known as the glans penis. Proximally, the corpus spongiosum forms the bulbous urethra.

Embryologically, during the third week of development, the mesenchyme from the primitive streak migrates around the cloacal membrane to form a pair of cloacal folds. At the cranial end, the folds fuse and unite to form the genital tubercle. At the caudal end, the cloacal folds subdivide into the urethral folds anteriorly and the anal folds posteriorly. At the same time, the genital swellings form on either side of the urethral folds. They will become the scrotum in boys and the labia majora in girls. After the sixth week, the fetal testes secrete androgens that begin differentiating the external genitalia, causing elongation of the pubic tubercle, which becomes the phallus. During this elongation, the phallus pulls the urethral folds forward to form the lateral walls of the urethral groove. This groove runs from the caudal end but does not completely reach the distal end at the glans. The lining of the groove is epithelial and originates from the endoderm. It becomes the urethral plate. By the end of the third month, the urethral folds close over the urethral plate, forming the penile urethra. This fusion occurs along the ventral midline of the phallus, but the newly created tube does not yet reach the tip of the phallus. Around the fourth month, the distal portion of the urethra is formed when ectodermal cells from the tip of the glans invaginate and form a short epithelial cord. This cord gradually thins and develops a lumen, forming the urethral meatus. The invaginating lumen from this cord meets the lumen of the penile urethra, establishing a continuous urethra (**Fig. 1**). The early developments set up the later ones, so, when an anomaly occurs, it usually results in a constellation of findings.

Natural History of Physiologic Phimosis

At birth, there is normally a physiologic phimosis, a natural inability to retract the foreskin (or prepuce) because of natural adhesions between the glans and the prepuce. During the first 3 to 5 years of life, as the penis develops, epithelial cells and natural oil accumulate to form smegma, which displaces the prepuce from the glans. Intermittent erections also distend the foreskin. The combination of these 2 factors ultimately allows the prepuce to be completely retractable. By age 3 years, most boys can retract their foreskins, and between the age of 5 and 7 years, nearly 90% can retract their foreskins. By 17 years of age, less than 1% have a persistent phimosis.[1]

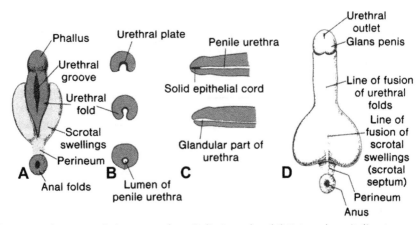

Fig. 1. Development of the external genitalia in males. (*A*) External genitalia at approximately 10 weeks. (*B*) Transverse sections through the phallus during penile urethra formation. (*C*) Development of the glanular urethra. (*D*) Normal newborn (prepuce not shown).

CONGENITAL CONDITIONS
Hypospadias

Definitions and anatomy

Hypospadias is a common congenital defect of the male external genitalia, occurring in approximately 1 in 250 newborn boys. Although commonly considered to be a low urethral opening, hypospadias is a spectrum of 3 conditions: (1) a low, abnormal position of the urethral meatus; (2) an abnormal development of the ventral penis resulting in curvature (also known as chordee); and (3) an abnormal formation of the foreskin. The urethral opening can be anywhere from the glans penis to the perineum beneath the scrotum. The degree of chordee ranges from nearly normal to the most severe form, which has a hooked penis. The foreskin in hypospadias is classically deficient ventrally and only well developed dorsally; this usually presents as hooded foreskin.[2]

Hypospadias is usually diagnosed during the newborn period. Mild cases or the rare variant with an intact foreskin may be discovered later in life.[3] There are other diagnoses that can be confused with a true hypospadias. Pseudo-hypospadias can be diagnosed if the glans is not fully visible. When newborns are being evaluated for circumcision, sometimes the foreskin is not completely retracted and becomes adherent near the meatus. If the complete meatus is not seen, the examiner may mistake it for a true hypospadias. However, once the foreskin is adequately retracted and the whole glans can be seen, then the urethral opening is found to be normal. Another possibility is a megameatus with an intact prepuce, which can confused with hypospadias. In this situation the meatus is sizable but it is located on the glans; often there is a strip of intact glans under lower edge of the meatus.[4]

Classification systems have been created to help describe hypospadias (**Fig. 2**).[5,6] The more distal meatal opening variants (glanular, coronal, subcoronal) comprise 50% to 70% of all cases of hypospadias.[7,8]

Embryology and causes

Recent reports suggest a multifactorial basis for hypospadias, possibly with a polygenic model. Factors such as endocrine disruptors from the environment, endocrinopathy, enzymatic or local tissue abnormality, or arrested development have been implicated.[9] The characteristic findings can occur as a result of abnormal androgen production from the fetal testis, limited androgen sensitivity in the developing external genitalia, or premature cessation or interruption of androgenic stimulation. Other possible causes include insufficient conversion of testosterone to dihydrotestosterone (caused by low 5α-reductase enzyme activity), or an androgen receptor defect. Several androgen insensitivity syndromes have been described as possible causes.[10]

Disruption of the normal androgen steroid pathway can lead to hypospadias.[11,12] Maternal progestin exposure has been supported and discounted.[11,13] There are markedly higher rates of hypospadias in boys conceived by in vitro fertilization, a process wherein progesterone is given early for pregnancy support, supporting the idea of endocrine disruption as a major cause of hypospadias.[14,15] A tenfold increase in hypospadias in the neonatal intensive care unit (ICU) population has been reported.[16] Poor intrauterine growth and advanced maternal age (35–40 years of age) have been implicated as possible factors.[17]

The currently accepted theory is based on the concept of arrest of development, whereby 1 or more of the possible causes discussed earlier disrupts an otherwise normal developmental pathway before the normal formation of the urethral and ventral phallus. This theory accounts for the simultaneous occurrence of all 3 findings characteristic of hypospadias: hypospadiac meatus, abnormal penile curvature, and deficient ventral foreskin.

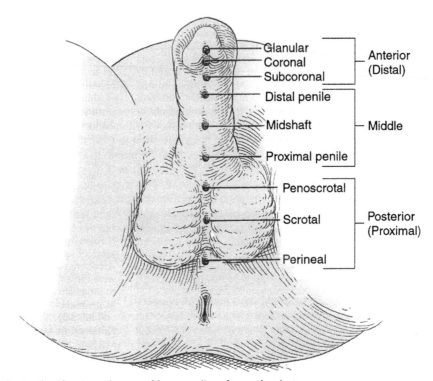

Fig. 2. Classification schemes of hypospadias after orthoplasty.

The rate of severe hypospadias has increased in 2 decades, from about 0.11 per 1000 male births to 0.27 to 0.55 per 1000 male births per year.[3,13,18] More frequent or early diagnosis of milder forms or more complete reporting have all been suggested as possible explanations. Although these reasons may be part of the increase they do not explain all of it. The ratio of minor to severe cases has been decreasing during this time, and the opposite would be expected if increased reporting of milder forms was the key factor.[19]

There is a strong familial association with hypospadias. Among boys with hypospadias, 6% to 8% of their fathers also have hypospadias. About 14% of male siblings will have hypospadias. Monozygotic twins have an 8.5-fold increased rate of hypospadias.[20,21] There are also more than 20 known syndromes in which hypospadias is an associated finding. Conditions linked with endocrinopathies comprise 78% of these conditions, such as micropenis, cryptorchidism, and scrotal abnormalities.[22]

Routine imaging of the urinary tract is not warranted for children with distal hypospadias. Preoperative imaging with voiding cystourethrography (VCUG) may be indicated for patients with a meatus located at the scrotal or perineal position.[23–25] Karyotyping is recommended for boys who have severe hypospadias and cryptorchidism, because about 20% will have an abnormal karyotype.[26,27] Disorders of sexual differentiation (DSD), formerly called intersex, are strongly associated with the finding of hypospadias and cryptorchidism.[28]

Treatment

Surgical correction is the primary treatment modality, with the main goals of creating a functional urethra and straightening out the phallus as much as possible. If possible, the glans and skin are reconstructed to achieve as normal an appearance as possible. In mild cases, an alternative to surgery is to do nothing. This is a reasonable choice when the patient has minimal to no chordee and a very distal meatus, the urinary stream is straight, and the patient can stand and void without difficulty.

Because of advances in pediatric anesthesiology, procedural improvements, and a concern for the psychological effects of genital surgery, surgery is usually scheduled between 6 and 12 months of age.[29] By this age, the penis is bigger and the child is physiologically more mature, which makes anesthesia better tolerated, so that the procedures can usually be carried out as an outpatient. Delaying the surgery until 18 months of age does not pose any significant risks or issues. However, delaying until much later in life (eg, 5 or 6 years of age, or even after puberty) is not recommended. There is a markedly higher rate of psychological effects and surgical complications in postpubertal patients.[30,31]

Hypospadias repair is carried out under general anesthesia. A caudal block or penile block can significantly reduce postoperative pain.[32,33] The child usually has a dressing and a urethral catheter for a few days to a week, although some distal repairs can be performed without a catheter.[34] Parents are advised to keep the child off all riding and straddling toys and to avoid rough play for about 4 weeks.

Although the details of surgical techniques are beyond the scope of this article, there are 2 broad classes of surgical methods. For patients with distal hypospadias, a single-stage operation is preferred.[22] For middle or proximal hypospadias, the longer length of tissue needed to construct the neourethra makes it necessary to rotate a flap of nearby tissue on a vascular pedicle or as a free graft. For proximal hypospadias, 2-stage procedures are common. First the phallus is straightened by an orthoplasty procedure. The prepuce is saved and, along with any other penile skin, it is rotated and secured ventrally. To allow the skin to form good vascular connections, a second procedure is carried out after at least 6 months. Using the now well-established skin, a neourethra can be created.[22] In some cases in which the available local skin is insufficient or has already been used for a prior surgery, it may be necessary to use a free graft. Scrotal skin, bladder epithelium, and oral mucosa have been used. The oral mucosa has the advantage of being easy to harvest, is not hair bearing, and heals well in the presence of moisture.

Androgen stimulation can be given briefly before surgery to temporarily increase penile size and make surgery easier to perform.[35–37] Studies to date have not shown any long-term adverse effects of such prepubertal androgen use.[38]

The major complications of hypospadias surgery are urethrocutaneous fistula, meatal stenosis, infection, bleeding, hematoma, urethral diverticulum, recurrent chordee, urethral stricture, and repair breakdown. Fistulas occur in less than 1% of distal hypospadias.[39,40] Bleeding is the most common complication. Diverticuli are uncommon and are typically associated with a distal stenosis. Infection is uncommon because of the good vascularity of the penis, but when it occurs, it can cause devastating breakdown of the entire repair.[41,42]

There are many techniques and each has particular nuances that may be advantageous in a particular patient, but not in others. Experience, training, and expertise are crucial to a good outcome. Because the best chance for a good outcome is with the first operation, it is recommended that the patient be evaluated and treated by an expert hypospadiologist at a center experienced with caring for these patients.[8,43]

Chordee without hypospadias

Chordee is the condition of ventral penile curvature and is most commonly associated with hypospadias. Some patients present with only chordee, a hooded foreskin, and a normally situated urethral meatus. There are 3 common causes: skin tethering, fibrotic dartos and Buck fascia, and corpora cavernosa disproportion. A congenitally short urethra is a rare cause. Repair techniques are similar to those for hypospadias. Releasing the skin tethering alone is effective in most cases. It is occasionally necessary to plicate the corpora cavernosal bodies. Plication sutures can safely be placed into the tunica albuginea along the dorsal midline, because the dorsal or 12-o'clock position is clear of nerves.[24] In more severely curved chordee, it may be necessary to add a free patch graft to the tunica albuginea ventrally, using de-epithelialized skin from the groin or tunica vaginalis tissue from the scrotum.[44,45] In mild cases, it is acceptable to do nothing if the patient can void effectively and, later in life, has a phallus that is straight enough for intercourse.

Long-term consequences of hypospadias

Patients who do well initially after hypospadias repair may still develop problems later in life. For primary care physicians who may encounter these patients later in adolescence or adulthood, several concerns should be kept in mind. If hair-bearing skin was used to form a neourethra, hair can grow inside the urethra, causing partial obstruction and discomfort. This is most commonly seen in patients repaired with older techniques that used scrotal skin. The patients present with dysuria and change in the force of stream. The treatment is endoscopic extraction of the hair. Laser ablation has also been described.[46] Strictures are also a common late problem, particularly in patients with proximal hypospadias. The patient may report a gradual decrease in the force of stream, dysuria, and straining with voiding. Internal urethrotomy under direct vision has been successful in only about 50% of cases. If there is a persistent or recurrent stricture, a patch graft may be needed.[47,48]

Some patients undergo multiple unsuccessful attempts at hypospadias repair. These patients are complex and challenging, and require extensive reconstruction.[49] They may present with persistent chordee, fistula, diverticuli, and poor cosmesis, and they often lack healthy tissue that can be used to perform reconstruction.[49] Referral to someone who is experienced with reoperative hypospadias repair is imperative. A staged approach is often needed.[50]

Penile Torsion

Penile torsion is a rotational defect of the penile shaft. In nearly all cases, the twist is in the counterclockwise direction (ie, to the left side). Usually penile size is normal, and the median raphe can be seen spiraling around the shaft. In general, it is of minor cosmetic significance, and correction is rarely necessary.[51]

OTHER CONGENITAL ANOMALIES
Micropenis

Micropenis is a normally formed penis that is at least 2.5 standard deviations less than the mean in length.[52] The length is measured from the pubic symphysis to the tip of the glans. In an obese child, the suprapubic fat pad must always be depressed completely to obtain an accurate measurement. Stretched penile length is used because it correlates with erectile length of the penis. The measurements should be compared with published standards for penile length.[53] In general, the penis of a full-term newborn should be at least 1.9 cm long. Typically, the ratio of shaft length to circumference in micropenis is normal. The scrotum is usually fused, but often small. The testicles are usually small and frequently undescended.

A true micropenis results from a hormonal abnormality that occurs after 14 weeks of gestation. The most common causes are hypogonadotropic hypogonadism, hypergonadotropic hypogonadism (primary testicular failure), and idiopathic.[54,55] Micropenis is often associated with major chromosomal defects, including Klinefelter syndrome (47,XXY), other X polysomy syndromes, and translocations, deletions, and trisomy involving chromosomes 8, 13, and 18.[52] Hypogonadotropic hypogonadism results from a failure of the hypothalamus to produce an adequate amount of gonadotropin-releasing hormone (GnRH). It may result from hypothalamic dysfunction, as in Kallmann syndrome (genital-olfactory dysplasia), Prader-Willi syndrome, Laurence-Moon-Biedl syndrome, or the CHARGE (Coloboma of the eye, Heart defects, Atresia of the nasal choanae, Retardation of growth and/or development, Genital and/or urinary abnormalities, and Ear abnormalities and deafness) association.[56,57] In other cases, there is an associated growth hormone deficiency or neonatal hypoglycemia secondary to congenital hypopituitarism. Congenital pituitary aplasia, midline brain defects, and primary testicular failure are other major causes. Micropenis secondary to hypergonadotropic hypogonadism may also result from gonadal dysgenesis or rudimentary testes syndrome.[54]

A karyotype should be performed in boys with micropenis. Consultation with pediatric endocrinology and genetics is helpful to determine the cause and to assess whether other abnormalities are present. Testicular function may be assessed by measuring serum testosterone levels before and after human chorionic gonadotropin (hCG) stimulation. Primary testicular failure produces an absent response and increased basal levels of luteinizing hormone (LH) and follicle-stimulating hormone (FSH). In some cases, a GnRH stimulation test is also carried out. Anterior pituitary screening tests should include serial measurements of serum glucose, sodium, potassium, and serum cortisol, and thyroid function tests. Magnetic resonance imaging of the head should be carried out to visualize the hypothalamus, the anterior pituitary, and the midbrain.

Androgen therapy is usually given to determine the penile response.[58] However, androgen treatment that results in penile growth to the normal range does not necessarily predict later growth at puberty. Until longer-term studies are available, exogenous androgen stimulation at birth and at puberty is reasonable.[59] In the past, when the penis did not respond to testosterone, gender reassignment was recommended. This approach has more recently been criticized, in large part because of the lack of long-term data regarding the risks and benefits of reassigning these patients to the female gender. In an important long-term retrospective study, 20 patients with a primary diagnosis of micropenis in infancy were assessed. Almost all had received androgen therapy during childhood. None of the adults had a penis within the normal range of size. All of the boys stood to urinate. Of the 12 patients in the adult group, 9 had a normal male appearance, and 3 appeared eunuchoid despite regular testosterone therapy. All had a strong male identity, although half had experienced teasing because of their genital appearance; 9 of the 12 patients were sexually active.[60] This study and others show that, although penile size may not reach what is considered a normal range, individuals born with micropenis have a male gender identity, and most can have satisfactory male sexual function.[61]

Webbed and Concealed Penis

Webbed penis is a condition in which the scrotal skin extends onto the ventrum of the penis. It is a congenital condition in which the penis, urethra, and scrotum are normal except for the webbing. This condition is corrected surgically by revising the shaft skin and its relationship with the scrotum. A concealed penis is a normally developed penis that is obscured by the suprapubic fat pad. This anomaly may be congenital or iatrogenic after circumcision (**Fig. 3**). Revision of the shaft skin by rotating more skin to the

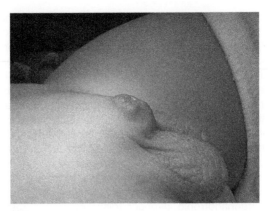

Fig. 3. Concealed penis.

ventral aspect and reconstructing the normal ventral penoscrotal angle is usually necessary.

In obese older children and adolescents, fat in the suprapubic region can raise the level of the surface skin. Recall that the phallic structures are fixed but the overlying skin is not. The rising surrounding skin displaces the penile shaft skin and can overtop the tip of the penis. Surgery is of limited value in this situation. Long-term resolution requires weight loss in the area.

Duplicated Urethra

Duplication of the urethra is a rare anomaly that can be dorsal or ventral. Some patients present with incontinence or infection, but most duplications are discovered in infancy on examination by the patient's parents or physician. Diagnosis of urethral duplication is confirmed with a voiding cystourethrogram. If the duplication is blind ending, a retrograde injection of contrast material and cystoscopy may be required to delineate the anatomy. Management of urethral duplication varies with symptoms and severity. No treatment is needed if the patient is free from infection and incontinence. Simple accessory duplicate urethras may be fulgurated and allowed to scar over. Others need to be excised to make the patient dry and to prevent infection.[62]

Ambiguous Genitalia (Disorders of Sexual Differentiation, Intersex)

DSD are complex conditions and typically present with ambiguous genitalia. This condition is usually diagnosed at birth when the gender of the child is unclear. There are many possible causes (congenital adrenal hyperplasia is the most common) and a full discussion is beyond the scope of this article. There are 2 critical issues for generalists who encounter this problem. The first concern is proper diagnosis with prompt recognition and treatment of any underlying metabolic issues (eg, salt wasting, hypertension). The second relates to gender assignment. The decision regarding gender assignment is not simple; straightforward gender-assignment rules do not exist. Gender is understood not to be simply genitalia,[63,64] nor is gender simply a matter of nurture or sex of rearing. The effect of fetal hormone exposure on the brain is now recognized as a major factor. This topic is controversial and evolving. The current approach is to involve a team, including pediatric urologists, general surgeons, geneticists, endocrinologists, psychologists, social workers, and the primary care physician, to present the findings of the evaluation to the parents and to help them make a decision.

ACQUIRED CONDITIONS
Common Penile Trauma

Zippers
Uncircumcised boys and adolescents will occasionally accidentally catch their foreskin in the zippers of their pants or other clothing (**Fig. 4**). Attempts at extraction by vigorous pulling and tugging are rarely successful. The most effective approach is to disassemble the zipper mechanism by cutting the median bar of the fastener, thereby separating the zipper into 2 parts, and releasing the entrapped skin.[65]

Toilet lid falling on penis
Young boys who are in the process of toilet training or who have only recently achieved control may be just tall enough to void into a standard toilet. They sometimes rest their penises on the seat, and the lid may accidentally fall on them. The injuries are usually limited to bruising and swelling. If the child is voiding and stable, further imaging is usually not required, unless there is a wound that suggests the urethra has been cut. Rest, antiinflammatories, and supportive care are typically all that is needed.[66]

Paraphimosis
Paraphimosis develops when the foreskin is retracted proximal to the coronal sulcus and becomes stuck in position (**Fig. 5**). Depending on the tightness of the foreskin, severe edema develops after several hours. Occasionally, paraphimosis occurs iatrogenically when the foreskin is retracted to place a catheter and is not returned to its normal position. Manual compression of the glans and edematous foreskin while pulling upward on the phallus usually allows reduction of the paraphimotic ring. This can be carried out under general or local anesthesia. Other treatments that have been reported include application of an iced glove for 5 minutes, or granulated sugar for 1 to 2 hours, in an effort to draw away the edema.[67] After successful reduction, formal treatment with circumcision or dorsal slit is advisable. Although technically feasible, it is prudent not to try to do a definitive treatment at the time of the original reduction. The edematous tissue may not heal as well, and a better cosmetic result will occur if the prepuce is allowed to return to normal.

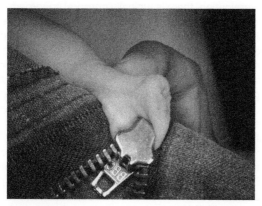

Fig. 4. Prepuce caught in zipper.

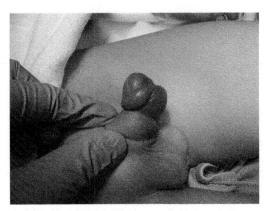

Fig. 5. Paraphimosis.

ERECTILE CONDITIONS
Priapism

Priapism is defined as being persistent erection of at least 4 hours in duration that continues beyond, or is unrelated to, sexual stimulation. Typically, only the corpora cavernosa are affected.[68,69] There are 3 subtypes: ischemic, nonischemic, and stuttering. Ischemic priapism is veno-occlusive, with little or no blood flow through the corpora cavernosa. The cavernosal blood is hypoxic, hypercapnic, and acidotic. The penis is rigid and tender to palpation. In contrast, nonischemic priapism is a result of arterial high flow of blood. There is a loss of regulation of inflow of arterial blood. The penis is usually not rigid or painful. Typically there is a history of an accident or fall as an inciting cause. The trauma creates a fistula between the cavernosal artery and the corpora cavernosa. Stuttering priapism is a recurrent form of ischemic priapism. Periods of painful erections are intermixed with periods of flaccidity and detumescence.

About 30% of boys with sickle cell disease develop ischemic priapism.[70] Sickling of red blood cells in the corpora cavernosa during normal erection causes venous stasis. This situation leads to decreased local oxygen tension and pH, which accelerates sickling and stasis.[71] Priapism typically develops during sleep, when a lower respiratory rate leads to lowered oxygen tension and pH in the corpora, causing ischemia and pain. On physical examination, there is typically corporal engorgement with sparing of the glans penis. Voiding may be impaired if there is spongiosal involvement. Evaluation includes complete blood count and serum chemistry, as well as hemoglobin electrophoresis if the patient's sickle cell status is unknown. If the history and physical examination are not sufficient to make a differentiation, corporal blood gas should be performed to distinguish between a high-flow and low-flow state. Usually, the P_{O_2} is less than 30 mm Hg, P_{CO_2} is more than 60 mm Hg, and pH is less than 7.25 in ischemic low-flow priapism.[69] Patients with nonischemic priapism will have corpora blood gases similar to arterial blood.

Priapism in adults in general is similar to that seen in children, but with a wider variety of causes.[71] About 20% of adult cases are caused by sickle cell disease. Leukemia and other blood dyscrasias are important causes of adult priapism; up to 50% of patients with chronic granulocytic leukemia will experience priapism.[72] Other causes include local and metastatic tumor invasion, brain tumors, brain and spinal cord trauma, and syphilis.[71,73,74] A long list of drugs can cause priapism, especially intracavernosal and intraurethral injectables and oral agents used for erectile dysfunction, as well as antipsychotics, selective serotonin reuptake inhibitors, and illicit drugs such as cocaine.[75–77] Accidental ingestion of these agents must be considered in children with priapism.[78]

Traditionally, priapism caused by sickle cell disease is managed primarily by medical therapy, including exchange transfusion, hydration, alkalinization, pain management with morphine, and oxygen. However, recent guidelines on priapism recommend concurrent intracavernosal aspiration and irrigation.[68,69,79] In many patients, general anesthesia or intravenous sedation will be necessary. Typically, a 19- or 21-gauge butterfly needle is inserted into one of the corporal bodies, and intracavernosal irrigation with a sympathomimetic agent (phenylephrine) is performed in conjunction with a local anesthetic. If priapism has been present longer than 48 hours, ischemia and acidosis can impair the intracavernosal smooth muscle response to sympathomimetics.[69] If irrigation and medical therapy are unsuccessful, a glanular shunt (or Winter shunt) should be considered. For stuttering priapism, administration of an oral α-adrenergic agent (pseudoephedrine, up to 60 mg) once or twice daily is first-line therapy. If this treatment is unsuccessful, an oral β agonist (terbutaline) or a GnRH analog plus flutamide can be used.[79]

Nonischemic, arterial, or high-flow priapism usually develops after perineal trauma that results in laceration of the cavernous artery, such as a straddle injury. The differential diagnoses include Fabry disease and sickle cell anemia.[80] In these cases, aspiration and corporal irrigation is diagnostic only. Injection of sympathomimetic agents may have significant adverse effects. Typically, the aspirated blood is bright red, and similar to arterial blood. Color Doppler ultrasonography will often show the fistula. Spontaneous resolution may occur. If not, angiographic embolization is indicated.[69,80,81]

Peyronie Disease

Peyronie disease is a poorly understood acquired penile problem, causing deformed erections, sometimes with penile pain during the initial stages of the disease. Affected men develop dense, palpable fibrous plaques of the tunica albuginea, leading to curvature of the erect penis, sometimes with flexure at the site of the plaque. These penile deformities may impair or prevent sexual penetration.

The cause of Peyronie disease is unclear. The onset of symptoms can sometimes be linked to penile trauma, although evidence is inconsistent.[82,83] The plaques seem to form as a result of an increased scar-forming tendency that may be genetic.[84] The penile pain, if present, usually resolves when the plaque stabilizes, typically within 6 to 18 months.[85] Peyronie disease is more common than previously reported, affecting about 3% to 10% of adult men.[86] Men of all ages can be affected, but the average age of diagnosis is about 55 years, and it is less common in men younger than 40 years.[87] The rate of erectile dysfunction seems to be increased in men with Peyronie disease.

There is no satisfactory nonsurgical treatment. Many different medicines have been tried, but evidence of benefit is unclear because of a lack of controlled studies and the spontaneous remission of about 10% to 15% of patients. Extended courses (6 months or more) of oral potassium paraaminobenzoic acid (Potaba), 3 g 4 times daily, may be helpful in some men,[88] but compliance is limited by cost and gastrointestinal side effects. Oral vitamin E is often tried, but likely provides no significant benefit.[89] Other oral medications being studied include colchicine and tamoxifen. Verapamil injections directly into the plaque have been studied with some success.[90] Intralesional collagenases showed slight benefit in 1 study.[91] Intralesional corticosteroids are currently not recommended because of unpredictable effects and local atrophy.

Erectile dysfunction in men with Peyronie disease can be treated with standard approaches. There are some reports of Peyronie disease occurring after trauma from vacuum erectile devices or after use of intracavernosal or intraurethral alprostadil, so oral phosphodiesterase type 5 inhibitors may be preferable.

Surgical treatment options for Peyronie disease include penile shortening procedures, lengthening procedures, and prosthesis implantation. Risks vary by procedure, but penile numbness and erectile dysfunction are more common in lengthening procedures, because of the risk of damaging the neurovascular bundle. The plaque and curvature should be stable for at least 6 to 12 months before surgical treatment is considered, to decrease the chance of continued progression of the plaque after surgery. For men with Peyronie disease and vascular insufficiency, prosthesis implantation is preferred. In general, surgical treatment is not recommended for men who have adequate erections and are able to continue intercourse.[92]

REFERENCES

1. Oster J. Further fate of the foreskin: incidence of preputial adhesions, phimosis, and smegma among Danish schoolboys. Arch Dis Child 1968;43:200–3.
2. Mouriquand PD, Persad R, Sharma S. Hypospadias repair: current principles and procedures. Br J Urol 1995;76(Suppl 3):9–22.
3. Boisen KA, Chellakooty M, Schmidt IM, et al. Hypospadias in a cohort of 1072 Danish newborn boys: Prevalence and relationship to placental weight, anthropometrical measurements at birth, and reproductive hormone levels at 3 months of age. J Clin Endocrinol Metab 2005;90(7):4041–6.
4. Hatch DA, Maizels M, Zaontz MR, et al. Hypospadias hidden by a complete prepuce. Surg Gynecol Obstet 1989;169(3):233–4.
5. Sheldon CA, Duckett JW. Hypospadias. Pediatr Clin North Am 1987;34(5): 1259–72.
6. Barcat J. Current concepts of treatment. In: Horton CE, editor. Plastic and reconstructive surgery of the genital area. Boston: Little Brown; 1973. p. 249–62.
7. Borer JG, Bauer SB, Peters CA, et al. Tubularized incised plate urethroplasty: expanded use in primary and repeat surgery for hypospadias. J Urol 2001; 165(2):581–5.
8. Duckett JW. The current hype in hypospadiology. Br J Urol 1995;76(Suppl 3):1–7.
9. Baskin LS. Hypospadias and urethral development. J Urol 2000;163(3):951–6.
10. Griffin JE. Androgen resistance—the clinical and molecular spectrum. N Engl J Med 1992;326:611–8.
11. Goldman AS, Bongiovanni AM. Induced genital anomalies. Ann N Y Acad Sci 1967;142(3):755–67.
12. Aaronson IA, Cakmak MA, Key LL. Defects of the testosterone biosynthetic pathway in boys with hypospadias. J Urol 1997;157(5):1884–8.
13. Paulozzi LJ. International trends in rates of hypospadias and cryptorchidism. Environ Health Perspect 1999;107(4):297–302.
14. Silver RI, Rodriguez R, Chang TS, et al. In vitro fertilization is associated with an increased risk of hypospadias. J Urol 1999;161(6):1954–7.
15. Silver RI. Endocrine abnormalities in boys with hypospadias. Adv Exp Med Biol 2004;545:45–72.
16. Hussain N, Chaghtai A, Herndon CD, et al. Hypospadias and early gestation growth restriction in infants. Pediatrics 2002;109(3):473–8.

17. Reefhuis J, Honein MA. Maternal age and non-chromosomal birth defects, Atlanta—1968–2000: teenager or thirty-something, who is at risk? Birth Defects Res A Clin Mol Teratol 2004;70(9):572–9.
18. Baskin LS, Himes K, Colborn T. Hypospadias and endocrine disruption: is there a connection? Environ Health Perspect 2001;109(11):1175–93.
19. Dolk H. Rise in prevalence of hypospadias. Lancet 1998;351(9105):770.
20. Roberts CJ, Lloyd S. Observations on the epidemiology of simple hypospadias. Br Med J 1973;1(856):768–70.
21. Sorber M, Feitz WF, de Vries JD. Short- and mid-term outcome of different types of onstage hypospadias corrections. Eur Urol 1997;32(4):475–9.
22. Borer JG, Retik AB, Hypospadias. In: Wein AJ, Kavoussi LR, Novick AC, et al, editors. Campbell & Walsh's urology (vol. 4). 9th edition. Philadelphia: WB Saunders; 2006. p. 3703–44. Available at: http://www.elsevier.com/wps/find/bookdescription.cws_home/709569/description#description. Accessed April 26, 2010.
23. Retik AB, Bauer SB, Mandell J, et al. Management of severe hypospadias with a 2-stage repair. J Urol 1994;152(2 Pt 2):749–51.
24. Baskin LS, Erol A, Li YW, et al. Anatomical studies of hypospadias. J Urol 1998;160(3 Pt 2):1108–15.
25. McArdle F, Lebowitz R. Uncomplicated hypospadias and anomalies of upper urinary tract. Need for screening? Urology 1975;5(5):712–6.
26. Aarskog D. Clinical and cytogenetic studies in hypospadias. Acta Paediatr Scand Suppl 1970;203(Suppl):1–61.
27. Aarskog D. Intersex conditions masquerading as simple hypospadias. Birth Defects Orig Artic Ser 1971;7(6):122–30.
28. Kaefer M, Diamond DA, Hendren WH, et al. The incidence of intersexuality in children with cryptorchidism and hypospadias: stratification based on gonadal palpability and meatal position. J Urol 1999;162(3 Pt 2):1003–6.
29. Kass E, Kogan SJ, Manley C. Timing of elective surgery on the genitalia of male children with particular reference to the risks, benefits, and psychological effects of surgery and anesthesia. American Academy of Pediatrics. Pediatrics 1996;97(4):590–4.
30. Lepore AG, Kesler RW. Behavior of children undergoing hypospadias repair. J Urol 1979;122(1):68–70.
31. Hensle TW, Kearney MC, Bingham JB. Buccal mucosa grafts for hypospadias surgery: long-term results. J Urol 2002;168(4 Pt 2):1734–6.
32. Chhibber AK, Perkins FM, Rabinowitz R, et al. Penile block timing for postoperative analgesia of hypospadias repair in children. J Urol 1997;158(3 Pt 2):1156–9.
33. Samuel M, Hampson-Evans D, Cunnington P. Prospective to a randomized double-blind controlled trial to assess efficacy of double caudal analgesia in hypospadias repair. J Pediatr Surg 2002;37(2):168–74.
34. Rabinowitz R. Outpatient catheterless modified Mathieu hypospadias repair. J Urol 1987;138(4 Pt 2):1074–6.
35. Koff SA, Jayanthi VR. Preoperative treatment with human chorionic gonadotropin in infancy decreases the severity of proximal hypospadias and chordee. J Urol 1999;162(4):1435–9.
36. Gearhart JP, Jeffs RD. The use of parenteral testosterone therapy in genital reconstructive surgery. J Urol 1987;138(4 Pt 2):1077–8.
37. Monfort G, Lucas C. Dehydrotestosterone penile stimulation in hypospadias surgery. Eur Urol 1982;8(4):201–3.
38. Baskin LS, Sutherland RS, DiSandro MJ, et al. The effect of testosterone on androgen receptors and human penile growth. J Urol 1997;158(3 Pt 2):1113–8.

39. Elbakry A, Shamaa M, Al-Atrash G. An axially vascularized meatal-based flap for the repair of hypospadias. Br J Urol 1998;82(5):698–703.
40. Elbakry A. Management of urethrocutaneous fistula after hypospadias repair: 10 years' experience. BJU Int 2001;88(6):590–5.
41. Horton CE Jr, Horton CE. Complications of hypospadias surgery. Clin Plast Surg 1988;15(3):371–9.
42. Zaontz MR, Kaplan WE, Maizels M. Surgical correction of anterior urethral diverticula after hypospadias repair in children. Urology 1989;33(1):40–2.
43. Duckett JW. Foreward: symposium on hypospadias. Urol Clin North Am 1981;8: 371–3.
44. Hendren WH, Keating MA. Use of dermal graft and free urethral graft in penile reconstruction. J Urol 1988;140(5 Pt 2):1265–9.
45. Ritchey ML, Ribbeck M. Successful use of tunica vaginalis grafts for treatment of severe penile chordee in children. J Urol 2003;170(4 Pt 2):1574–6.
46. Crain DS, Miller OF, Smith LJ, et al. Transcutaneous laser hair ablation for management of intraurethral hair after hypospadias repair: initial experience. J Urol 2003;170(5):1948–9.
47. Baskin LS, Duckett JW. Buccal mucosa grafts in hypospadias surgery. Br J Urol 1995;76(Suppl 3):23–30.
48. Wessells H, McAninch JW. Current controversies in anterior urethral stricture repair: freegraft versus pedicled skin-flap reconstruction. World J Urol 1998; 16(3):175–80.
49. Horton CE, Devine CJ Jr. A one-stage repair for hypospadias cripples. Plast Reconstr Surg 1970;45(5):425–30.
50. Bracka A. A versatile two-stage hypospadias repair. Br J Plast Surg 1995;48(6): 345–52.
51. Fisher PC, Park JM. Penile torsion repair using dorsal dartos flap rotation. J Urol 2004;171:1903–4.
52. Aaronson IA. Micropenis: medical and surgical implications. J Urol 1994;152:4–14.
53. Feldman KW, Smith DW. Fetal phallic growth and penile standards for newborn male infants. J Pediatr 1975;86:395–8.
54. Lee PA, Houk CP. Outcome studies among men with micropenis. J Pediatr Endocrinol Metab 2004;17:1043–53.
55. Lee PA, Mazur T, Danish R, et al. Micropenis: I. Criteria, etiologies and classification. Johns Hopkins Med J 1980;146:156–63.
56. Walsh PC, Wilson JD, Allen TD, et al. Clinical and endocrinological evaluation of patients with congenital microphallus. J Urol 1978;120(1):90–5.
57. Ragan DC, Casale AJ, Rink RC, et al. Genitourinary anomalies in the CHARGE association. J Urol 1999;161:622–5.
58. Choi SK, Han SW, Kim DH, et al. Transdermal dihydrotestosterone therapy and its effects on patients with microphallus. J Urol 1993;150:657–60.
59. Tietjen DN, Uramoto GY, Tindall DJ, et al. Micropenis in hypogonadotropic hypogonadism: response of the penile androgen receptor to testosterone treatment. J Urol 1998;160:1054–7.
60. Reilly JM, Woodhouse CRJ. Small penis and the male sexual role. J Urol 1989; 142:569–71.
61. Wisniewski AB, Migeon CJ. Long-term perspectives for 46, XY patients affected by complete androgen insensitivity syndrome or congenital micropenis. Semin Reprod Med 2002;20:297–304.
62. Woodhouse CR, Williams DI. Duplications of the lower urinary tract in children. Br J Urol 1979;51:481–7.

63. Reiner WG. Gender identity and sex-of-rearing in children with disorders of sexual differentiation. J Pediatr Endocrinol Metab 2005;18(6):549–53.
64. American Academy of Pediatrics: Committee on Genetics: evaluation of the newborn with developmental anomalies of the external genitalia. Pediatrics 2000;106(1 Pt 1):138–42.
65. Nolan JF, Stillwell TJ, Sands JP Jr. Acute management of the zipper-entrapped penis. J Emerg Med 1990;8:305–7.
66. Gazi MA, Ankem MK, Pantuck AJ, et al. Management of penile toilet seat injury–report of two cases. Can J Urol 2001;8(3):1293–4.
67. Mackway-Jones K, Teece S. Ice, pins, or sugar to reduce paraphimosis. Emerg Med J 2004;21:77–8.
68. Huang Y-C, Harraz AM, Shindel AW, et al. Evaluation and management of priapism: 2009 update. Nat Rev Urol 2009;6(5):262–71.
69. Montague DK, Jarow J, Broderick GA, et al. American Urological Association guideline on the management of priapism. J Urol 2003;170(4 Pt 1):1318–24.
70. Mantadakis E, Cavender JD, Rogers ZR, et al. Prevalence of priapism in children and adolescents with sickle cell anemia. J Pediatr Hematol Oncol 1999;12: 518–22.
71. Nelson JH, Winter CC. Priapism: Evolution of management in 48 patients in a 22-year series. J Urol 1977;117:455–8.
72. Morano SG, Latagliata R, Carmosino I, et al. Treatment of long-lasting priapism in chronic myeloid leukemia at onset. Ann Hematol 2000;79:644–5.
73. Bruno D, Wigfall DR, Zimmerman SA, et al. Genitourinary complications of sickle cell disease. J Urol 2001;166(3):803–11.
74. Munro D, Horne HW Jr, Paull DP. The effect of injury to the spinal cord and cauda equina on the sexual potency of men. N Engl J Med 1948;239:903–11.
75. Lomas GM, Jarow JP. Risk factors for papaverine-induced priapism. J Urol 1992; 147:1280–1.
76. Lue TF. Priapism after transurethral alprostadil. J Urol 1999;161:725–6.
77. Lue TF, Hellstrom WJG, McAninch JW, et al. Priapism: a refined approach to diagnosis and treatment. J Urol 1986;136:104–8.
78. Cantrell FL. Sildenafil citrate ingestion in a pediatric patient. Pediatr Emerg Care 2004;20:314–5.
79. Maples BL, Hagemann TM. Treatment of priapism in pediatric patients with sickle cell disease. Am J Health Syst Pharm 2004;61:355–63.
80. Volkmer BG, Nesslauer T, Kraemer SC, et al. Prepubertal high flow priapism: incidence, diagnosis and treatment. J Urol 2001;166:1018–22.
81. Kuefer R, Bartsch G Jr, Herkommer K, et al. Changing diagnostic and therapeutic concepts in high-flow priapism. Int J Impot Res 2005;17:109–13.
82. Devine CJ, Somers KD, Jordan SD, et al. Proposal: trauma as the cause of the Peyronie's lesion. J Urol 1997;157(1):285–90.
83. Zargooshi J. Trauma as the cause of Peyronie's disease: penile fracture as a model of trauma. J Urol 2004;172(1):186–8.
84. Hellstrom WJG, Bivalacqua TJ. Peyronie's disease: etiology, medical, and surgical therapy. J Androl 2000;21(3):347–54.
85. Mulhall JP, Schoff J, Guhring P. An analysis of the natural history of Peyronie's disease. J Urol 2006;175:2115–8.
86. Greenfield JM, Levine LA. Peyronie's disease: etiology, epidemiology and medical treatment. Urol Clin North Am 2005;32:469–78.
87. Levine LA, Estrada CR, Storm DW, et al. Peyronie disease in younger men: characteristics and treatment results. J Androl 2003;24:27–32.

88. Weidner W, Hauck EW, Schnitker J. Potassium paraaminobenzoate (Potaba) in the treatment of Peyronie's disease: a prospective, placebo-controlled, randomized study. Eur Urol 2005;47:530–6.
89. Gelbard MK, Dorey F, James K. The natural history of Peyronie's disease. J Urol 1990;144:1376–9.
90. Levine LA, Goldman KE, Greenfield JM. Experience with intraplaque injection of verapamil for Peyronie's disease. J Urol 2002;168(2):621–5.
91. Gelbard MK, James K, Riach P, et al. Collagenase versus placebo in the treatment of Peyronie's disease: a double-blind study. J Urol 1993;149(1):56–8.
92. Gholami SS, Gonzalez-Cadavid NF, Lin C-S, et al. Peyronie's disease: a review. J Urol 2003;169:1234–41.

Male Reproductive Health and Infertility

Keith A. Frey, MD, MBA

KEYWORDS

- Male infertility • Preconception care
- Men's health • Men's preventive healthcare

OPTIMIZING MALE REPRODUCTIVE HEALTH

Little attention has been given to male reproductive health. Preconception care for men is important for improving family planning and pregnancy outcomes, preparing men for fatherhood, and enhancing the reproductive health and health behaviors of men and women. Preconception care offers an opportunity, similar to the opportunity it presents to women, for disease prevention and health promotion in men.[1]

In 2005, the Centers for Disease Control and Prevention (CDC) and 35 partner organizations convened a national summit and issued a set of recommendations to promote preconception care in the United States. Although passing recognition was given to the importance of preconception health promotion "among both men and women," the focus was on women.

There are at least 5 distinct reasons why preconception care for men is important[1]:

1. To ensure that all pregnancies are planned and wanted.
2. To enhance men's biologic and genetic contributions to the pregnancy.
3. To provide improved reproductive health biology, health practices, and outcomes for women.
4. To improve men's capacity for parenthood and fatherhood.
5. To enhance the health of men through access to primary health care.

PRECONCEPTION CARE FOR MEN

As defined by the CDC Select Panel, preconception care is a set of interventions that aims to identify and modify biomedical, behavioral, and social risks to women's health or reproductive outcomes through prevention and management. This definition can also be applied to preconception care for men, with the basic components consisting of risk assessment, health promotion, and clinical and psychosocial interventions.

No internal or extramural funding support.
Department of Family Medicine, Mayo Clinic in Arizona, 13737 North 92nd Street, Scottsdale, AZ 85260, USA
E-mail address: frey.keith@mayo.edu

Prim Care Clin Office Pract 37 (2010) 643–652
doi:10.1016/j.pop.2010.04.005
0095-4543/10/$ – see front matter © 2010 Elsevier Inc. All rights reserved.

Risk Assessment

The primary objective of risk assessment is to identify ongoing problems that need to be addressed. Risk assessment has 8 main parts:

Reproductive life plan

Risk assessment begins with evaluation of the couple's reproductive life plan: a set of goals, based on their values and resources, for having or not having children, and their plan to achieve those goals.[1,2] The patient is asked whether he plans to have any (more) children, and if so, how long he and his partner plan to wait. If they plan to wait less than a year, he should return for a full preconception assessment. If they plan to wait more than a year, he should continue to receive recommended age-appropriate preventive health services. He and his partner should be encouraged to use effective contraception and update their reproductive life plan at every routine visit.

Past medical and surgical history

The primary care physician should periodically review the patient's medical and surgical history, including any ongoing medical conditions that may impair his reproductive health. Several medical conditions have been associated with reduced sperm quality, including obesity, diabetes mellitus, varicocele, and sexually-transmitted infections. Men with diabetes mellitus type I generally have lower semen volume, diminished sperm motility, and poorer morphology than controls. Additionally, all diabetic men with unsatisfactory glycemic control tend to have lower sperm count, motility, velocity, and viability characteristics than men with satisfactory glycemic control.[3]

Medications

Past and current medication use, including prescription, nonprescription, and herbal products should be reviewed. Any medication use, including over-the-counter medications, should be guided by a risk-benefit evaluation, weighing benefits for the man's health against known or potential risks to his offspring. Several medications can affect sperm count and quality, including calcium channel blockers, cimetidine, colchicine, corticosteroids, erythromycin, finasteride, methadone, nitrofurantoin, phenytoin, spironolactone, sulfasalazine, and tetracycline.

Family history and genetic risks

A man's genetic risk assessment should be based on family history, age, and ethnicity. A three-generation family history of genetic disorders should be obtained, because certain disorders (autosomal recessive or sex-linked) may skip generations. Several genetic disorders, such as cystic fibrosis, Klinefelter syndrome, Kartagener syndrome, and polycystic kidney disease, may impair fertility and sperm quality.[1] Discussion of paternal age-related decline in sperm quality may help inform the couple's reproductive life planning, because many men are not aware of the growing body of evidence linking paternal age to schizophrenia in the offspring.[4,5] If the patient belongs to an ethnic group at increased risk for certain genetic disorders (eg, Ashkenazi Jews, African Americans, Southeast Asians, and those of Mediterranean origin), he should be offered screening if his partner's genetic screen is positive or unknown. In general, the partner at increased genetic risk should be screened first.

Social history

The patient's social history, including potential occupational exposures, should be reviewed. Ongoing exposure to metals, solvents, endocrine disruptors, and pesticides can impair sperm quality, which may lead to infertility, miscarriage, and birth defects (see later discussion on avoidance of harmful exposures). The patient may obtain a copy of the Material Safety Data Sheet of any chemical exposure at work from his employer to be reviewed for potential reproductive toxicity.

Risk behaviors

The patient's major and potential risk behaviors, including hobbies and tobacco, alcohol, and drug use, should be reviewed. Tobacco use has been associated with decreased sperm count and abnormal sperm morphology, motility, and fertilizing capacity. Recent evidence suggests that nicotine and other chemicals in cigarettes can also induce oxidative damage to sperm DNA. The effects of alcohol use on sperm quality are unclear. Some studies have shown that moderate drinking may protect against DNA damage, perhaps, in part, due to the antioxidant effect of some alcoholic beverages.[6] Other studies have shown that alcohol may be damaging to sperm DNA.[7] The CAGE questions can be used to screen for alcohol abuse,[8] and include these 4 questions that begin "Have you ever: (1) felt the need to *cut* down your drinking; (2) felt *annoyed* by criticism of your drinking; (3) had *guilty* feelings about drinking; and (4) taken a morning *eye* opener?"

Several recreational drugs have also been linked to male infertility, including marijuana, cocaine, and anabolic steroids. Marijuana has been shown to reduce testosterone production, sperm count, and semen quality. Cocaine has been associated with decreased sperm count and abnormal sperm morphology and motility, and the effects of cocaine can linger for up to 2 years from the last use. Anabolic steroids can reduce testosterone level and sperm quality.[1] A study of anabolic steroid use and semen quality in bodybuilders found that men using steroids exhibited lower sperm concentrations and lower amounts of morphologically normal spermatozoa compared with a control group.[9] CAGE questions can also be used to screen for recreational drug use.

Certain hobbies may expose the patient to reproductive hazards. Hobbies that involve refinishing furniture, repairing cars, painting, building models, or anything that requires the use of strippers, degreasers, or nonwater-based glues or paints may expose the patient to organic solvents. Hobbies that involve painting, pottery, making stained glass windows, or handling, shooting, or cleaning guns may expose the patient to lead or other heavy metals.

Nutrition

There is a national epidemic of obesity. In 2003 to 2004, 62.2% of men aged 20 to 39 were overweight or obese, categorized as having a body mass index of 25 or higher.[10] Men who are overweight or obese have been associated with lower testosterone level, poorer sperm quality, and reduced fertility, compared with those who are not overweight or obese. The risk of infertility increases by 10% for every 20 lbs overweight.[11] Nutritional screening should review current dietary patterns and use of restrictive diets. Zinc and folate have antioxidant properties that can counteract reactive oxygen species and may protect sperm against oxidative stress and DNA damage. In a randomized controlled trial of 99 fertile and 94 subfertile men, daily administration of 66 mg zinc sulfate and 5 mg folic acid significantly increased sperm concentration of the subfertile men, suggesting the importance of multiple nutrients impacting fertility. The study authors also found an increase in the median percentage of abnormal spermatozoa from 80% to 84%.[12] A study of 33 subfertile men from a male infertility clinic who received an intervention consisting of twice daily oral 220 mg zinc sulfate for 3 months significantly increased mean percentage progressive and total motility of sperm.[13] In a randomized controlled trial giving 250 mg zinc sulfate twice a day, investigators found that for asthenozoospermic men, 3 months of zinc therapy yielded increases in progressive motility of sperm, sperm count, and sperm membrane integrity while decreasing the percentage of nonmotile sperm.[14]

Other supplements have also been used to treat male infertility, including vitamin C, vitamin E, selenium, glutathione, ubiquinol, carnitine, and carotenoids. However, the safety and efficacy of such treatment have not been clearly established. In one study, the combination of vitamins C and E at high doses resulted in sperm DNA damage in vitro, raising concerns about the potential harm of high-dose antioxidant supplementation.[15]

Mental health
Routine screening for mental health disorders should be performed. Estimates of the lifetime risk of major depression for men range from 1.4% to 11%. Recent evidence suggests that depression of a father during the postnatal development of his children can significantly affect the children and is associated with poor childhood emotional and behavioral outcomes, even after adjusting for maternal depression and paternal depression during a different developmental stage of the child.[16] Furthermore, depressed fathers can have a negative impact on mother-child interaction behaviors, and these fathers are less likely to engage in certain father-child interactions, such as playing outdoors with their children.[17] On the other hand, fathers with good mental health have been shown to reduce the impact of a mother's depression on the child.[18]

Physical examination and laboratory testing
Physical examination and laboratory testing should be guided by clinical history. For example, men at increased risk for sexually transmitted infections should be offered screening for HIV, syphilis, and other sexually transmitted infections (STIs). The US Preventative Services Task Force recommends screening all adult men for high blood pressure and obesity; men aged 35 years and older for lipid disorders; men with hypertension or hyperlipidemia for type 2 diabetes mellitus; and men aged 50 years and older for colorectal cancer.[19] Routine screening for testicular cancer in asymptomatic men is not recommended. Screening for prostate cancer in men aged 50 to 75 years may be considered.

INFERTILITY
Definitions and Epidemiology

Infertility is a common condition seen in primary care practices and is defined as one year of unprotected intercourse in which a pregnancy has not been achieved. Fifteen to twenty percent of all couples in the United States are infertile, with higher rates seen in older couples.[20,21] This rate has remained stable since the early 1980s. For a normal couple younger than 35 years, the probability of achieving a pregnancy within one menstrual cycle is approximately 25%. Infertility is considered primary if neither partner has ever achieved a successful pregnancy. Secondary infertility includes couples in whom there has previously been a pregnancy but there is current difficulty with conception. It is estimated that approximately 25% of women will have an episode of infertility during their childbearing years.[20] In recent years, there has been an increase in demand for infertility services. This increased demand seems to be related to a societal trend toward delayed marriage and childbirth, greater awareness of treatment options, and increased societal acceptance of infertility as a medical condition.

Etiology

The causes of infertility include abnormalities of any portion of the male or female reproductive system. A specific cause can be identified in approximately 80% of couples, with a third due to female factors alone, a third due to male factors alone, and a third due to a combination of problems. Unexplained infertility, in which no specific cause is identified, occurs in approximately 20% of infertile couples.[20,22,23] When possible, it is advisable to meet individually with each partner and with the couple together. The physician should arrange a meeting with the couple early in the diagnostic workup. This provides an important opportunity to review reproductive biology and the rationale for subsequent laboratory test results. The optimal frequency of intercourse is every 1 to 2 days around the time of expected ovulation. The commercially available lubricants can be spermatotoxic and should be used sparingly. Additionally, infertility is often associated with intense emotional issues for couples. The primary care physician should anticipate and discuss the range of emotional responses, including depression, anxiety, anger, and marital discord.[20,24]

Diagnostic Evaluation of the Man

Because infertility may arise from one or more areas of the reproductive system, it requires a comprehensive diagnostic evaluation. The initial assessment consists of a thorough history and physical examination and appropriate laboratory tests. For the female partner, the content of this evaluation has been well documented in previous review articles.[20–22] For the male partner, the areas requiring extra attention in the medical history are identical to those outlined earlier for the preconception risk assessment.

Specific areas of attention in the male physical examination include the hair pattern (consistent with appropriate virilization), breast examination (gynecomastia, nipple discharge), focal neurologic findings (anosmia, visual fields cuts), and genitalia. The examination of the male genitalia should note a normal location for the urethral meatus, a normal prostate without tenderness or nodules, bilaterally descended testes of normal size (≥ 4 cm in long axis or ≥ 20 cm^3 volume), presence of a palpable vas deferens on each side, and evaluation for a varicocele (standing and with a Valsalva maneuver).[20,21,24]

Laboratory Tests

The first test should be a semen analysis, with a workup algorithm outlined in **Fig. 1**. The laboratory used for the semen analysis must at least follow the World Health Organization (WHO) criteria (http://www.who.int/reproductivehealth/publications/infertility/9789241547789/en/index.html). If the semen analysis is entirely normal, it is unlikely that any other laboratory testing will be needed or useful.[20] If the semen analysis is abnormal, a repeat semen analysis should be performed. If severe oligospermia or azoospermia is found, then testing for serum testosterone, luteinizing hormone, follicle-stimulating hormone, and prolactin is warranted. Other laboratory tests (eg, complete blood count, urinalysis, screening for sexually transmitted diseases, and sensitive thyroid-stimulating hormone) should be done if indicated by risk factors in the medical history. Patients with abnormalities should be treated or referred for further evaluation to the appropriate specialist. Abnormal semen analysis presentations could include oligospermia or azoospermia, disorders of sperm function or motility (asthenospermia), and abnormalities of sperm morphology (teratospermia).[20,24] The incidence of chromosomal abnormalities in men is approximately 7%, with Klinefelter syndrome being the most common. The most commonly encountered

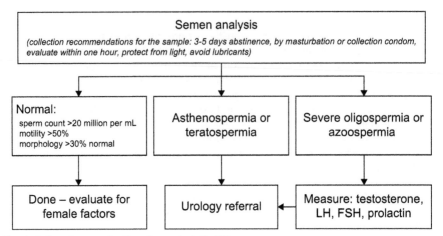

Fig. 1. Laboratory evaluation for male infertility.

physical finding associated with male infertility is a varicocele, a network of palpably distended veins of the pampiniform plexus of the spermatic cord. Studies suggest that palpable varicoceles have a greater impact on fertility.[25] Approximately 7% of men with nonobstructive azoospermia have been shown to have Y-chromosome microdeletions. Men with a congenital bilateral absence of the vas deferens have an approximately 70% chance of being carriers of cystic fibrosis mutations.[26,27]

Treatment

Infertility may arise from one or more areas of the reproductive system, and therefore requires a comprehensive diagnostic evaluation. This diagnostic survey can and should be completed for most couples within 6 to 12 months. Each couple's evaluation must be individualized, based on history and physical examination findings. However, an initial survey of each major reproductive factor is necessary in all couples and can be coordinated by the primary care physician.[20,21,24]

Infections of the male genitourinary tract (such as prostatitis and epididymitis) are treated as usual with the indicated antibiotics. Abnormalities of sperm count or motility associated with a palpable varicocele can improve following a varicocelectomy,[25] and a urology referral is warranted. Other causes of oligospermia require referral to an infertility specialist for consideration of intrauterine insemination or advanced reproductive technology, such as intracytoplasmic sperm injection, a technique in which a single sperm is injected directly into the oocyte.[20]

Prognosis

The exact prognosis for an infertile couple is difficult to define because of the multiple potential causes of infertility. For most causes, conception will not be achieved without specific treatment. However, with specific therapy, subsequent pregnancy rates have been studied and the results are favorable. Unexplained infertility is the persistent inability to conceive after a comprehensive diagnostic assessment of the couple fails to establish a specific diagnosis. Couples with infertility of 4 years or more tend to have a poor prognosis.[22,24] If a comprehensive diagnostic workup fails to identify a cause or if the appropriate treatment at the primary care level is unsuccessful, the physician should refer the patient to an infertility subspecialist for further evaluation and consideration of advanced reproductive techniques.

PROMOTING MEN'S REPRODUCTIVE HEALTH: ROLE OF THE PRIMARY CARE PHYSICIAN

Healthy Weight and Nutrition

An important objective of preconception care is to achieve a healthy weight before conception. Clinical guidelines have been established for the identification, evaluation, and treatment of overweight and obesity. Men should be encouraged to set weight loss goals, to develop a plan to reach those goals, and to exercise at least 30 minutes a day on most days of the week. A referral to a nutritionist or a structured weight loss program may be useful. After successful weight loss, the likelihood of weight loss maintenance is enhanced by a program consisting of dietary therapy, physical activity, and behavior therapy, which should be continued at least until pregnancy.[1]

Stress Reduction and Enhancing Resilience

The impact of chronic stress on men's cardiovascular health has been well demonstrated; much less is known about the impact of chronic stress on men's reproductive health. Stress can disrupt hypothalamic-pituitary-gonadal functions, resulting in decreased steroidogenesis and spermatogenesis. Stress can also increase susceptibility to infection and inflammation, which may cause oxidative damage to sperm. However, the literature on stress and semen quality has been inconsistent. Stress has been shown to negatively impact semen quality variables for patients having in vitro fertilization and those visiting andrology clinics,[10,28–31] but in other studies, stress has been shown to have no impact on semen quality for these patients.[32] Weekly time at job and stress have been shown to negatively impact sperm quality variables for fertile men, but job strain and stress have also shown no impact on sperm for infertile men and those of unknown fertility.

It seems prudent to recommend steps that promote stress reduction and resilience in the context of male preconception care. Elements to consider include regular exercise, adequate sleep, and balanced nutrition. Activities that strengthen social support, including friendship, team sports, and volunteer, civic, and church activities, should be encouraged.

Inflammation and Immunization

Chronic inflammation can cause oxidative damage to sperm. Sources of chronic inflammation include chronic untreated infections, such as periodontal disease or STIs, stress, diet, and exposure to harmful substances. Screening for such disorders or exposures should be included as a routine part of health promotion during preconception care.

The immunization status of men should be reviewed as part of a preconception evaluation, and appropriate vaccines should be offered. Immunization recommendations are updated annually by the CDC, the American College of Physicians , and the American Academy of Family Physicians.

Avoidance of Harmful Exposures

An increasing number of environmental exposures, including phthalates (a type of plasticizer used in food-can linings and many household products), acrylamide (produced during frying, baking and overcooking), and pesticides and dioxins, have been shown to cause sperm DNA damage. According to the National Institute for Occupational Safety and Health, male reproductive health can be negatively affected by the following workplace exposures: lead, dibromochloropropane, carbaryl, toluenediamine, dinitrotoluene, ethylene dibromide, plastic production (styrene and acetone), ethylene glycol monoethyl ether, welding, tetrachloroethylene, mercury vapor, heat, military radar, insecticides such as Kepone (in large doses), bromine vapor (in large doses), radiation (in large doses), carbon disulfide, and herbicides such as 2, 4-dichlorophenoxyacetic acid.[33] Additional substances have been identified as potential causes of male infertility, including beta-chloroprene (used to make Neoprene), lead azide, lead II thiocyanate, manganese, manganese tetroxide, tetraethyl lead, and tetramethyl lead.[34] Physical exposures like heat, sedentary work positions, and radiation have the potential to affect male fertility, though the evidence supporting a direct effect remains unclear.[35] The most up-to-date information about potential environmental exposures may be found at the Center for the Evaluation of Risks to Human Reproduction Web site (http://cerhr.niehs.nih.gov/common/index.html).

Support

Preconception and infertility care offer an opportunity to address the psychosocial needs of men before pregnancy and parenting. Three types of psychosocial services should be made available to men during preconception care: (1) social services, (2) clinical support, and (3) partner and parenting support. Social services may include financial literacy training or assistance with job placement to help men get ready to start a family. The preconception care visit can offer a platform for accessing these services. Men who have mental health problems, including depression, could benefit from some forms of psychological support and therapy. Many men can use guidance on how to provide emotional support to their partners, with emphasis on strengthening their capacities for communication and nurturance. Similarly, most men can use some lessons to help them prepare for fatherhood, and preconception is a good time to start.[1]

As noted earlier, the evaluation, diagnosis, and treatment of infertility can precipitate intense emotional reactions. The primary care physician should discuss with and provide support to the couple for such emotions as anger, guilt, self-doubt, depression, and grief. Additional steps that may prove beneficial include helping the couple understand their motives for parenting, assisting them in the development of mutual support and an adaptive coping style, and encouraging them to broaden their support systems,[20] including self-help groups such as Resolve, Inc (see RESOLVE National Home Page at http://www.resolve.org).

SUMMARY

Primary care physicians have an essential role and opportunity in positively impacting the reproductive health of men. Although men are less likely than women to consistently seek preventive services, an office visit for any reason should be seen as an opportunity to introduce the idea of reproductive health. The recommendation for a subsequent office visit for a physical examination, with a focus on health promotion, disease prevention, and reproductive assessment as outlined earlier, is strongly encouraged.[1,36] Additionally, the primary care physician can and should initiate the diagnostic infertility survey for couples in their practices.[20,21,24]

REFERENCES

1. Frey KA, Navarro SM, Kotelchuck M, et al. The clinical content of preconception care: preconception care for men. Am J Obstet Gynecol 2008;199(6 Suppl 2): S389–95.
2. Dunlop AL, Jack B, Frey K. National recommendations for preconception care: the essential role of the family physician. J Am Board Fam Med 2007;20(1):81–4.

3. Padrón R, Dambay A, Suárez R, et al. Semen analyses in adolescent diabetic patients. Acta Diabetol 1984;21:115–21.
4. Sipos A, Rasmussen F, Harrison G, et al. Paternal age and schizophrenia: a population based cohort study. BMJ 2004;329:1070.
5. Malaspina D, Harlap S, Fennig S, et al. Advancing paternal age and the risk of schizophrenia. Arch Gen Psychiatry 2001;58:361–7.
6. Marinelli D, Gaspari L, Pedotti P, et al. Mini-review of studies on the effect of smoking and drinking habits on semen parameters. Int J Hyg Environ Health 2004;207:185–92.
7. Muthusami KR, Chinnaswamy P. Effect of chronic alcoholism on male fertility hormones and semen quality. Fertil Steril 2005;84:919–24.
8. Ewing JA. Detecting alcoholism: the CAGE questionnaire. JAMA 1984;252(14): 1905–7.
9. Torres-Calleja J, Gonzalez-Unzaga M, De- Celis-Carrillo R, et al. Effect of androgenic anabolic steroids on sperm quality and serum hormone levels in adult male bodybuilders. Life Sci 2001;68:1769–74.
10. Ogden CL, Carroll MD, Curtin LR, et al. Prevalence of overweight and obesity in the United States, 1999–2004. JAMA 2006;295:1549–55.
11. Sallmen M, Sandler DP, Hoppin JA, et al. Reduced fertility among overweight and obese men. Epidemiology 2006;17:520–3.
12. Wong WY, Merkus HM, Thomas CM, et al. Effects of folic acid and zinc sulfate on male factor subfertility: a double-blind, randomized, placebo-controlled trial. Fertil Steril 2002;77:491–8.
13. Kynaston HG, Lewis-Jones DI, Lynch RV, et al. Changes in seminal quality following oral zinc therapy. Andrologia 1988;20:21–2.
14. Omu AE, Dashti H, Al-Othman S. Treatment of asthenozoospermia with zinc sulphate: andrological, immunological and obstetric outcome. Eur J Obstet Gynecol Reprod Biol 1998;79:179–84.
15. Donnelly ET, McClure N, Lewis SE. The effect of ascorbate and alpha-tocopherol supplementation in vitro on DNA integrity and hydrogen peroxide-induced DNA damage in human spermatozoa. Mutagenesis 1999; 14:505–12.
16. Ramchandani P, Stein A, Evans J, et al. ALSPAC Study Team. Paternal depression in the postnatal period and child development: a prospective population study. Lancet 2005;365:2201–5.
17. Paulson JF, Dauber S, Leiferman JA. Individual and combined effects of postpartum depression in mothers and fathers on parenting behavior. Pediatrics 2006;118:659–68.
18. Kahn RS, Brandt D, Whitaker RC. Combined effect of mothers' and fathers' mental health symptoms on children's behavioral and emotional well-being. Arch Pediatr Adolesc Med 2004;158:721–9.
19. US Preventative Task Force. Guide to clinical preventive services, 2007: recommendations of the US Preventative Services Task Force. AHRQ Publication No. 07–05100. Rockville (MD): Agency for Healthcare Research and Quality; 2007. Available at: http://www.ahrq.gov/clinic/pocketgd07/. Accessed April 29, 2010.
20. Frey KA, Patel KS. Initial evaluation and management of infertility by the primary care physician. Mayo Clin Proc 2004;79(11):1439–43.
21. Jose-Miller AB, Boyden JW, Frey KA. Infertility. Am Fam Physician 2007;75(6): 849–56.
22. Whitman-Elia GF, Baxley EG. A primary care approach to the infertile couple. J Am Board Fam Pract 2001;14:33–45.

23. Speroff L, Glass RH, Kase NG. Clinical Gynecologic Endocrinology and Infertility. 5th edition. Baltimore (MD): Williams & Wilkins; 1994. p. 809–964.

24. Frey KA. Infertility. Prim Care Rep 2003;9:109–15.

25. American Urological Association, American Society for Reproductive Medicine. Infertility: report on varicocele and infertility. Available at: http://www.asrm.org/Media/Practice/Report_on_varicocele.pdf. 2008. Accessed April 29, 2010.

26. Kolettis PN. Evaluation of the subfertile man [published correction appears in Am Fam Physician 2003;68:1266]. Am Fam Physician 2003;67:2165–72.

27. American Urological Association, American Society of Reproductive Medicine. Infertility: report on evaluation of the azoospermic male. Available at: http://www.asrm.org/Media/Practice/Evaluation_of_the_azoospermic.pdf. 2008. Accessed April 29, 2010.

28. Harrison KL, Callan VJ, Hennessey JF. Stress and semen quality in an in vitro fertilization program. Fertil Steril 1987;48:633–6.

29. Pook M, Tuschen-Caffier B, Krause W. Is infertility a risk factor for impaired male fertility? Hum Reprod 2004;19:954–9.

30. Clarke RN, Klock SC, Geoghegan A, et al. Relationship between psychological stress and semen quality among in-vitro fertilization patients. Hum Reprod 1999;14:753–8.

31. Ragni G, Caccamo A. Negative effect of stress of in vitro fertilization program on quality of semen. Acta Eur Fertil 1992;23:21–3.

32. Pellicer A, Ruiz M. Fertilization in vitro of human oocytes by spermatozoa collected in different stressful situations. Hum Reprod 1989;4:817–20.

33. National Institute of Occupational Safety and Health. The effects of workplace hazards on male reproductive health. Centers for Disease Control and Prevention. DHHS (NIOSH) Publication No. 96–132. Available at: http://www.cdc.gov/niosh/malrepro.html. Accessed April 29, 2010.

34. Brown JA. Haz-map database. Infertility, male. Available at: http://hazmap.nlm.nih.gov/index.html. Accessed April 29, 2010.

35. Jensen TK, Bonde JP, Joffe M. The influence of occupational exposure on male reproductive function. Occup Med (Lond) 2006;56:544–53.

36. Files JA, David PS, Frey KA. The patient-centered medical home and preconception care: an opportunity for internists. J Gen Intern Med 2008;23(9):1518–20.

Index

Note: Page numbers of article titles are in **boldface** type.

Prim Care Clin Office Pract 37 (2010) 653–672
doi:10.1016/S0095-4543(10)00063-1
0095-4543/10/$ – see front matter © 2010 Elsevier Inc. All rights reserved.

primarycare.theclinics.com

Printed and bound by CPI Group (UK) Ltd, Croydon, CR0 4YY

03/10/2024

01040460-0005